PRACTICAL CARDIOVASCULAR PATHOLOGY

Mary Sheppard MD MRCPath

Senior Lecturer and Honorary Consultant in Histopathology,
Royal Brompton National Heart and Lung Hospital,
London, UK

Michael J. Davies MD FRCP FRCPath

Professor and Honorary Consultant in Cardiovascular Pathology,
British Heart Foundation Cardiovascular Pathology Unit,
St George's Hospital,
London, UK

A member of the Hodder Headline Group
LONDON • SYDNEY • AUCKLAND
Co-published in the USA by Oxford University Press, Inc., New York

First published in Great Britain in 1998 by
Arnold, a member of the Hodder Headline Group,
338 Euston Road, London NW1 3BH

Co-published in the United States of America by
Oxford University Press, Inc.,
198 Madison Avenue, New York, NY10016
Oxford is a registered trademark of Oxford University Press

Whilst the advice and information in this book is believed to be true and
accurate at the date of going to press, neither the authors nor the publisher
can accept any legal responsibility or liability for any errors or omissions that
may be made

British Library Cataloguing in Publication Data
A catalogue record for this book is available from the British Library

Library of Congress Cataloging-in-Publication Data
A catalog record for this book is available from the Library of Congress

ISBN 0 340 67749 X

Publisher: Georgina Bentliff
Production Editor: James Rabson
Production Controller: Sarah Kett
Cover designer: Terry Griffiths
Composition by Scribe Design, Gillingham, Kent
Colour reproductions by DP Graphics, Holt, Wiltshire
Printed by Tenon & Polert Colour Scanning Ltd

CONTENTS

PREFACE

Our decision to write this book was based upon the recognition that pathologists dealing regularly with cardiovascular material need a concise and practical bench book. Cardiovascular disease is the commonest cause of sudden death and also one of the commonest causes of morbidity in the community, and therefore the general pathologist dealing with autopsies must have a practical and detailed knowledge of cardiovascular disease, particularly the heart. In addition, intervention procedures for cardiovascular disease are increasing in number, and the pathologist has to deal with post-operative complications and deaths that may occur. As a result, we have emphasised anatomy, practical approaches to dissection of the heart, post-operative deaths and sudden deaths, as well as specific disease entities. We have not covered transplant pathology since this is going to be dealt with in a companion book. In addition, we have not dealt with peripheral vascular disease since this encompasses many systems and is dealt with in other textbooks. We set out to write a book that was practical and accessible, helping pathologists to answer immediate problems faced in the course of their work both in diagnostic and autopsy material.

We both have large referral practices in which many hearts are sent to us, either because the pathologist has not been able to establish a cause of death or because it is a complex operative case, and have found that a detailed knowledge of cardiac anatomy as well as operative procedures, together with a practical and variable approach to the dissection itself, is essential. It is important for the pathologist to know the normal as well as the abnormal changes microscopically within the myocardium. In cardiovascular pathology, much is learned from detailed macroscopic examination and the taking of appropriate tissue. We hope this book will help the pathologist in his or her approach to the examination of the heart on a daily basis.

We wish to thank Mrs Patricia McKinnon, for help with the manuscript, and Mr Dean Jansen, for help with the photography.

MJ Davies
MN Sheppard

CARDIAC EXAMINATION AND NORMAL CARDIAC ANATOMY

The heart lies in the middle of the inferior mediastinum mainly to the left of the midline behind the second to the sixth costal cartilage (Fig. 1.1). On each side the heart abuts the lungs and the pleural cavity overlies the right side of the heart as far as the midline. On the left side, the lung and pleura are pushed to the left and in the area of the cardiac notch, the surface of the heart comes to lie directly against the rib cage, separated from it only by the pericardium. Anatomically, because of its rotated position within the chest, the right border of the heart is occupied by the right atrium while the inferior and anterior surface is formed by the right ventricle, lying on the diaphragm. The left ventricle only comes to the anterior surface as a thin strip between the anterior interventricular groove and the obtuse margin of the heart. The left atrium is a completely posterior structure lying close to the oesophagus. That is why transoesophageal echocardiography gives such excellent views of the left side of the heart. The tips of the right and left atrial appendages can be seen at the upper right and left margin of the heart (Fig. 1.1).

The pericardium encloses and protects the heart. It forms a tough fibrous sac with a serosal lining, the parietal layer and there is also an inner serosal layer firmly adherent to the heart forming the visceral layer. A thin film of fluid lies between the two surfaces and allows movement of the heart within. 20–50 ml of clear straw-coloured fluid is normal. The vagus and phrenic nerves run anteriorly and posteriorly respectively to the pulmonary hilum on either side and are in close proximity to the pericardium.

TECHNIQUES FOR EXAMINING THE HEART *IN SITU*

After removal of the sternum it is extremely important to examine the pericardium in the intact state to assess tamponade. The pericardium will be distended and full to touch if tamponade is present. Great care must be exercised in removal of the intact pericardium in these cases. A longitudinal cut is made through the anterior aspect of the pericardial sac and the amount of blood, either fresh or collected by suction into a container, should be in the region of 500–1000 ml. If the blood has clotted it should be weighed. The mere presence of blood in the pericardium does not indicate tamponade. The blood must distend the sac. In purulent pericarditis the amount of pericardial fluid is measured and its character noted. If indicated, a pericardial fluid sample is taken by needling through an area of pericardium which has been seared for sterilisation. The surface of the visceral as well as parietal pericardium is examined for exudates,

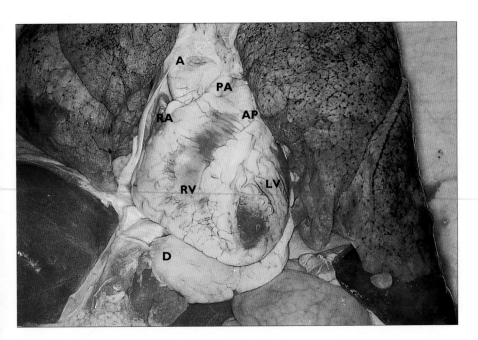

Figure 1.1
Opened thorax with sternum removed. Right atrium (RA) is at the upper right margin abutting the parietal pericardium. Right ventricle (RV) occupies the right and inferior margin of the heart lying on the diaphragm (D). Left ventricle (LV) margin lies on the left lung while tip of the left atrial appendage (AP) can be seen just to the left of the pulmonary artery (PA). Aorta (A) lies behind and to the right of the main pulmonary artery.

adhesions, tumour nodules or dense fibrosis associated with constrictive pericarditis which can follow infections such as tuberculosis or previous cardiac operations or may be idiopathic. Samples of the thickened pericardium from cases of constrictive pericarditis are often sent for analysis. All the tissue should be processed to look for necrotising granulomas in tuberculosis or rheumatoid nodules in cases of rheumatoid arthritis. Usually the samples show dense fibrosis and non-specific chronic inflammation and the aetiology in these cases is believed to have been viral. A short longitudinal incision 2 cm above the pulmonary valve will enable a check for thromboemboli in the main pulmonary trunk and two main branches *in situ*. Needle the right atrium after searing at its junction with the inferior vena cava to obtain a sample of heart blood for culture if required. Congenital heart disease can go undetected clinically well into old age. Check for patent ductus arteriosus, coarc-

tation of the aorta and persistent left superior vena cava. Check azygous and hemiazygous veins as well as the superior and inferior vena cava *in situ* in order to check for anomalous pulmonary venous drainage. Always keep the heart and lungs intact if any congenital abnormalities are detected in order to check the arterial and venous connections between the heart and lungs as well as any collaterals which may develop especially in tetralogy of Fallot, where pulmonary valve obstruction may be severe. Dissect the superior vena cava into the innominate and right azygous veins to check for thrombus or stenosis. Check the aorta for coarctation at the isthmus.

REMOVAL OF THE HEART

The heart is removed by first cutting both great vessels, the aorta and the pulmonary trunk, transversely 2 cm

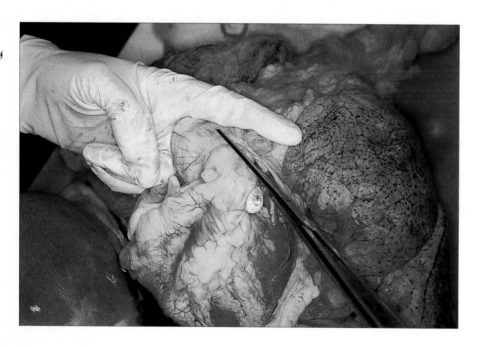

Figure 1.2
The aorta and pulmonary artery are cut across by inserting finger behind them into the transverse sinus and cutting through well above the position of both valves.

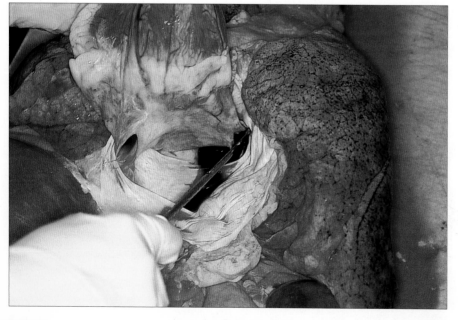

Figure 1.3
The heart has been moved up towards the head to expose the diaphragmatic surface and the posterior aspect of the left atrium with attached veins which have been cut across with release of blood.

above the semilunar valves by inserting the index and middle finger into the transverse sinus of the pericardial cavity and cutting both vessels across (Fig. 1.2). If a dissecting aneurysm is suspected, leave the aorta intact and dissect it out complete with abdominal aorta down to the iliofemoral junction. Then cut the inferior vena cava just above the diaphragm and lift the heart by the apex, reflecting it anteriorly and upwards to facilitate exposure of the pulmonary veins at their pericardial reflection. After confirming that the left and right pulmonary veins enter normally into the left atrium, the pulmonary veins are cut (Fig. 1.3). Then the superior vena cava is opened to check for thrombosis or occlusion and opened up into the left and right brachiocephalic veins before being cut across. Following removal of the heart from the pericardial cavity and before weighing the specimen, post mortem blood clot should be removed manually. If one sees aneurysmal dilatation of the right ventricular wall, particularly the posterior wall, be aware of the possibility of right ventricular dysplasia. Aneurysm formation in the left ventricle is usually associated with a previous infarct. Flexibility is called for when dissecting the heart since each disease process requires a different approach.

The epicardial surface of the heart normally contains fat. The amount varies with the nutrition of the person and increases with age. Normally it fills the atrioventricular groove and extends along the anterior and posterior interventricular sulci towards the apex (Figs 1.1 and 1.2). When a patient is obese it may completely envelop the epicardial surface of all chambers especially along the course of the coronary blood vessels. Fat also spreads into the myocardium along the intramyocardial vessels, particularly in the right ventricle and the interatrial septum. The right ventricular wall is thinnest and contains most fat where it meets the interventricular septum, particularly in elderly patients. It is this area which is most likely to be ruptured during catheterisation procedures. The wall needs to be completely

replaced by fat, dilated and attenuated to consider right ventricular dysplasia and then it affects particularly the infundibulum and the posterior wall below the tricuspid valve. Fat may also be seen partly replacing the left ventricular wall, particularly on the epicardial surface in this condition. The external surface of the heart is examined visually and by palpation. The location and size of the four heart chambers are assessed as are abnormalities of chamber size. Any focal or diffuse disease process that has affected the epicardium should also be apparent. Discolouration and haemorrhage on the surface will point to acute infarction or possible rupture. Evidence of rupture may be subtle with a small area of haemorrhage into fat on the surface and not a gaping hole. Careful probing in this area is required. White patches of epicardium (soldier's patches) are common, especially over the anterior surface of the right ventricle and have been attributed to mechanical trauma or to healed pericarditis, but there is no definite histological evidence for either of these processes. Swelling around the root of the aorta may point to a sinus of Valsalva aneurysm, a root abscess in aortic valve endocarditis, or an aneurysm of the proximal coronary arteries. A careful methodical approach is needed to dissect out these structures in order to determine the origin of any swelling in this area. A cut across the aorta above the cusps of the aortic valve will usually expose the valve architecture in order to look for abnormalities, and also to show the ostia of the coronary arteries. At this stage in the fresh heart, a detailed examination of the coronary arteries is undertaken in routine autopsies.

Examination of coronary vessels

To obtain the best analysis of the coronary vessels as regards the lumen and degree of stenosis, it is best to perfuse fix the heart from the aorta with a pump which will (via a tube placed in the aorta) under pressure of 100 mm Hg force open the coronary vessels and fix the heart over a period of 24 hours (Thomas and Davies,

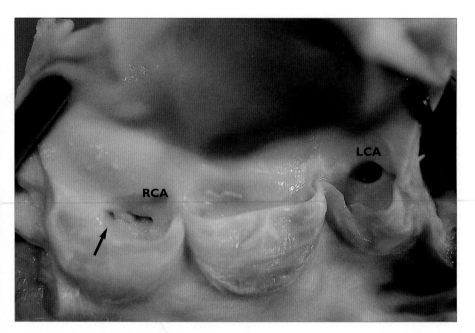

Figure 1.4
Aorta has been opened to show the outflow tract from the left ventricle. A long incision has been made through the anterior wall of the left ventricle between the right anterior and left lateral leaflet to show the rounded orifice of the left coronary artery (LCA) at the sinotubular junction while the right coronary artery (RCA) shows an ellipitical opening below the sinotubular junction with an additional orifice for a conal artery branch (arrow).

1985). The coronary vessels will maintain their lumen as in life and there will not be the overestimation of narrowing which can be seen when hearts are simply fixed in formalin where the coronaries often will contract down after death. Always check the origin of each artery within the respective sinus. While the majority arise within the sinus, there is great variation in the exact location as we have shown in normal individuals with the ostia being at, above and below the sinotubular junction. The majority are below the junction, but do not exceed 2 mm below it (Muriago *et al.*, 1997). Usually there is only one ostium on the left (Fig. 1.4), but in 1% of hearts an additional ostium for the circumflex can be identified. In the right coronary sinus, multiple ostia are common (74% of cases in our study) and give rise to branches supplying the right ventricle with a branch to the conus or infundibulum being particularly frequent (Fig. 1.4). The shape of the ostium can be round, ellipitical or crescentric. It is essential to look at the ostia and origin of both coronary arteries in the coronary sinuses. Thus anomalous origin of the coronary arteries will not be missed.

In specialist centres the coronary arterial system is injected with a barium–gelatin mixture and studied in radiographs. Polyethylene tubing, the tips of which may be flared in a flame, are used to cannulate each coronary ostium. The tubes are secured by a ligature at the origin of the coronary arteries, as close to the aorta as possible. The free end of each tube is attached to a hypodermic needle (size 16) on the barrel of a disposable syringe (30 ml). The pressure of injection may be gradually increased to 100–120 mm Hg and maintained for 10–15 minutes. Following injection, the cannulae are pulled out and the ligatures tightened and knotted quickly. The heart is then fixed for 24 hours in formaldehyde. After washing the fixed specimen in water, radiographs are made in anteroposterior as well as left and right anterior oblique positions. A superior view can also be done after the ventricles have been transversely sliced in a 'bread-loaf' manner.

In routine autopsies, the pathologist will simply cut across the main vessels at 5 mm intervals in the fresh heart and assess the presence of dilatation, atherosclerotic plaque formation, thrombosis, stenosis or dissection. The coronary arteries are cut transversely with a sharp scalpel blade using a gentle sawing motion – not firm pressure – to confirm any sites of narrowing and to evaluate the pathology directly (Fig. 1.5). It is generally agreed that cutting the vessels longitudinally can destroy thrombi/emboli and make the estimation of stenosis impossible. The vessels that are usually examined in all hearts include the four major epicardial coronary arteries, the left main, the left anterior descending, the left circumflex, and the right coronary arteries. However, attention must also be directed to smaller branches, such as the left diagonals, the left obtuse marginals, the intermediate, and the posterior descending coronary arteries. If the coronary arteries are heavily calcified, they are removed intact and following dissection of the vessels from the epicardial

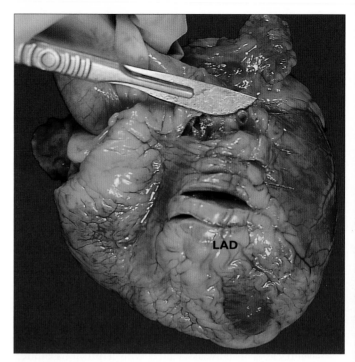

Figure 1.5
Fresh heart showing scalpel cuts across the left anterior descending (LAD) artery at 5 mm intervals demonstrating an atherosclerotic plaque which does not cause significant stenosis.

surface, each coronary artery is carefully trimmed of excess fat and the intact arterial tree is placed in a container of formic acid for slow decalcification over 12–18 hours. Decalcification of isolated segments of vessel may be sufficient for cases in which the coronary arteries are only focally calcified. Calcification bears no relation to the severity of coronary artery disease. The areas of maximal narrowing are noted by specifying the degrees of reduction of the cross-sectional area of the lumen (e.g. 0–25%, 26–50%, 51–75%, 76–90%, and 100%). Most cardiologists agree that, in the absence of other cardiac disease, significant coronary artery narrowing is that exceeding 75%.

The coronary anatomy

There are two major coronary arterial branches which arise from two of the three sinuses of Valsalva, the right coronary and left coronary sinuses respectively. The two coronary arteries have major differences in their branching patterns once they have emerged from their sinuses.

The right coronary artery after arising from its sinus, runs around the orifice of the tricuspid valve in the interventricular groove (Fig. 1.6). In this initial course it usually gives off the sinus nodal artery into the atrial musculature and the infundibular (or conal) artery into the right ventricular muscle mass. The conal/infundibular branch commonly anastomoses with a small branch of the left coronary artery to form the anastomotic ring (of Vieussens). These branches and the ring are sometimes very considerably enlarged in atherosclerosis

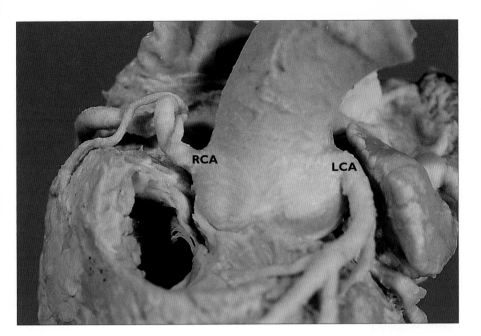

Figure 1.6
Aortic sinuses which balloon out from the aortic wall at its origin and show the origin of right coronary artery (RCA) with infundibular branch to the right ventricle and left coronary artery (LCA).

when there is distal disease in the right coronary artery. The artery then runs to the acute margin of the heart where it gives rise to the acute marginal artery of the right ventricle and usually a lateral atrial artery. Continuing around the tricuspid orifice it gives off a varied number of smaller ventricular branches before, in the majority of hearts, it ends in the posterior interventricular groove (Fig. 1.7). The area of junction of the posterior interventricular and the atrioventricular grooves is generally called the crux of the heart. The posterior interventricular (descending) artery is given off at this point. Before it forms the posterior descending branch the right coronary artery itself makes a U-turn into the area of atrioventricular muscular septum and gives off the artery to the atrioventricular node from the apex of the U. It then continues onto the diaphragmatic surface of the left ventricle as the posterior descending artery which is often grafted in ischaemic coronary artery disease. The foregoing describes the anatomy to be found in the majority of people (i.e. that the artery supplying the posterior descending branch is the right coronary artery). This arrangement is called right coronary dominance. Although the left coronary artery always supplies a greater mass of muscle than does the right, it is not usually dominant. Left dominance (posterior descending branch is the continuation of the circumflex) is found in only about 15% of people.

The left coronary artery originates in the left (antero-lateral) aortic sinus and passes undivided for up to 2.5 cm as the left main coronary artery between the aorta and the left atrial appendage (Fig. 1.6). It generally bifurcates into anterior descending and circumflex branches, but in about a third of individuals it trifurcates (Fig. 1.8). The branch between the anterior descending and circumflex branches is called the intermediate branch. The anterior descending branch passes in the anterior interventricular sulcus towards the apex. During its course it gives a variable number of branches

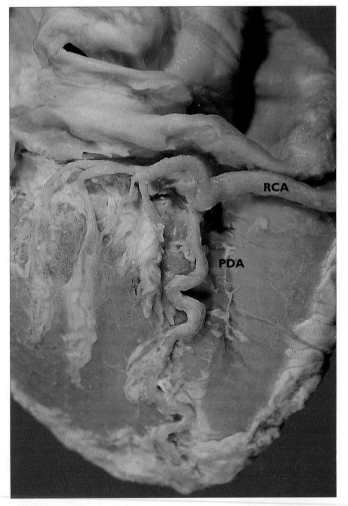

Figure 1.7
This shows the diaphragmatic surface of the heart with right coronary artery (RCA) extending to the crux and leading into the posterior descending artery (PDA). Note that the right coronary artery continues across the midline to supply branches to the left ventricle.

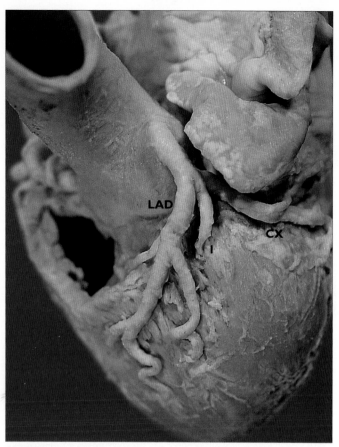

Figure 1.8
Left main stem of left coronary artery divides into anterior descending (LAD), intermediate (I) and circumflex (CX) arteries. Note diagonal branches of the LAD to the left ventricle.

muscle for part of its length. When the left coronary artery trifurcates this first diagonal branch is replaced by the intermediate branch. In addition to the diagonal branches passing to the left ventricle, there are smaller branches passing to the right ventricle. These infundibular branches to the outflow component of the right ventricle often anastomose with branches from the right coronary artery. In addition to the diagonal and right ventricular sprigs, the anterior descending branch of the left coronary artery also gives a number of branches passing from its underside (epicardial aspect), vertically downwards into the anterior ventricular septum. These important arterial branches are the septal branches, sometimes also called the septal perforators or perforating branches. They are variable in number and site of origin, except for the first branch. The 'first septal' artery is a relatively large branch (1–2 mm in diameter in normal people) which takes origin from the anterior descending branch close to the origin of the first diagonal branch. This branch can become greatly enlarged in coronary artery disease. It is also the branch which is selectively occluded by alcohol injection to induce infarction in the upper septum in left outflow obstruction associated with hypertrophic cardiomyopathy.

The course of the circumflex artery is more variable than the other coronary arteries. In some hearts, it terminates almost immediately and often gives off the atrial circumflex artery which runs in the atrial myocardium around the mitral orifice. More usually, the circumflex artery continues to the obtuse margin of the left ventricle and breaks up into the obtuse marginal arteries which are often embedded within the muscle of the left ventricle (Fig. 1.9). The circumflex branch of the left coronary artery runs in the left atrioventricular groove and the obtuse marginal branches are often sites for vein grafts. The circumflex artery itself is not graftable because of its inaccessibility in the left atrioventricular groove. In 70% of people the circumflex branch terminates as an obtuse marginal branch at

(diagonal branches) to the left ventricle (Fig. 1.8). These, together with their parent branch, are important for arterial and vein grafting. The first diagonal branch is a major vessel which originates in the proximal third of the anterior descending branch. It may reach the apex of the heart, and is quite often submerged in

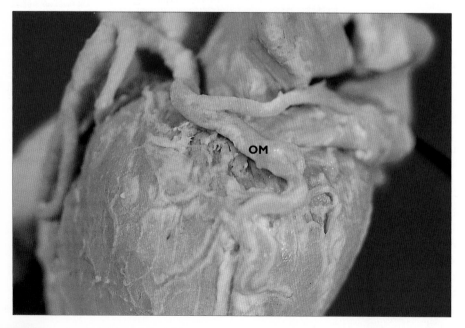

Figure 1.9
Circumflex branch of the left coronary artery with obtuse marginal (OM) branches. Main stem continues around the atrioventricular junction to the posterior left ventricle.

or near the obtuse margin of the heart. In a small proportion of hearts, the circumflex artery continues all the way around the mitral orifice and hugs closely the atrioventricular groove (Fig. 1.9). It may then gives rise to both the posterior interventricular artery and the artery to the atrioventricular node. This arrangement is called left dominance, in contrast to the much more common pattern of right dominance. In still other hearts, both the right and circumflex arteries may supply the diaphragmatic surface without there being a prominent posterior interventricular artery. This arrangement is termed a balanced circulation.

Cardiac veins

The coronary veins run with the major arteries and return the blood to the coronary sinus, forming a major channel in both the interventricular and the atrioventricular grooves. A large vein is formed in the anterior interventricular groove and is termed the great cardiac vein. It runs around the mitral orifice and expands to form the body of the coronary sinus in the left atrioventricular groove (Fig. 1.10). At the crux, the coronary sinus receives the blood from the middle cardiac vein, which runs up the posterior interventricular groove and the small cardiac vein (Fig. 1.10). The small cardiac vein initially accompanies the acute marginal artery and then runs round the orifice of the tricuspid valve in the right atrioventricular groove before terminating in the coronary sinus at the crux. It is important to examine these veins when retrograde cardioplegia is used in cardiac operations to look for complications such as rupture or thrombosis.

The heart is supplied by a rich plexus of lymphatics. The lymphatic channels run along with the veins and drain the lymph to the pulmonary hilar lymph nodes and also directly into the thoracic duct and the left lymphatic channel.

DISSECTION OF THE HEART

Dissection methods are learnt by personal experience and vary with the individual pathologist. In 1959 Levy and McMillan reviewed the methodologies used by previous pathologists and came to the conclusion that the inflow–outflow trans-valvular incisions originally described by Oppenheimer in 1912 were the best approach to dissection, since they preserved the conduction system as well as allowing rapid diagnosis and selection for microscopic slides. This is a common method still used by many pathologists for examining the heart with the opening each of the four chambers according to the flow of blood. The right atrium is opened from the inferior vena cava to the tip of the atrial appendage. The right ventricle is opened along its attachment to the ventricular septum from the tricuspid annulus through to the pulmonary outflow tract. The left atrium is opened by cutting across the roof of the atrium between the left and right pulmonary veins and the left ventricle is opened laterally between the anterior

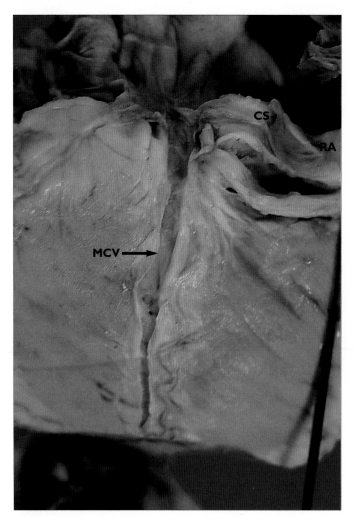

Figure 1.10
Middle cardiac vein (MCV) running alongside the posterior descending artery and joining the great cardiac vein to form the coronary sinus (CS) draining into the right atrium (RA).

and posterior papillary muscles to the apex and then cut along the anterior wall adjacent to the ventricular septum through the aortic outflow tract. The first incision in the right atrium is made 2 cm above and parallel to the atrioventricular groove. It passes from 1 cm anterior to the ostium of the inferior vena cava to the tip of the right atrial appendage. This incision is preferable to one that joins the superior and inferior vena cavae, which will destroy the valve of the inferior vena cava, making it impossible to determine if a Chiari network is present, and it also will often destroy the sinoatrial node which lies just to the right of the entry of superior vena cava into the atrium at the top of the atrial crest. It may sometimes be visible especially in infants or non-fatty hearts from older subjects. After viewing the interior of the right atrium, look at the tricuspid valve, which will normally admit the middle three fingers. If the tricuspid valve or any valve should prove to be diseased or abnormal, the valve ring should be left intact and the heart opened by incising the chamber distal to the valve. If vegetations are seen they should be sampled in a sterile manner for culture. The next incision is made along the acute (right) margin of the heart and extends from the first atrial incision to the right ventricular apex and cuts through the posterior tricuspid leaflet exposing the inflow tract, the tricuspid valve and its tensor apparatus. A third incision is made parallel to and 1 cm to the right of the interventricular septum, from the right ventricular apex to the transected end of the main pulmonary artery, keeping the knife edge vertical to the heart wall. Another approach is to cut from the end point of the second incision, keeping the knife anterior to the anterior papillary muscle. The triangular flap created will be joined to the septum by the moderator band which joins the base of the anterior papillary muscle from the distal end of the interventricular septum.

In another review of cardiac dissection methods, Chapman (1964) disagreed with this and pointed out that using the trans-valvular blood flow slicing technique (which he attributed to Mallory and Wright, 1897) could miss anomalies within the valves or chambers. The shape of the heart is better preserved by lateral inflow incisions along the acute and obtuse borders than by paraseptal incisions that Chapman attributed to Virchow. Obviously the technique to use will depend on the type of abnormality in the heart itself (Silver and Freedom, 1991; Anderson and Becker, 1993).

We generally find that after careful dissection of the coronary arteries, serial sections along the short axis of both ventricles will reveal abnormalities of the chambers such as acute infarction, hypertrophy, scarring, thinning, fatty replacement, nodules, pericardial or endocardial thickening as well as papillary muscle abnormalities. The myocardium is best examined for the presence or absence of acute or healed myocardial infarction by slicing the ventricles in this bread-loaf manner. To evaluate the specimen, a series of short-axis cuts are made through the ventricles from apex to base. This method is best accomplished using a long sharp knife on the intact fixed specimen, following examination of the coronary arteries. With the anterior aspect of the heart downward (against the cutting board), the cuts are made parallel to the posterior atrioventricular sulcus at 1–1.5 cm intervals from the apex of the heart to a point approximately 2 cm caudal to the sulcus (Fig. 1.11). The result is a series of cross sections through the ventricles including papillary muscles with the atrioventricular valve apparatus left intact in the remainder of the specimen. The location and extent of any pathology is noted. Location may be stated using terms relating to the standard anatomic frame of reference (e.g. anteroseptal, posterolateral, and so forth). The extent of disease may be described in terms of circumference of the ventricle subtended and longitudinal portion of the ventricle involved (e.g. basal third, middle third, and apical third). The distribution within the wall is also described (e.g. transmural or subendocardial). The gross pathological appearance of the myocardium must be confirmed by histological examination. We routinely take full thickness samples from all areas of the right and left ventricle, usually in

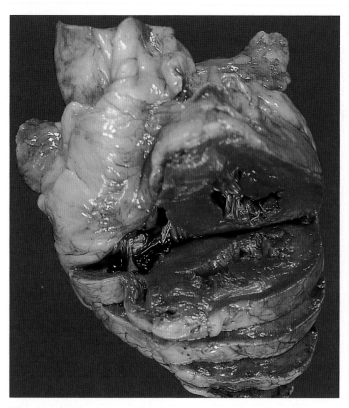

Figure 1.11
Serial 5 mm transverse sections through the left and right ventricles up close to the atrioventricular junction.

the middle third of both chambers even in the absence of gross pathology. These blocks include the free wall of the right ventricle, infundibulum, anteroseptal right ventricular wall, the posteroseptal wall of the right ventricle, interventricular septum, the anteroseptal wall of the left ventricle, anterior wall, lateral wall, posterior wall and the posteroseptal wall of the left ventricle, making ten blocks in total.

Examination of the heart valves

The cuts extend up as far as the atrioventricular valve orifices. If an atrioventricular valve lesion is suspected, then an incision is made into both atria to gain access and inspect the valves from above in order to assess the degree of stenosis or floppy change that may be present, as well as the possibility of vegetations and perforations with infection. If chordal or papillary muscle rupture is suspected which is usually seen in the mitral valve, first cut transversely at the apex and locate the origin of both papillary muscles, then cut upwards on the obtuse margin between them in order to expose the whole tensor apparatus and assess the possibility of rupture.

The valves are best studied intact. Both aspects of each valve – atrial and ventricular aspects of the atrioventricular valves, and ventricular and arterial aspects of the semilunar valves – are examined. Thus, the tricuspid valve is exposed by a lateral incision through the right atrium from the superior vena cava to 1 cm above the valve annulus. Similarly, the mitral valve may be studied following the opening of the left atrium via an incision

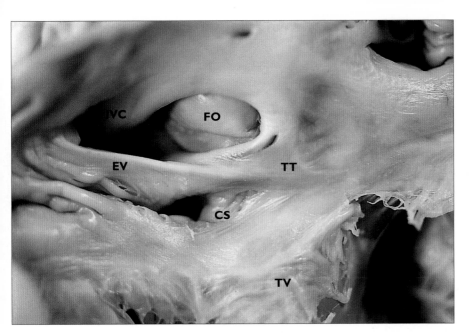

Figure 1.12
Opened right atrium demonstrating the fossa ovalis (FO) below which there is the opening of the coronary sinus (CS) and tricuspid valve leaflets (TV). Note the opening of the inferior vena cava (IVC) from which the Eustachian valve (EV) extends down to merge with the thebesian valve of the coronary sinus to form the tendon of Todaro (TT) which extends to the septal leaflet of the tricuspid valve to outline the triangle of Koch.

extending from one of the left pulmonary veins to one of the right pulmonary veins and another incision continuing through the atrium laterally to a point 1 cm above the annulus. If a valve abnormality requires closer inspection, the atria, including interatrial septum may be removed 1 cm above the atrioventricular valves. The ventricular aspects of the atrioventricular valves may be viewed following removal of the serial slices of ventricle as described above. The semilunar valves are best studied after removal of the aorta and main pulmonary artery above the coronary ostia or valve annulus. In selected cases, the valvular pathology may best be visualised using a four-chamber cut in the plane including both the acute and obtuse margins of the heart posteriorly. The aortic valve area can be demonstrated by a left ventricular long-axis cut passing from the apex through the outflow tract (ventricular septum and anterior mitral valve leaflet) and aortic valve. Similarly the pulmonary valve and infundibulum may be visualised with a long-axis cut to the right ventricle. Measurements of the circumference of valves is not useful in valve stenosis, but can be useful for incompetence. Examination of the heart valves should document the type and severity of the ventricular disease and its effect on the cardiac chambers. In cases where histology of a valve may be helpful, the leaflets are sectioned together with a portion of the adjacent chambers and/or vessel walls. For example, the posterior leaflet of the mitral valve is sectioned including a portion of left atrium and left ventricular free wall: the anterior leaflet includes ventricular septum and non-coronary cusp of the aortic valve. In cases of rheumatic heart disease, sections of the atrial appendages are submitted for histological examination because the incidence of Aschoff bodies is highest in these structures.

Right atrium

The normal right atrium possesses a smooth-walled component (the venous sinus) which receives the

superior and inferior caval veins along with the coronary sinus, a vestibule which surrounds the right atrioventricular junction, a septal surface with the fossa ovalis (Fig. 1.12) and a prominent broad based triangular appendage. The atrial wall thickness is usually 2 mm. When viewed internally, the opening of the superior caval vein is bound medially by the superior rim of the oval fossa and laterally by the terminal crest which is a prominent muscular ridge which runs down to the lateral boundary of the inferior caval vein. Externally the ridge is marked by the terminal groove which is an important landmark because it contains the sinus node. The most constant feature of the morphologically right atrium and hence the best marker of its morphological rightness is the shape of the appendage together with the anatomy of its junction with the smooth walled atrium. The appendage has the shape of a broad based triangle. Its junction with the venous component is marked internally by the prominent terminal crest from which arise the pectinate muscles. The pectinate muscles in the right atrium extend all round the atrioventricular junction and reach the coronary sinus beneath the orifice of the inferior caval vein, this area being called the sinus septum.

The wall of the inferior caval vein often runs directly in to the oval fossa (Fig. 1.12) but in many hearts, a fold of tissue (Eustachian valve) springs from the crest in this area that is a remnant of the more extensive valve which in fetal life, serves to direct the richly oxygenated placental blood from the inferior caval vein, into the left atrium through the oval foramen. The true atrial septum consists only of the fossa ovalis. Dissection shows that most of the rest of what appears to be septum is really composed of infoldings of the atrial wall or atrioventricular septum. The septum secundum which is the rim of the oval fossa is a characteristic feature of the right atrial septal surface and is made up predominantly of the infolded atrial roof. In up to 25% of normal hearts, the floor of the fossa ovalis has failed to fuse with this rim anteriorly resulting in a probe-patent fossa ovalis which is of no significance. The posterior aspect of the oval fossa is the wall of the inferior caval vein (Fig. 1.12). The inferior border is mainly atrioventricular septum where atrial and ventricular septal structures overlap in a small area where the tricuspid and mitral valves are attached opposite each other. This area of overlap constitutes the atrioventricular septum and separates the cavity of the right atrium from the left ventricle. It has two components, muscular and membranous. The muscular septum exists because the proximal attachment of the septal leaflet of the tricuspid valve is considerably further towards the ventricular apex than the attachment of the leaflets of the mitral valve in the left ventricle. In the muscular atrioventricular septum lies the atrioventricular node within the triangle of Koch which is defined inferiorly by the attachment of the septal leaflet of the tricuspid valve, superiorly by the tendon of Todaro and posteriorly by the mouth of the coronary sinus (Fig. 1.12). The opening of the coronary sinus occupies the most posteroinferior corner of the right atrium separated by the sinus septum from the oval fossa. It is also guarded in foetal life by a valve (thebesian valve). When persisting in postnatal life, this valve extends on to the atrioventricular septum and joins with the Eustachian valve to form the tendon of Todaro which is the marker for the superior margin of the triangle of Koch already described. More extensive remnants of the valves of the venous sinus often extend in filigree fashion across the cavity of the right atrium to attach to the superior portion of the terminal crest; these are called Chiari networks. They are of no functional significance unless present as a solid sheet. Although usually small in comparison with the orifices of the caval veins, the mouth of the coronary sinus can be large when it drains a persistent left superior caval vein. Such a venous channel is present during early foetal life, but usually becomes absorbed and attenuated during development. Its site is marked by the oblique ligament of the left atrium.

Right ventricle

Both ventricles have three components. These are the inlet component, the apical trabecular component and the outlet component. They are particularly well seen in the right ventricle. The inlet component extends from the atrioventricular junction to the distal attachments of the tendinous cords (chordae tendineae) of the tricuspid valve (Fig. 1.13). The outlet component is the smooth walled tube of muscle which supports the three semi-lunar leaflets of the pulmonary valve. The apical trabecular component extends out from these two parts and reaches to the apex. The apex is coarsely trabeculated and exhibits on its septal surface, the particularly prominent and characteristic muscular structure which is called the septomarginal trabeculation.

In addition to its own coarse trabeculations, the ventricle also possesses a series of septoparietal trabeculations which extends from the anterior surface of the septomarginal trabeculation on to the parietal (free) wall of the ventricle. Another muscle bundle, the moderator band carrying the right bundle branch of the conduction system, is prominent and crosses from the septomarginal trabeculation of the interventricular septum to the anterior papillary muscle and thence to the free right ventricular wall. The major feature of the outlet of the right ventricle is that it is a complete muscular structure known as the conus. Measurement of the thickness of the right ventricle is best made here since it avoids erroneous inclusion of trabeculae which are thick and coarse in the right ventricle. Measurements are taken 1.5 cm below the pulmonary valve, and 3–5 mm is normal. Because the pulmonary outlet is a complete muscular structure, the pulmonary valve can be removed and used as an autograft to be inserted into the aortic position, while a homograft replaces the pulmonary valve (Ross procedure).

The muscular shelf which separates the tricuspid and pulmonary valves in the roof of the ventricle is called

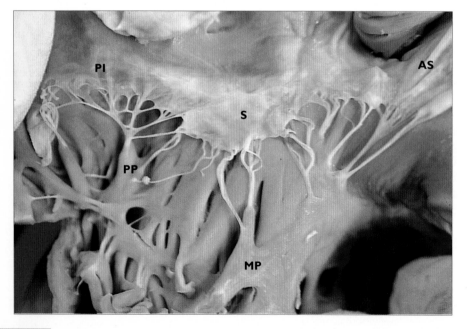

Figure 1.13
Tricuspid valve with anterosuperior leaflet (AS), septal leaflet (S) and posteroinferior leaflet (PI) supported by the chordae tendineae and showing also the middle papillary muscle (MP) and the smaller bundles of the posterior papillary muscle (PP). The coarse trabeculations of the right ventricle are seen also as well as the septomarginal trabeculation.

the supraventricular crest and is made up of the inner curvature of the heart wall; it is also known as the ventriculo-infundibular fold. The septomarginal trabeculation extends up and divides in the roof of the ventricle into two limbs which clasp the supraventricular crest, and this is the area where ventricular septal defects most commonly occur.

Because of the low attachment of the tricuspid valve, the right atrium directly abuts the left ventricular wall and the septal leaflet of the tricuspid valve divides the membranous septum into supra- and infra-tricuspid components. The supra-tricuspid component separates the left ventricle from the right atrium and is therefore the atrioventricular membranous septum. The infra-tricuspid component of the membranous septum is known as the interventricular membranous septum. Below this is the crest of the muscular interventricular septum; this is important because it is where the conduction system divides into left and right bundles. Below it is the muscular interventricular septum which extends down to the ventricular apices.

Tricuspid valve

The morphologically tricuspid valve has three leaflets in the anterosuperior, septal and posteroinferior position (Fig. 1.13). The diameter of the annulus ranges from 110–130 mm. The posteroinferior leaflet takes its origin exclusively from the diaphragmatic parietal wall of the ventricle and is often called the mural leaflet.

The leaflets are separated from each other by commissures, which defined literally are simply junctions. Each commissure has by convention been defined in terms of its support by a prominent papillary muscle topped by a fan-shaped commissural cord. However, in the tricuspid valve, they are not always supported by the corresponding papillary muscle, and they are better considered as breaches in the leaflet skirt extending from the central point of closure of the valve to its circumferential margin. In terms of muscular support, the anterior muscle is the largest and usually springs directly from the body of the septomarginal trabeculation. The complex of cords supporting the anteroseptal commissure is dominated by the medial papillary muscle (of Lancisi), a relatively small muscle which springs either as a single band or as a small sprig of cords from the posterior limb of the septomarginal trabeculation (Fig. 1.13). The inferior muscle, the most insignificant, is usually single but may be represented by several small muscles (Fig. 1.13). The most characteristic and distinguishing feature of the tricuspid valve is the direct attachment of cords from the septal leaflet to the septum (Fig. 1.13) which can be seen at echocardiography. These chordal attachments to the septal surface are never seen in the morphological left ventricle, except when the tricuspid valve straddles and inserts on to the left ventricular septal aspect in atrioventricular septal defects. The reason for this complex arrangement of chordae tendineae is that the atrioventricular valves must close during systole and the chordae prevent them ballooning into the atria. The atrioventricular valves are open and ventricles fill during diastole, while the ventriculoarterial valves are closed.

Pulmonary valve

This is similar in structure to the aortic valve and usually measures 75–85 mm in circumference. It has three semilunar shaped cusps separated by three commissures. They are the right, left and posterior leaflets. Each cusp is thinner and more transparent than the aortic valve, but has basically the same structure. Always check for anomalous origin of a coronary artery from the pulmonary sinuses.

Left atrium

To gain access, incise parallel to the atrioventricular groove, 1 cm proximal to it and extend the incision to the tip of the atrial appendage. The mitral valve is

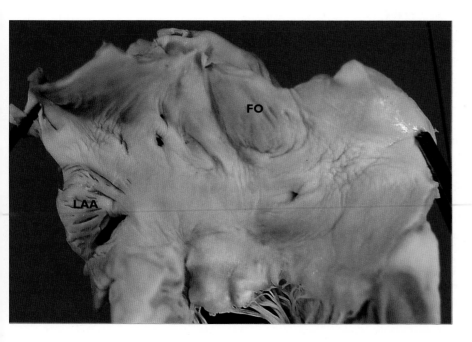

Figure 1.14
Opened smooth walled left atrium. The fossa ovalis (FO) is seen as a depression on this side. Note the ridges and blind-ending sacs in the left atrial wall as well as the pectinate muscle at the mouth of the left atrial appendage (LAA).

examined and usually admits two fingers. Like the right atrium, the left atrium possesses a venous component, a vestibule leading to the atrioventricular junction, a septal surface and the appendage. The thickness is usually 3 mm. Again it is the appendage which is the most constant feature on the left side (Fig. 1.8). The left appendage is a tubular structure with several bends along its length. It has a narrow junction with the smooth walled atrium. This junction is not marked by a terminal crest or groove as in the right atrium. The pectinate muscles in the left atrium are confined within the appendage. The largest part of the left atrium is formed by the extensive venous component anchored at its corners by the connections of the four pulmonary veins (Fig. 1.14). The four pulmonary veins normally connect to the morphologically left atrium in a constant fashion, each entering a different corner of the posterior atrial wall so that together they enclose a substantial area (Fig. 1.3). The oblique ligament (or a persistent left superior caval vein, if present) always runs between the left pulmonary veins and the left atrial appendage. The septal surface comprises the flap valve of the oval fossa. Typically there are several rough ridges along the atrial roof (Fig. 1.14).

The left ventricle

Normally the fifth incision is through the mitral annulus and along the obtuse margin of the heart to the apex, carefully palpating between the two papillary muscles and guiding the knife between them. As with the right ventricle the left ventricle is described in terms of inlet, apical trabecular and outlet components. The inlet component contains the mitral valve (Fig. 1.14) and extends from the atrioventricular junction to the attachments of the prominent papillary muscles. The valve has two leaflets of markedly dissimilar shape and circumferential length. The most anteriorly located leaflet is square in shape and takes up only one-third of the annular circumference. Because of the obliquity of location of the valve, the leaflet is not strictly anterior. Its most characteristic feature is its fibrous continuity with the leaflets of the aortic valve (Fig. 1.15). The other leaflet is long and thin, making up two-thirds of the annular circumference. It is attached throughout its length to the diaphragmatic wall of the ventricle and is described as the mural or posterior leaflet. The commissure between the leaflets is orientated in a posteromedial and anterolateral position. Its two ends are traditionally described as separate commissures, which are supported by prominent anterior and posterior papillary muscles which have their origins very close together (Fig. 1.15). A characteristic feature is that the mitral valve never possesses chordal attachments to the septum in contrast to the tricuspid valve. The apex of the left ventricle has fine trabeculae which is characteristic, and the septal surface is smooth with no septomarginal trabeculation or a moderator band (Fig. 1.15). The left ventricular wall thickness is best measured along the obtuse free wall approximately 1.5 cm below the posterior leaflet of the mitral valve; 12–15 mm thickness is normal and should not include trabeculae. The last incision opens the

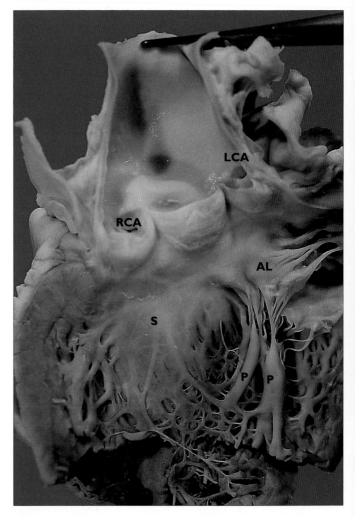

Figure 1.15
Outflow track with aortic valve. Note that the anterior leaflet (AL) of the mitral valve is in direct continuity with the aortic valve. There are some lipid rich plaques on the mitral valve leaflet and also in the aorta. The left bundle branch extends out as pale strands beneath the endocardium from beneath the membranous septum onto the septal surface (S) of the left ventricle which is smooth. Note also the close proximity of both papillary muscles (P) to each other and the fine trabeculations of the left ventricular wall. Note the orifices of the left coronary artery (LCA) and right coronary artery (RCA).

ventricular outflow tract and is made from the apex to the aorta parallel to and 1 cm to the left of the interventricular septum. It passes between the pulmonary artery to the right and the left atrial appendage to the left and up the left side of the aorta dividing the coronary cusp, close to the left coronary ostium (Fig. 1.15). The outlet from the left ventricle leads to the aortic valve. There is no muscular ventricular-infundibular fold in the left ventricle which separates the mitral and aortic valve so that they are in direct continuity with each other and disease of one can easily lead to disease in the other. Another method of exposing the aortic valve, is to cut through the anterior leaflet of the mitral valve, but this destroys the leaflet.

Aorta

The aorta is distinguished from the pulmonary trunk by its branching pattern. It takes origin usually behind and to the right of the pulmonary trunk at the base of the heart. The origin at the ventriculoarterial junction is characterised by the three sinuses which support the semilunar attachments of the aortic valve (Fig. 1.4, 1.6 and 1.15). In the normal heart, it is the sinuses facing the pulmonary trunk that usually give rise to the coronary ostia, the so-called right and left facing sinuses. The ascending portion of the aorta in the normal heart gives rise to the brachiocephalic (innominate) artery followed by the left common carotid and the left subclavian arteries. The aortic arch then continues as the isthmus which extends to the junction of the aortic arch with the arterial duct (ductus arteriosus). The duct is a wide channel in the foetus and the newborn, but closes rapidly shortly after birth. It is represented subsequently by the attachment of the arterial ligament to the underside of the arch. The aorta then continues as the descending thoracic aorta, which gives rise to the bronchial and intercostal arteries before piercing the diaphragm to become the abdominal aorta. Always check the aorta for dilatation, aneurysm formation, evidence of intimal thickening in aortitis and dissection.

The pulmonary trunk

The pulmonary trunk arises in front of and to the left of the aorta (Fig. 1.2) and has a very simple branching pattern, dividing into the left and right pulmonary arteries. The trunk in the foetus continues as the arterial duct into the descending aorta, the right and left pulmonary arteries being side branches from the flow pathway from the duct to the aorta. After birth with closure of the arterial duct, the site is marked by the arterial ligament with the recurrent laryngeal nerve passing around it. Always check the pulmonary trunk for thromboemboli and atherosclerosis pointing to pulmonary hypertension.

THE CONDUCTION TISSUES

Examination of the conduction system

For cases in which conduction disturbances are suspected clinically, histological examination of the cardiac conduction tissues can be rewarding in terms of documenting a structural basis for the problem. Many pathologists are intimidated by the prospect of doing conduction system studies because the pertinent tissues cannot be visualised grossly. Yet, with practice and careful attention to anatomical landmarks, these structures can be dissected and removed for histological examination.

Sinoatrial node

In most humans the sinoatrial node is a cigar shaped structure lying immediately sub-epicardially within the terminal groove on the lateral aspect of the junction of the superior vena cava and the right atrium (Fig. 1.16a). In some patients, it is a horseshoe-shaped structure wrapped across the superior aspect of the cavoatrial junction. Histologically, the node consists of relatively small diameter, haphazardly orientated atrial muscle cells admixed with connective tissue (Fig. 1.16b). Often, the artery to the sinoatrial node can be identified in or around the nodal tissue. Because the sinus node is not visible grossly, the entire block of tissue from the suspected area should be taken and serially sectioned, either in the plane perpendicular to the sulcus terminalis (parallel to the long axis of the superior vena cava) or in the plane containing the sulcus (perpendicular to the vessel). In small infants, it is preferable to section the entire cavoatrial junction serially. The artery supplying the sinus node is a branch of the right coronary artery in 50% of people and from the left circumflex coronary artery in the other 50%.

Atrioventricular node

The atrioventricular node is arranged as a continuous axis which extends from the atrioventricular muscular septum, penetrates the atrioventricular membranous septum and divides on the crest of the muscular interventricular septum. The atrial component of the atrioventricular axis is contained exclusively within the triangle of Koch already described (Fig. 1.12). The atrioventricular node lies in the atrial subendocardium and the axis passes through the atrioventricular membranous septum at the apex of the triangle of Koch, as the penetrating atrioventricular bundle (of His). The apex of the triangle anteriorly is the membranous septum and denotes the point at which the common bundle of His penetrates the membranous septum to reach the left ventricle (Fig. 1.15). It then emerges in the subaortic outflow tract beneath the commissure between the non-coronary and right coronary leaflets of the aortic valve (Fig. 1.15). The axis branches immediately in the normal heart, usually on the crest of the muscular septum but sometimes to its left side. The left bundle branch then fans out on the smooth aspect of the septum in a continuous cascade, splitting into three divisions: anterior, septal and posterior towards the ventricular apex (Fig. 1.15). The right bundle branch turns back through the interventricular septum as a cord-like structure before crossing in the moderator band and ramifying into the right ventricular myocardium. There is no anatomical evidence for the existence of specialised pathways between the sinoatrial and atrioventricular node. Thus, the tissue excised for study of the conduction system must include the atrioventricular septum, the membranous septum and the crest of the interventricular septum. It must be remembered that removal of the conduction system involves extensive removal and mutilation of the heart, so one must have carried out a detailed study of the cardiac chambers and coronary arteries before removal of the sinus and atrioventricular nodes. From the opened right atrioventricular aspect, excess right and left ventricular muscle is removed so that the atrioventricular septal area and membranous septum can be laid flat with the aortic outflow tract flat to the cutting surface on the bench. The block to be excised reaches from the anterior margin of the coronary sinus to the medial papillary muscle of the right ventricle, including 1 cm of atrium and ventricle on either side of the valve

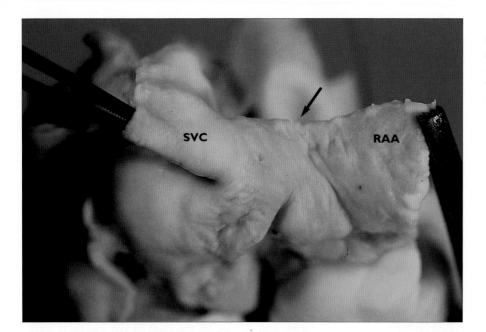

Figure 1.16a
Superior vena cava (SVC) entering the right atrium with attached right atrial appendage (RAA). In the groove between the SVC and the appendage lies the sinoatrial node (arrow).

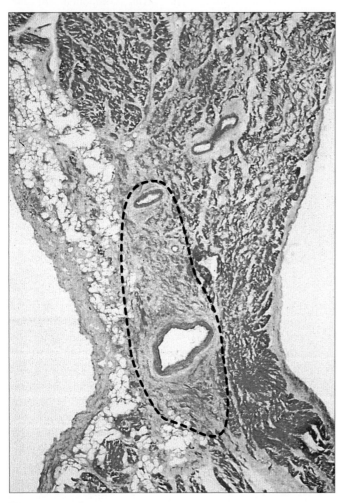

Figure 1.16b
Masson trichrome stain showing the sinonodal artery with surrounding pale bundles of myocytes around the artery which is the sinoatrial nodal tissue with connective tissue and collagen (note outline).

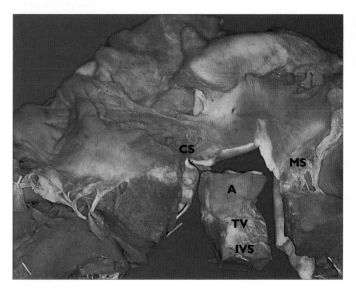

Figure 1.17a
Block taken for histology of the atrioventricular node from the right atrial aspect in the fresh heart. This block extends from the mouth of the coronary sinus (CS) to the membranous septum (MS) beneath the septal leaflet of the tricuspid valve (TV) and includes atrium above (A) and interventricular tissue (IVS) below.

(Fig. 1.17a). Often we have found that taking a good block of muscular atrium above, and ventricle below the triangle of Koch, enables cutting of the blocks more evenly and parallel to each other. It is often quite difficult to dissect out, because the membranous septum is thin and cutting it evenly as a thin membrane between two muscle blocks can be challenging with twisting and oblique cuts. The blocks will include the membranous septum through which the bundle of His passes, the septal leaflet of the tricuspid valve and anteror leaflet of the mitral valve (Fig. 1.17b). One has to have a relatively large block, immobilise it by pinning it out on a cutting surface and use a very sharp knife and even parallel cuts. One can also approach the atrioventricular conduction system from the left ventricle. In the left ventricular outflow tract which is again laid flat with removal of excess cardiac muscular tissue, the block can

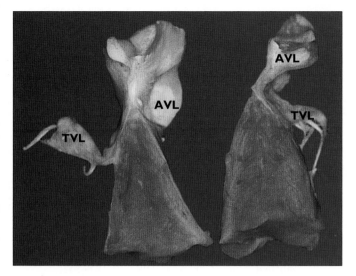

Figure 1.17b
Close up of blocks taken for histology of the atrioventricular node. Block on the left shows the tricuspid valve leaflet (TVL) with aortic valve leaflet (AVL) on the other side and membranous septum in between containing the penetrating bundle. The right block is from a more posterior position in the right atrium near the coronary sinus and shows the tricuspid valve leaflet (TVL) in continuity with the aortic valve leaflet (AVL) and atrioventricular septum containing the node.

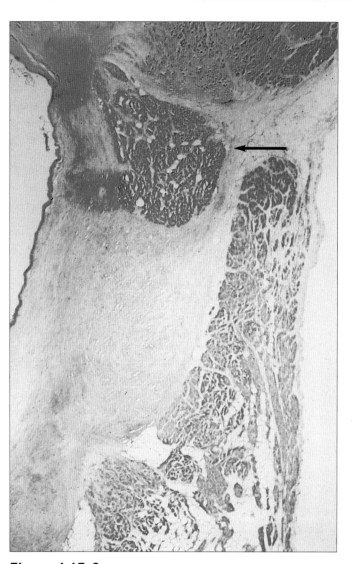

Figure 1.17c2
Haematoxylin and eosin stained section showing the penetrating bundle (arrow) in the collagen of the membranous septum.

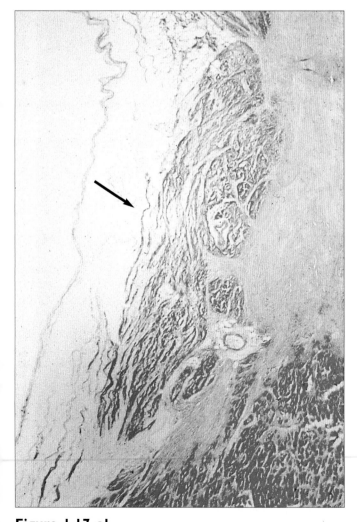

Figure 1.17 c1
Haematoxylin and eosin stained slide showing the atrioventricular node (arrow) beneath the endocardium in the atrioventricular septum.

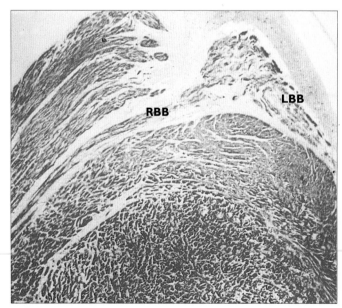

Figure 1.17c3
Haematoxylin and eosin stained section showing the bundle dividing into left bundle branch (LBB) and right bundle branch (RBB) at the crest of the muscular interventricular septum.

be cut with aorta above and interventricular septum below with non-coronary sinus and valve leaflet in between. The other cut is perpendicular to the aortic valve from the margin of the attachment of the anterior leaflet of the mitral valve to the left edge of the membranous septum. The block should include the non-coronary cusp of the aortic valve and the crest of the ventricular septum. In either case the block of tissue removed should be divided in the plane, from posterior to anterior and should be marked with India ink, so that orientation can be maintained throughout the embedding process. Mark the non-cutting surface of each block, as the block is embedded, to give uniformity of face for each block. In the adult heart the entire tissue should be ideally step-sectioned, and every 25th or 50th section stained with Masson's trichrome. Alternatively, one or two sections can be cut from each block which will generally enable you to view the atrioventricular node, the penetrating bundle, the dividing bundle, and proximal right and left bundle branches (Fig. 1.17c); however, focal lesions may be missed if all the blocks are not serially sectioned. The Masson trichrome stain is the most useful for delineating the myocardium, nodal tissues and membranous septum. For infant hearts the entire block of tissue should be serially sectioned with each fifth 10 μm-thick section stained with Masson's trichrome initially.

References

Anderson RH, Becker AE. Normal cardiac anatomy. In: Anderson RH, Becker AE, Robertson WB (eds). *The cardiovascular system. Part A: General considerations and congenital malformations.* Edinburgh: Churchill Livingstone, 1993;3–26.

Chapman CB. On the study of the heart. A comment on autopsy techniques. *Arch Intern Med* 1964;**113**:318–24.

Levy M, McMillan JB. A semiquantitative histopathologic method for the study of the entire heart for clinical and electrographical correlations. *Am Heart J* 1959;**58**:140–52.

Muriago M, Sheppard MN, Yen Ho S, Anderson RH. Location of the coronary arterial orifices in the normal heart. *Clin Anat* 1997;**10**:297–302.

Silver MM, Freedom RM. Gross examination and structure of the heart. In: Silver MD (ed). *Cardiovascular pathology.* New York: Churchill Livingstone, 1991;1–42.

Thomas AC, Davies MJ. The demonstration of cardiac pathology using perfusion-fixation. *Histopathol* 1985;**9**:5–19.

THE CORONARY ARTERIES – ATHEROSCLEROSIS AND ISCHAEMIC HEART DISEASE

ATHEROSCLEROSIS AS A PROCESS

Introduction

The great majority of ischaemic damage to the myocardium is the result of coronary atherosclerosis. Atherosclerosis is an intimal disease of medium to large arteries including the aorta, carotid, coronary and cerebral arteries. Some medium-sized arteries such as the internal mammary are spared, as are veins. In the absence of pulmonary hypertension the pulmonary arteries are also spared.

Atherosclerosis is a focal intimal disease – each discrete lesion being called a plaque (Table 2.1). Within each plaque there are combinations of extracellular lipid, intracellular lipid contained within foam cells (predominantly of macrophage origin) and collagen with other connective tissue matrix components produced by smooth muscle cells. Many plaques undergo calcification. Lipid is an essential component of the atherosclerotic disease process; atherosclerosis can only be produced in animal models by inducing hyperlipidaemia. Plaques can be considered as an inflammatory-repair response to lipid within the intima.

Table 2.1

Characteristics and plaque components of atherosclerosis

Atherosclerosis	
Characteristics	**Plaque components**
Arterial intimal focal lesions (plaques)	Smooth muscle cells
	Connective tissue matrix
	Macrophages
	Lipid – intracellular
	Lipid – extracellular
	T-lymphocytes
	Basophils

Smooth muscle proliferation is one component of plaques, but is also a ubiquitous response of the vessel wall to any injury. Disease processes which solely consist of smooth muscle proliferation should not be called atherosclerosis. For this reason post-angioplasty stenosis, intimal thickening following experimental endothelial damage, hypertensive changes and age-related intimal thickening should not be called atherosclerosis.

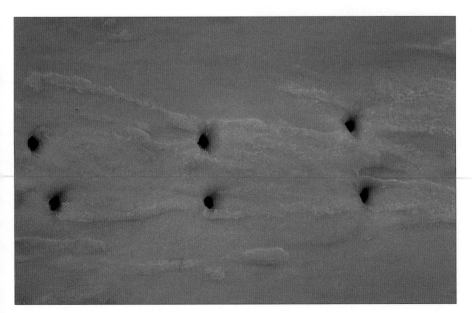

Figure 2.1
Aortic fatty streaks. The aorta has been opened and pinned out to display the intimal/endothelial surface. There is a series of yellow longitudinal streaks which are barely raised above the intimal surface. While some fatty streaks are situated at the openings of the intercostal arteries many are not.

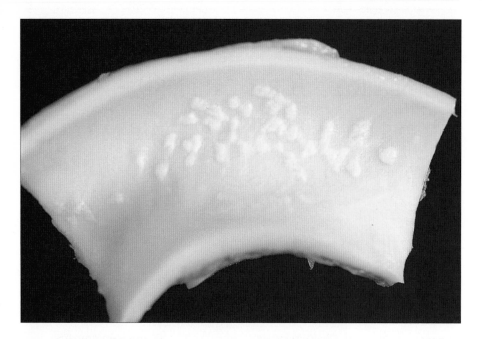

Figure 2.2
Aortic fatty dots. In the ascending aorta in particular, but also in the rest of the aorta, small yellow dots are found. Their histology is identical to that of fatty streaks.

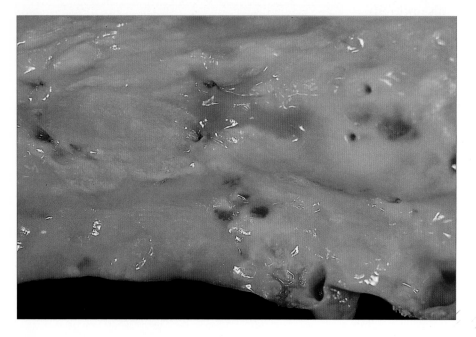

Figure 2.3
Aortic atherosclerotic plaques. There are some fatty streaks and dots on the intimal surface; in addition there are some larger more elevated yellow lesions which are intermediate type plaques. The large raised white lesions are fully formed fibrolipid plaques. There is also a flat reddish brown gelatinous lesion.

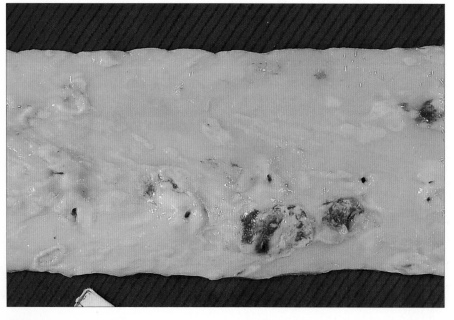

Figure 2.4
Aortic atherosclerotic plaques. The intimal surface shows some fatty streaks and dots as well as some white raised fibrolipid plaques around the orifices of the intercostal arteries. In addition two plaques show ulceration with their surface covered by a mixture of yellow lipid and thrombus.

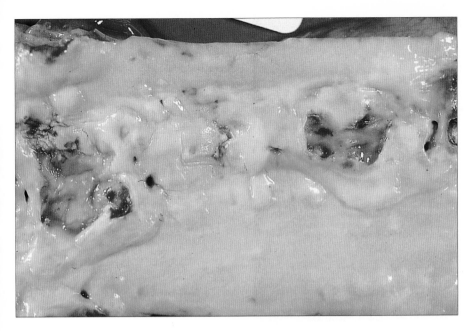

Figure 2.5
Aortic atherosclerotic plaques. Two large fibrolipid plaques are shown in the healing phase after plaque ulceration and thrombosis. The plaques contain central craters with flat floors on which there is a small amount of residual thrombus. The cholesterol of the original core has been washed out and embolised into the lower limb arteries.

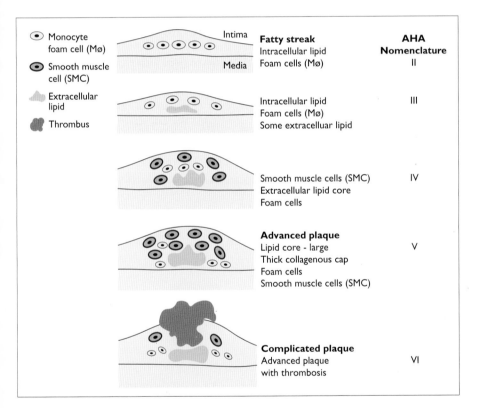

Figure 2.6
Plaque evolution. The sequence of plaque evolution with the cellular and lipid composition alongside the AHA nomenclature is shown.

Atherosclerosis is a biphasic disease. Virtually all individuals in the countries of the developed world will have some plaques, but only a minority will at some point in their life enter the second phase of atherosclerosis and develop clinical symptoms.

The lesions of atherosclerosis

Examination of the intimal surface of the human aorta opened longitudinally at autopsy shows plaques with considerable variation in their macroscopic appearances (Figs 2.1–2.5). Studies of cohorts of individuals of different ages who die from non-cardiac disease allows inferences to be made about the temporal sequence of the development of the different forms of plaque. The earliest lesion which is visible by naked eye examination is the fatty streak. This is a flat yellow dot or streak on the intima. Fatty streaks are the only lesions found in children up to 10 years of age. Although it seems likely that not all fatty streaks progress, they are considered the starting point in sequential plaque development (Fig. 2.6). Histologically the fatty streak consists of a focal collection of lipid filled macrophages over which

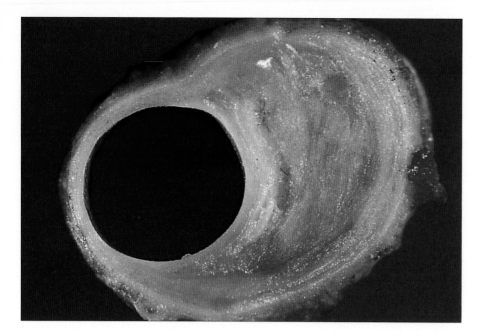

Figure 2.7
Coronary advanced fibrolipid plaque. When seen in cross-sections of arteries which have been fixed by perfusion with formalin the lumen is round in shape; the plaque is situated to one side of the artery leaving a segment of normal arterial wall opposite the plaque. The tissue slice has been treated with oil red O to show the lipid in the core. The core is separated from the arterial lumen by the fibrous cap of the plaque which is pearly grey in colour due to its high collagen content.

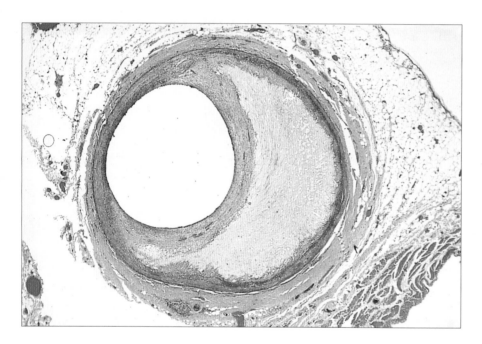

Figure 2.8
Coronary advanced fibrolipid plaque. In this perfused fixed artery the lumen is round and there is a large eccentrically situated plaque. The core is very large occupying most of the area of the plaque cross-section. The cap stains a deeper pink in H&E stained sections due to its high content of collagen and smooth muscle cells (H&E ×22.75).

there is an intact endothelial surface. This lesion has been called Stage II by the American Heart Association (AHA) Committee on plaque nomenclature (Stary *et al.* 1994; 1995). Stage I is the adhesion of monocytes to the intact endothelial surface through which they subsequently move to enter the intima and become the foam cells of the fatty streak.

Stage III lesions look very like Stage II macroscopically, apart from being somewhat larger. Histologically they are marked by the presence of droplets of extracellular lipid and smooth muscle cells just beneath the endothelium.

The next stage of plaque evolution is the development of lesions which are elevated above the intimal surface as smooth oval humps. Such raised fibrolipid or advanced plaques may be yellow or white.

Histologically at this stage the plaque has a central core of acellular lipid-containing cholesterol crystals. This core is surrounded by lipid-filled foam cells of macrophage origin and contained within a capsule of collagen. The core is separated from the lumen by a portion of the collagenous capsule which is known as the plaque cap (Figs 2.7–2.9).

In the AHA classification Type IV plaques have a thin cap while in Type Va the cap is much thicker. The external colour of the raised fibrolipid plaque is basically yellow due to the carotenoid pigment in the lipid core, but if the plaque cap is thick the external colour is white.

The later stages of plaque evolution comprise complications such as calcification (AHA Type Vb) and thrombosis (Type VI).

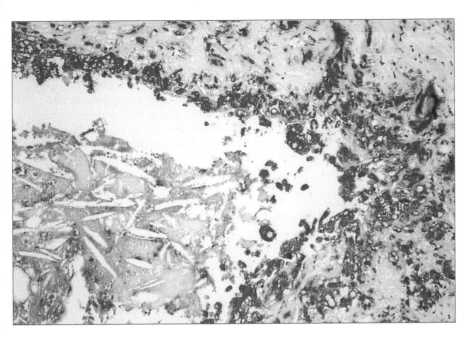

Figure 2.9
Macrophages in relation to lipid core. The slide shows immunohistochemistry using the alkaline phosphatase method and an antibody to the macrophage antigen CD68. The core is acellular and contains numerous cholesterol clefts. At the margins of the core there are numerous brightly stained macrophage foam cells. The core stains faintly with the antibody. This staining is a constant feature and suggests the core contains macrophage cytoplasmic material and is created by death of macrophages. The CD68 antibodies are the most reliable for staining foam cells both in frozen and paraffin embedded formalin fixed material.

In adults the aorta at autopsy usually contains all these morphological types of plaque suggesting the sequence of development continues to be initiated throughout life. There is good epidemiological evidence from large numbers of autopsies in different ethnic and geographic populations that not all fatty streaks progress (Wissler 1995; Restrepo and Tracy 1975). In Caucasian populations fatty streaks first develop in sites such as the proximal left anterior descending coronary artery; it is at the same site that raised plaques first appear (Strong 1992; Tejada *et al.* 1968). In populations such as the South African Bantu where there is very little atherosclerosis present in later age groups, there are often numerous fatty streaks in children which seem to have vanished in adults (Tejada *et al.* 1968).

Mechanisms of plaque formation

Animal models of atherosclerosis are either induced by feeding diets very rich in lipid to cause hypercholesterolaemia (Faggiotto *et al.* 1984; Faggiotto and Ross 1984; Kaplan *et al.* 1993; Small *et al.* 1984) or by genetic defects which lead to hyperlipidaemia such as the Watanabe (Shiomi *et al.* 1995) or the St. Thomas' rabbit. Some species such as rabbits, primates and pigs are susceptible to the induction of atheroma; others such as rats and mice are very resistant.

There is consensus that the first stage in atherogenesis is adhesion of circulating monocytes to the intact endothelial surface followed by their migration between endothelial cells to reach the intima (Ross 1993). In the intima the monocytes take up lipid and become foam cells. The adhesion and migration of the monocytes is invoked by the induction of a number of adhesion molecules and cytokines. On the endothelial cells intercellular adhesion molecule (ICAM-1. CD54), endothelial adhesion molecule (ELAM.E-selectin.CD62E) and vascular cell adhesion molecule (VCAM.CD106) are all expressed – the last is thought to be the most important in monocyte migration. The monocytes are

acting under the chemoattractant MCP-1. Within the intima macrophage colony stimulating factor (MCSF) is important in maintaining monocytes and allowing mitotic division.

The unexplained aspect of atherosclerosis for many years was why monocytes migrated into the intima, and there was also a paradox because monocytes do not have the low density lipoprotein (LDL) receptor, yet they take up LDL in the intima. This is now explained (Fig. 2.10). Low density lipoprotein (LDL) from the plasma freely moves in, and out, of the intima, and invokes no response. Within the intima, or on the endothelial surface however, a small proportion of the LDL undergoes minor modification and then oxidative change (Steinberg *et al.* 1989). The minimally modified LDL acts as an inflammatory stimulus and invokes both adhesion molecule expression by endothelial cells monocyte migration and cytokine production. Once oxidised, the LDL can be taken up by the macrophage scavenger receptors. Some of these receptors do not down-regulate, and lipid uptake continues until the cytoplasm is packed with lipid to form the foam cell. Smooth muscle cells may also take up some lipid via the conventional LDL receptor and by low levels of expression of a scavenger receptor, but seldom form classic foam cells.

Extracellular lipid in the core of the advanced plaque is thought to be derived in large part from the cytoplasm of dying macrophages (Ball *et al.* 1995) and contains a high proportion of oxidised lipid and ceroid pigment. A component of the extracellular lipid may be derived directly from LDL which becomes bound to proteoglycans in the intima (Guyton and Klemp 1993).

For many years, central core necrosis was thought to be due to macrophage death due to the direct toxicity of hydroxylipids in the core, but it is being increasingly recognised that it is also due to apoptosis (Hegyi *et al.*

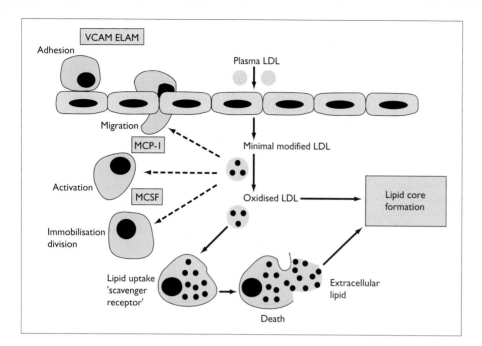

Figure 2.10
Lipid core formation in plaques. Plasma LDL enters the intima and undergoes modification to become an inducer of adhesion molecules and cytokines by endothelial cells. LDL is then further oxidised. Monocytes enter the intima, take up oxidised LDL to become foam cells and then die by apoptosis and necrosis to release oxidised lipid into the developing core.

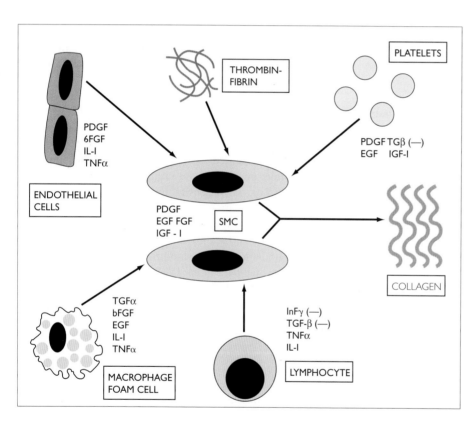

Figure 2.11
Factors inducing smooth muscle cell proliferation. Many factors as shown potentially drive smooth muscle proliferation and the production by smooth muscle cells of collagen and other matrix proteins. Other factors inhibit these processes. [PDGF – platelet derived growth factor; bFGF – basic fibroblast growth factor; EGF – epidermal growth factor; TGF – transforming growth factor; TNFα – tumour necrosis factor; IGF – insulin like growth factor, InFγ – interferon γ]. The main inhibitors are marked (–).

1996; Geng and Libby 1995). The trigger for this is not known but may be a reduction in growth factors such as MCSF-1 or induced by tumour necrosis factor α (TNFα). Associated with the macrophages surrounding the lipid core are T-lymphocytes, a proportion of which are capable of cytotoxic function containing granzyme and perforin. Within the plaque itself B-lymphocytes are absent, but a very heavy adventitial inflammatory cell infiltrate containing numerous T- and B-lymphocytes and plasma cells is common. In part this is an autoimmune response to oxidised LDL released from within the plaque and circulating humoral antibodies are

generated. Such antibodies may bind to lipid in the plaque further enhancing macrophage uptake.

The inflammatory processes which are a major component of the plaque are in part responsible for the smooth muscle proliferation (Ross 1993; Raines and Ross 1993) which produces the collagenous skeleton of the plaque (Fig. 2.11). The smooth muscle proliferation is driven by a large number of putative growth factors. Very many of these have been demonstrated to be present within human plaques and their receptors have been shown to be present on the smooth muscle cell.

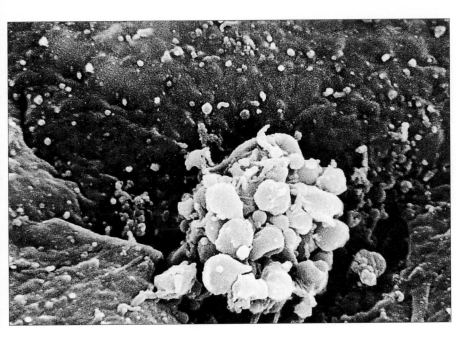

Figure 2.12
Platelet thrombi over human coronary plaque. A single endothelial cell has been lost and in this discrete area platelets adhere to the underlying exposed connective tissue matrix. Scanning electron microscopy (×11 900).

Which are the dominant or rate-limiting growth factors is unclear. Smooth muscle cells themselves also produce growth factors in an autocrine stimulation system.

The mode of action and interplay between the different growth factors stimulating smooth muscle cells is very complex. The best characterised is platelet-derived growth factor stored in the alpha granules of platelets, but also produced by endothelial cells and macrophages. Smooth muscle cells and fibroblasts have receptors for PDGF, which induces both smooth muscle cell proliferation and migration. Transforming growth factor β may either be stimulatory or inhibitory depending on the level of other cytokines, but along with interferon γ is usually regarded as the main inhibitory mechanism. Fibroblast growth factor released by damaged smooth muscle cells is important in the response to mechanical trauma to the vessel wall.

Fibrinogen also readily passes into the intima and within the plaque may be converted to fibrin by thrombin produced by macrophages; thrombin/fibrin complexes are a potent stimulus to smooth muscle cell growth (Bini *et al.* 1989). Within the plaque many of the macrophages are activated and show a wide range of phenotypic expressions. Tissue factor is produced by many of the macrophages which surround the lipid core (Annex *et al.* 1995). A range of metalloproteinases including gelatinase B, collagenase and stromelysin are also expressed within plaques (Galis *et al.* 1994).

The plaque is therefore becoming increasingly recognised as a site of intense activity in which collagen deposition and collagen removal are occurring (Libby 1995; Davies 1996). If collagenolysis is dominant the core increases in size and the cap thins; if deposition predominates the plaque becomes more fibrous. This activity may be phasic and plaques which are relatively acellular probably represent an end stage burnt out process.

Endothelial status over atheromatous plaques

Both in animal models and in human coronary arteries there is consensus that the endothelium over fatty streaks is intact and that no platelet adhesion occurs (Davies *et al.* 1988; Burrig 1991). Thus, platelets can play no part in plaque initiation. Once advanced plaques are present however, loss of individual or groups of endothelial cells is almost ubiquitous. This loss of endothelial cells exposes the subendothelial matrix and allows platelets to react with collagen via the platelet lb receptor. A monolayer of platelets form (Fig. 2.12). The process is on far too small a size scale to cause clinical symptoms but may stimulate smooth muscle proliferation via platelet-derived growth factor.

Complications of advanced plaques – thrombosis

Thrombosis and calcification are the complications which affect types IV and Va plaques. Thrombosis is the most important being responsible for a range of acute manifestations of ischaemic heart disease including myocardial infarction, unstable angina and sudden death. The advent of thrombosis converts a type IV or Va plaque to VI in the AHA system.

Thrombosis develops over plaques because of two different processes (Fig. 2.13). The first is superficial intimal injury in which there are large areas of endothelial loss and intimal erosion over a plaque (van der Wal *et al.* 1994). Thrombus forms which is entirely superimposed onto the luminal surface of the plaque. The underlying cause of this type of injury is inflammation below the endothelium in which numerous activated macrophages are present and adjacent smooth muscle cells express Class II MHC antigens (Fig. 2.14). Endothelial death may be the result of apoptosis triggered by cytokines such as TNFα. The evolution of the thrombus is dependent initially on the interaction of the platelet 1a/1b complex with collagen and Von Willebrand Factor. Further deposition on the initial

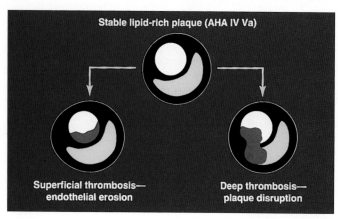

Figure 2.13

Mechanisms of coronary thrombosis. In endothelial erosion the thrombus is adherent to the luminal surface of the plaque. In plaque disruption the cap of a plaque tears allowing blood to enter the core where thrombus forms deep within the plaque and then protrudes into the arterial lumen.

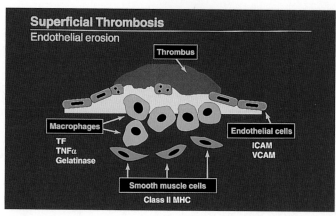

Figure 2.14

Endothelial erosion. The loss of endothelial cells is associated with large numbers of activated macrophages and local accumulation of tissue factor, TNFα and other pro-inflammatory cytokines.

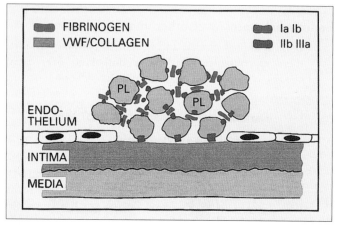

Figure 2.15

Platelet adhesion mechanisms. Following endothelial denudation injury platelets adhere to the exposed collagen by the 1a/1b receptor complex. Further build-up of a thrombus depends on platelet to platelet adhesion using the 2b/3a receptor complex and fibrinogen.

monolayer of platelets depends on the 2b/3a receptor which binds platelets to platelets via interactions with fibrinogen (Fig. 2.15). The 2b/3a receptor is expressed at relatively low levels in circulating platelets but is upregulated very strikingly in activated platelets. Good antibodies are commercially available to the 2b/3a receptor allowing ready identification of activated platelets in tissue sections by immunohistochemistry. While many of the coronary thrombi related to endothelial erosion over a plaque are small, a minority are larger and can lead to significant mural thrombi or even complete occlusion (Figs 2.16, 2.17).

In deep intimal injury or plaque disruption the cap of a plaque with a lipid core tears. The interior of the core is exposed to blood which enters from the arterial lumen. The interior of the plaque contains tissue factor, and is intensely thrombogenic; thrombus forms within the core itself due to activation of both platelets by the

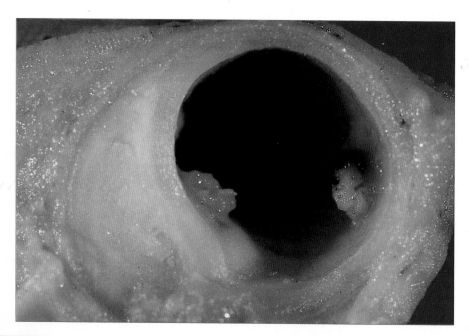

Figure 2.16

Coronary thrombus – endothelial erosion. Two small mural thrombi are adherent to the luminal surface of a coronary artery in relation to a plaque which is intact without any evidence of disruption.

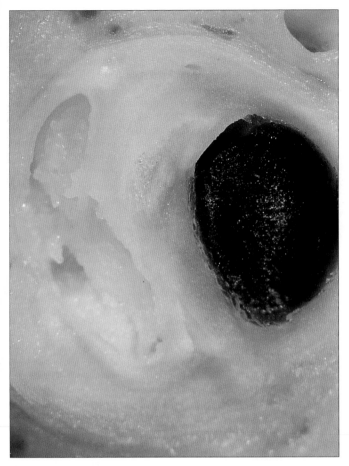

Figure 2.17
Coronary thrombus – endothelial erosion. There is a large plaque with a lipid core but no evidence of disruption and no thrombus within the core. The lumen is occluded by dark red thrombus.

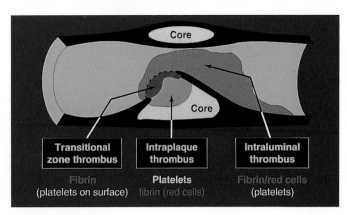

Figure 2.18
Thrombosis in plaque disruption. The thrombus within the core is rich in platelets; in a transitional zone within the cap tear there is densely packed fibrin covered by a layer of activated platelets. The final occluding thrombus is rich in red cells and fibrin. Distal propagating thrombus is very venous in type, i.e. rich in red cells.

occludes the lumen it is richer in fibrin and red cells (Fig. 2.18). The complexity of the different areas of the thrombus means that a series of sections have to be taken through the thrombus rather than a single histological slide if the structure is to be appreciated.

Plaque disruption has a wide spectrum of severity (Figs 2.19–2.22). Small tears may have only an intraplaque component of thrombus. At the other extreme the cap may be lost over several millimetres in the coronary artery and the whole bed of the core exposed with extrusion of the lipid contents. In the aorta or carotid arteries where both the plaques and the vascular lumen are much larger chronic ulcers filled with thrombus develop as the result of disruption (Fig. 2.5).

Coronary thrombi are dynamic and not immutable and undergo a repair and organisation process leading to reversion to a stable lesion with or without some

1b and 2b/3a receptors and the generation of thrombin. The thrombus within the plaque may then extend through to tear in the cap and extend into the lumen. There is a transitional zone in the tear itself in which both platelets and fibrin are present while if thrombus

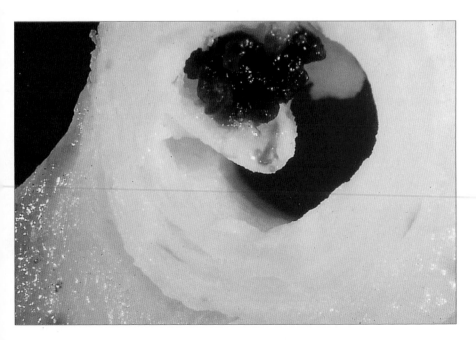

Figure 2.19
Coronary thrombus – plaque disruption. The plaque cap is torn and projects upward into the arterial lumen. The core contains a mass of mural thrombus which projects into but does not occlude the lumen.

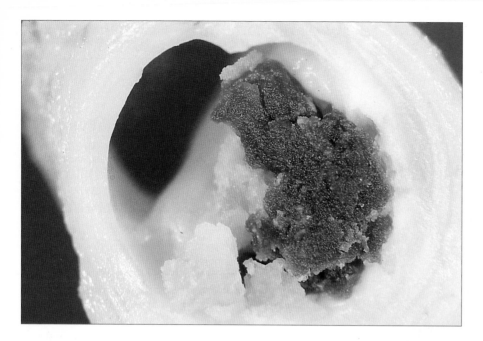

Figure 2.20
Coronary thrombosis – plaque disruption. The whole of the original lipid core is filled with a large mass of thrombus which has expanded the plaque from within and also projects into but does not occlude the lumen.

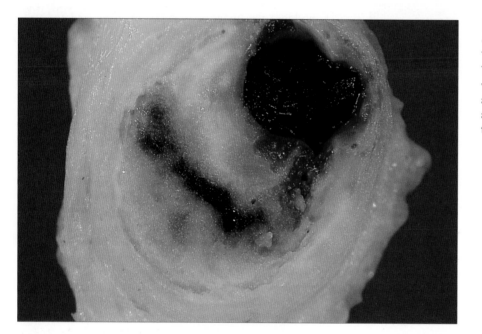

Figure 2.21
Coronary thrombosis – plaque disruption. The plaque was causing high grade stenosis. The cap has torn leading into a long fissure which extends down into the core. There is a moderate amount of intraplaque thrombus and thrombus has extended from the fissure to occlude the lumen.

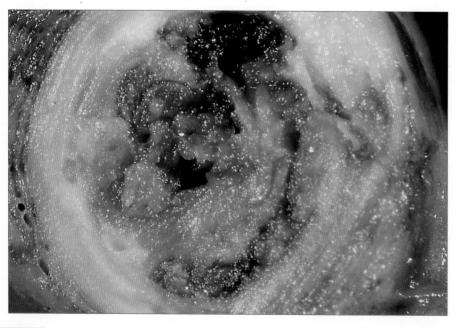

Figure 2.22
Coronary thrombosis – plaque disruption. The lumen is occluded by a mass of lipid and thrombus and there is no recognisable plaque remaining. This is the extreme end of the spectrum of disruption and occurs following complete disintegration of a very lipid rich plaque.

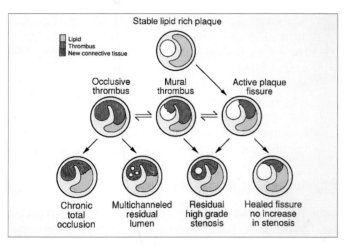

Figure 2.23
Outcome of coronary thrombosis. Thrombus is labile and mural and occlusive lesions pass from one to the other as a result of natural fibrinolytic activity. If thrombus is not lysed it is ultimately replaced by collagen produced by incoming smooth muscle cells. The end result can be anything from chronic total occlusion, recanalisation with multiple new smaller lumens or just a stenotic lesion.

restoration of the lumen (Fig. 2.23). Fibrinolysis, whether natural or therapeutically induced with streptokinase, is often effective at removing part or all of the intraluminal thrombus which is a loose network of fibrin and restoring some antegrade flow. Thrombus within the plaque is more resistant or less accessible. Thrombotic material which is not lysed invokes a florid smooth muscle cell proliferation response ultimately leading to fibrous replacement. The fibrous tissue contains many new capillary vessels and if the thrombus has remained occlusive ultimately there is the formation within the original lumen of a number of new vascular channels.

Plaque calcification

Calcification is a common factor in atherosclerotic plaques, increasing steadily in degree with both the extent of plaque formation and with age. Two distinct patterns occur. In one, nodular masses of calcium form within the lipid core, in the other plates of calcification develop in the connective tissue deep in the intima close to the medial/intimal junction. While formerly regarded as a passive precipitation of calcium phosphate crystals, plaque calcification is now recognised as a regulated process in which osteopontin, osteonectin, and osteocalcin are involved. Both macrophages and smooth muscle cells are involved in the production of these bone-promoting substances. Evidence of osteoclast and osteoblast like differentiation occurs in plaques and bone may be laid down. The question is whether calcification plays any more major role than hindering dissection by surgeons and pathologists. The current view is that the extent of calcification very roughly relates to the amount of atherosclerosis, but not to the degree of arterial narrowing. Calcification has no direct causal link to thrombosis with one exception. In old age (>75 years) diffuse intimal atherosclerosis and calcification is often associated with diffuse ectasia (dilatation) of the coronary arteries. Intimal tears at the margins of plates of calcium due to shear stress may then cause thrombosis.

THE PATHOLOGICAL CONSEQUENCES OF CORONARY ATHEROSCLEROSIS

An understanding of how coronary atherosclerosis will produce clinical disease must be based on knowledge of the anatomy, histological structure and physiology of the coronary arteries themselves.

Figure 2.24
Coronary artery anatomy and nomenclature. The coronary arteries arise from the two forward facing aortic sinuses which are called the right and left (RC, LC). The pulmonary valve lies between the left and right coronary arteries.

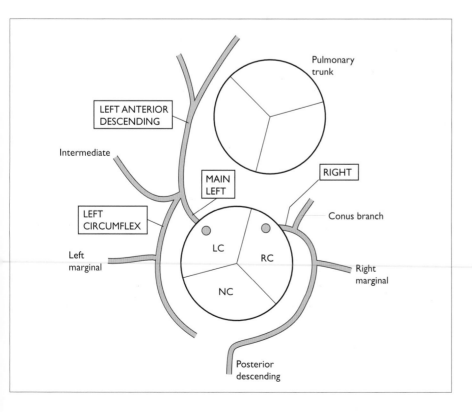

Normal coronary artery anatomy and histological structure

The two coronary arteries arise from the root of the aorta close to the sino-aortic junction. The orifices may be round in shape but occasionally are more slit-like with an overhanging shelf of aortic wall. These variants are of no functional significance and ostial stenosis (see below) is not present if a 2 mm probe can be passed easily at autopsy. A small subsidiary coronary orifice in up to 50% of normal individuals lies close to the right coronary artery; this small subsidiary vessel supplies the conus of the right ventricle. When a separate orifice is absent, the conus is supplied by the first branch of the right coronary artery. The nomenclature of the aortic cusps in relation to the coronary orifices is shown in Fig. 2.24.

While there are anatomically two coronary arteries, in functional terms there are three. These are the right, the left anterior descending and the left circumflex coronary arteries; these last two arise from the short main left coronary artery. The most important artery, because it supplies up to 50% of the total left ventricular mass, is the left anterior descending. This artery supplies the whole anterior wall of the left ventricle and the anterior two-thirds of the interventricular septum. It runs down the anterior wall of the heart to reach the apex of the left ventricle. Penetrating branches run backwards into the interventricular septum. The right coronary artery runs in the right atrioventricular groove supplying branches to the right ventricle and ultimately reaches the posterior wall where the posterior descending coronary artery runs down to the apex of the heart. Penetrating branches run into the ventricular septum to meet the longer penetrating branches of the anterior descending artery. The right coronary artery supplies 30–40% of the left ventricular mass. The left circumflex coronary artery runs in the left atrioventricular groove being obscured to view by the overhanging left atrial appendage. It gives origin to a major branch running down the lateral margin of the left ventricle (left marginal artery) and then passes round the atrioventricular ring to meet the right coronary artery on the posterior wall of the left ventricle. The left circumflex artery supplies approximately 20% of the myocardial mass.

The three coronary arteries are functionally regional in that there is virtually no overlap between the myocardial segments they supply. Occlusion leads to an area of ischaemia colocalising with the myocardial region supplied.

There is considerable variation in the anatomy of the human coronary artery supply superimposed on the basic pattern described above. Dominance refers to the contribution made by the right and left circumflex arteries to the blood supply of the posterior wall of the heart. Dominance can be used in a simple binary fashion. Right dominance is when the right coronary artery gives rise to the posterior descending coronary artery and this is found in more than 80% of normal hearts. Left dominance is when the left circumflex gives rise to the posterior descending coronary artery. This usage of the word dominance is the one adopted by most pathologists. Clinicians often apply a more relative usage of the word based on the extent to which the right coronary artery crosses the midline posteriorly to supply the posterior wall of the left ventricle before reaching the territory of the left circumflex artery.

Physiology of coronary flow

The epicardial coronary arteries have a well-developed medial coat containing very little elastic and numerous smooth muscle cells. Medial tone can vary and significantly alter lumen calibre. On exercise in normal subjects without atherosclerosis the epicardial coronary arteries dilate. The epicardial coronary arteries send numerous branches down into the myocardium. These intramyocardial arteries also have well-developed medial muscle. Two systems are present; one has straight vessels which do not branch until they give rise to a subendocardial plexus. The other system begins to branch immediately the myocardium is entered. The majority of intramyocardial arteries have an external diameter of 30–100 µ and are the resistance vessels where vascular tone controls intramyocardial flow. The pathophysiology of the blood flow to the myocardium is unique in that it does not occur in systole when the left ventricle is contracting. The epicardial arteries fill in systole but flow into the myocardium cannot begin until diastole. As the ventricular myocardium relaxes blood is sucked in from the epicardial arteries and aortic root above the closed aortic valve. Intramyocardial blood flow therefore depends on the difference between the aortic root pressure in diastole and the left ventricular cavity diastolic pressure. Any factors which conjointly cause a fall in diastolic aortic pressure and a rise in diastolic left ventricular cavity pressure will impair overall coronary blood flow.

Detailed vascular pathology of acute ischaemic syndromes

Unstable angina

Unstable angina is clinically characterised by transient episodic myocardial ischaemia manifesting as pain and ECG changes (ST segment depression) at rest. Angiographic studies show that there is a culprit coronary artery lesion characterised by a stenosis with ragged outlines and overhanging edges indicating a disrupted plaque. The thrombotic process seems arrested at a stage when thrombus is projecting into the lumen (Figs 2.19, 2.20) and has an active surface covered by platelets but antegrade blood flow is still occurring. Microemboli of platelets into the distal vascular bed (Fig. 2.25) are responsible for the episodic chest pain and also cause small microscopic foci of necrosis (Davies *et al.* 1986; Falk 1985). The thrombotic process in the artery ultimately resolves or progresses to totally occlude the artery.

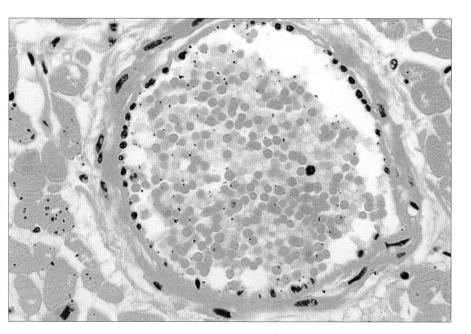

Figure 2.25a

Platelet intramyocardial emboli. H&E stained section of a small intramyocardial artery. The lumen contains red cells some of which are ghosts. They are much the same size as the white blood cells.

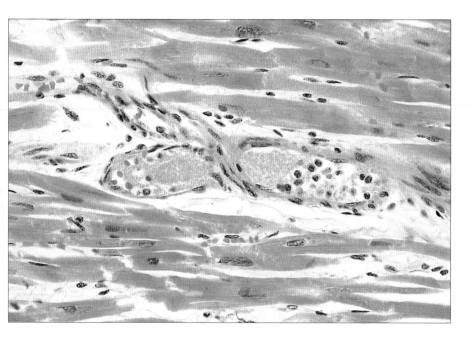

Figure 2.25b,c

Platelet intramyocardial emboli. In H&E stained sections, platelet clumps within small intramyocardial arteries can be recognised by their appearance as small punctate eosinophilic bodies contrasting with the much larger red cells. The use of techniques such as immunohistochemistry (c) using antibodies to the 2b/3a receptor, however, makes their recognition far easier. In this slide this alkaline phosphatase method shows a small artery within the myocardium occluded by a large mass of platelets.

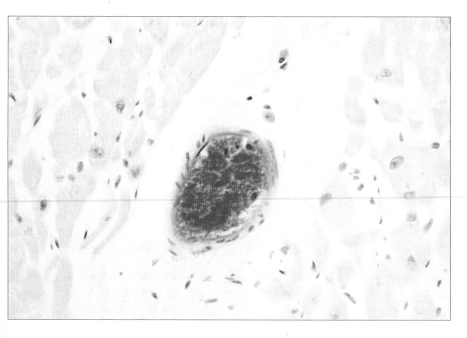

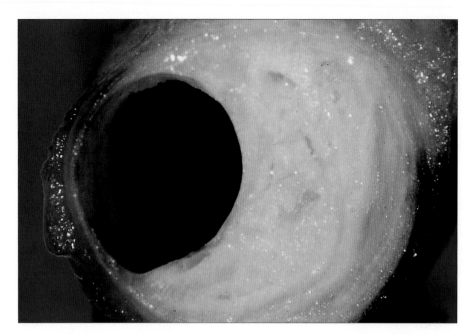

Figure 2.26
Eccentric lipid rich coronary plaque. The plaque has a very large lipid core which is extending up close to the lumen with a very thin cap in one area. The lipid was soft and could be easily expressed from the plaque by pressure. Opposite the plaque is a segment of normal arterial wall.

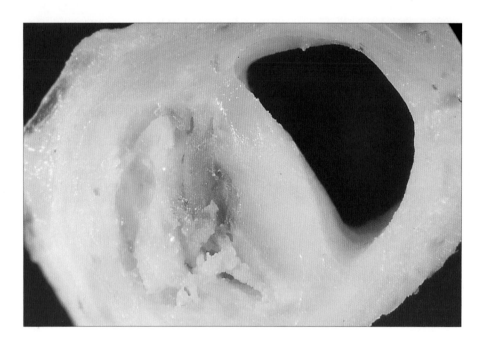

Figure 2.27
Eccentric lipid rich plaque. This plaque has a large crumbling lipid core but there is more collagenous fibrous tissue and the cap is thick.

Acute myocardial infarction

The blood supply of the human myocardium is regional in that each branch of the epicardial coronary arteries supplies a specific segment of myocardium from the endocardial to the epicardial surface. In the normal heart there is no functional overlap between adjacent arteries. In animal models the only way of producing a regional infarct is to occlude a coronary artery for at least 6 hours.

The same principles apply to human pathology and the presence of a regional infarction means that flow had ceased for at least some hours in the subtending artery. It is mandatory for a pathologist to find the cause when a regional infarct is found. The great majority (at least 99%) of infarcts are caused by thrombosis over an atherosclerotic plaque (Figs 2.17–2.22). Rare causes include spontaneous dissection and emboli; if there is no visible cause, spasm has to be considered but is a diagnosis made by exclusion. Provided that heavy calcification is absent, cross-sections of the coronary arteries made at 2–3 mm intervals will reveal thrombi. These may not be totally occlusive due to recanalisation or lysis, but it is usually easy to recognise thrombus within the plaque. Major disruptions lead to the lumen being occluded by a mixture of thrombus and extruded lipid (Fig. 2.22).

Vascular pathology of stable angina

Angiography in life shows that patients with stable exertional angina have segments of chronic high-grade stenosis in one or more of the coronary arteries.

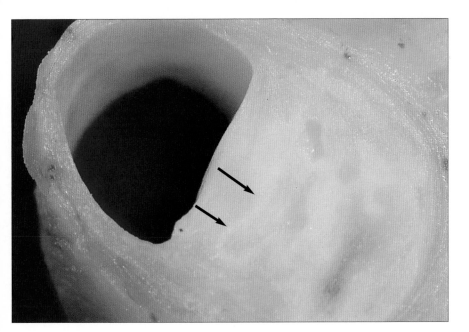

Figure 2.28
Eccentric atherosclerotic coronary plaque.
The plaque contains a lot of pearl grey
collagenous tissue and a small lipid core.
The lesion is also calcified (arrows).

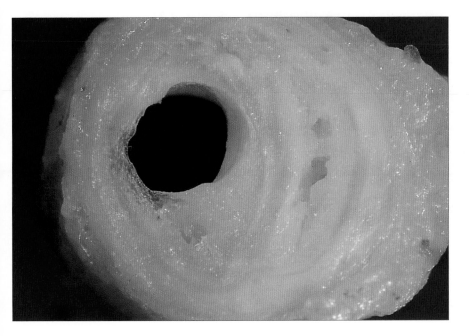

Figure 2.29
Multilayered coronary plaque. The plaque
contains several layers of yellow lipid and
the most superficial zone consists of semi-
translucent collagen. Although the lumen of
the artery is not central relative to the long
axis of the vessel, the segment of arterial
wall opposite the plaque shows considerable
intimal thickening.

Pathology series (Hangartner *et al.* 1986) confirm this view, although as expected are biased toward multi-vessel involvement. Significant coronary stenosis means that the lumen at the stenotic point is reduced by 50% in diameter (75% by cross-sectional area). This is the degree of narrowing which begins to reduce flow in experimental models and appears to be applicable in clinical practice.

Morphological forms of stenosis in stable angina

There is considerable diversity in the plaques causing high-grade stenosis (Figs 2.26–2.32). Some are relatively simple type Va plaques with a lipid core and a cap where the plaques have caused stenosis by primary atherogenesis, i.e. lipid and collagen formation. The size of the plaque core relative to overall size is very variable. Many relative simple plaques are eccentric,

leaving an arc of normal media on the opposite side of the vessel wall. Some plaques may be total solid and fibrous (Type Vc). High-grade stenoses are often very complex with multi-layered plaques, some with more than one core (Type Vb). Plaques may form opposite each other and involve the whole circumference of the intima. Circumferential fibrous thickening of the intima often occurs distal to high grade stenosis. Replacement of the lumen by several smaller channels indicates recanalisation of an occluding thrombus (Roberts and Virmani 1984). Such arterial segments may or may not be related to healed infarcts.

Coronary anastomoses

Functionally there are no connections between adjacent coronary artery beds. If one coronary artery develops high-grade stenosis, however, a pressure gradient exists

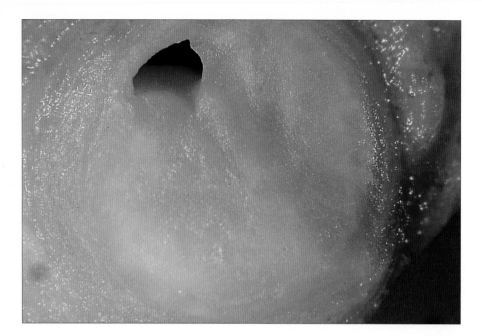

Figure 2.30
Lipid rich plaque causing high-grade stenosis.
The whole plaque is yellow due to lipid but
there is no discrete lipid core and cap. This
form of plaque is typical of very severe
hypercholesterolaemia and diabetes. The
lumen is reduced to a pin point.

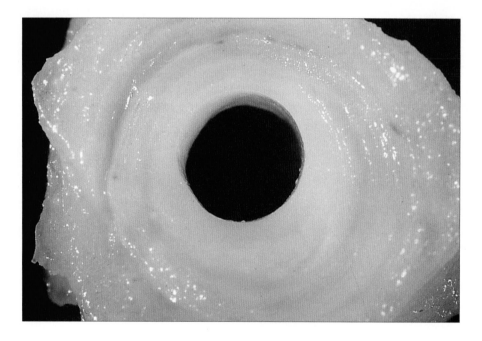

Figure 2.31
Concentric fibrous plaque. The plaque
completely surrounds the lumen and is solid
and fibrous with just a few flecks of yellow
lipid.

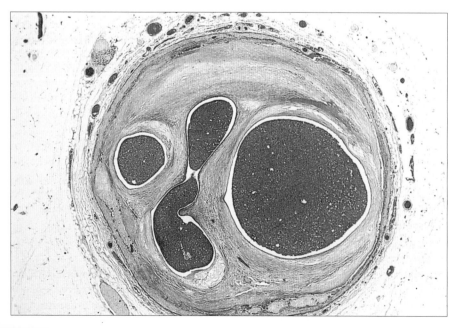

Figure 2.32
Recanalisation of coronary artery. The
coronary artery shows four separate new
lumens within the original lumen. The
vessels contain post mortem angiographic
medium.

between the two beds. Under these circumstances previously existing small vessels enlarge and allow collateral flow. These anastomotic vessels can only be assessed by *in vivo* or post mortem coronary arteriography and are not visible by ordinary macroscopic examination. Collaterals develop at three levels. In the adventitia of coronary artery segments with high-grade stenoses vessels enlarge and bridge the narrowed segment. While these can be recognised very easily in angiograms, their functional significance is minimal. Second, large vessels on the pericardial surface of the heart or atrial branches may enlarge and have a characteristic corkscrew pattern in angiograms; these arterial anastomoses are of functional significance. Finally, in diffusely scarred left ventricles, a plexus of subendo-cardial thin-walled vessels appears, which fills readily throughout the ventricle following injection of dye into one coronary artery. This form of intramyocardial collateral flow is most common in subjects with diffuse triple vessel disease who have not had large regional infarcts.

Measurement of coronary stenosis

The complexity of trying to measure coronary stenosis at autopsy must not be underestimated. In angiograms in living patients, the lumen diameter at the stenotic segment is compared with that of the nearest apparently normal segment of artery. This method has proven moderately effective in clinical practice as a guide to judging the need to insert coronary artery bypass grafts or perform angioplasty. Angiography is however, very insensitive for the detection of plaques unless they are encroaching on the lumen. Intravascular ultrasound in life shows clearly that angiographically normal segments of artery can contain large plaques (Mintz *et al.* 1995; Tuzcu *et al.* 1995). In effect there is no direct relation between plaque size and stenosis. The explanation of this paradox lies in remodelling of the vessel wall. In one form of remodelling, the media behind an eccentric plaque thins (Crawford and Levene 1953) and the elastic lamina breaks, allowing the plaque to bulge outward rather than inward. Seen in cross-section, the artery wall has an eccentric outline. The second form of remodelling lies in a reorganisation of the medial muscle. As the plaque develops, the external diameter of the vessel increases to accommodate the plaque without needing to reduce the lumen dimensions (Glagov *et al.* 1987; Ge *et al.* 1993; LoSordo *et al.* 1994). The phenomenon of remodelling has serious implications for pathologists and the traditional method of measuring stenosis in which the cross-sectional area or diameter of the lumen is compared with the dimensions of the vessel *at the same point*. This method inherently overestimates diameter stenosis by a factor of up to 30% when compared with an angiographic method (Mann and Davies 1996). Because the degree of remodelling differs from plaque to plaque the error is not constant but can range from 0 to 50%.

Practicalities of assessing coronary disease at autopsy

Slitting the coronary arteries open longitudinally and inspecting the intima enface to assess the percentage of the intima covered by plaques is a standard method used in large geographic studies, but gives no information on the degree of stenosis other than indicating that where the scissors will not pass a particular point, there might be high-grade stenosis.

The preferred method is to cut multiple cross-sections at 2–3 mm intervals along all the three major arteries. Visual assessment can be made of the degree of stenosis seen at different sites. Simple visual impressions of the degree of stenosis (Fig. 2.33) can with practice become very reproducible by a single observer and even between observers. This must not, however, be allowed to hide the fact that the method has very serious limitations when used for correlation with angiograms carried out in life, or used to indicate clinical significance. Pathologists will innately tend to overestimate the degree of narrowing. The reasons for this are multiple and include the fact that any method which compares the lumen to the size of the vessel *at the same point* has ignored the remodelling that occurs. The external size of the vessel at this point is larger than normal and the degree of stenosis will be exaggerated. A second factor is that pathologists are examining collapsed and empty arteries in which the lumen is often slit-like (Figs 2.34). In plaques which are eccentric leaving a segment of normal vessel wall when the artery is distended the lumen becomes round, but when empty is slit-like causing a spurious impression of stenosis (Fig. 2.35). The final factor is that calcification will hinder the

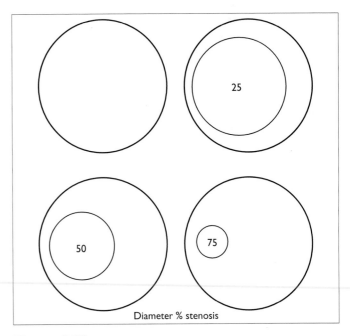

Diameter % stenosis

Figure 2.33
Visual assessment of coronary stenosis. In this diagram the different degrees of diameter stenosis are shown. The higher the grade of stenosis the greater the degree of certainty that the figure would reflect significant stenosis in life.

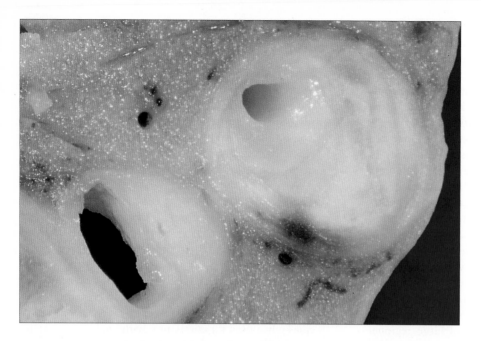

Figure 2.34
Coronary stenosis. In the two arteries shown one has a pin-point lumen indicating well over 75% diameter stenosis and can be confidently said to have produced obstruction and would have been seen on angiography. The other vessel has an elongated oval lumen with an eccentric plaque retaining an arc of normal vessel wall. It is not possible accurately to predict what the lumen size was in life when the vessel was distended.

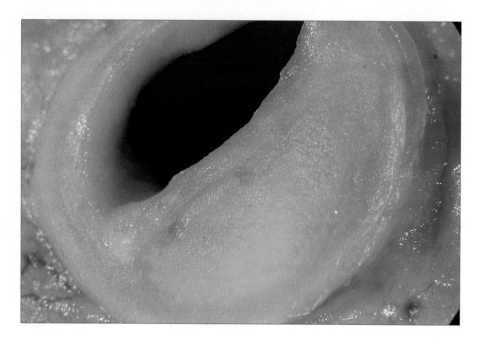

Figure 2.35
Coronary stenosis. There is a plaque with a large core and a cap. The plaque is eccentrically situated and the lumen is oval in shape due to the lumen collapsing. Visual assessment of the stenosis would require the mental ability to convert this irregular shape to the area of a circle with the same perimeter.

cutting of cross-sections without completely distorting the tissues.

Pathologists are regularly called on to assess coronary atherosclerosis at autopsy, despite the difficulties inherent in the methods used to quantify stenosis. The first factor to consider is the reason for, and importance of, such an examination. The techniques used will need to vary according to these reasons. For general autopsy work it is sufficient to cut cross-sections and visually assess the number and site of segments which show stenosis of more than 75% by diameter. Such pin-point lumens indicate that high-grade stenosis must have been present in life. Lesser degrees of stenosis based on visual assessment can be made, but will reflect coronary flow in life with far less certainty. If there is going to be any question of the degree of stenosis being used in legal cases or in the audit of cardiac surgical work, more

sophisticated techniques are needed. This will mean decalcifying the coronary arteries before making the cross-cuts. Segments of the major coronary arteries several centimetres long can be removed from the heart and decalcified for 24 hours. In such segments the degree of stenosis can be accurately assessed by comparing the vessel lumen at the narrowest point compared with the lumen at the closest point in the artery in which the wall appears relatively normal. Use of this external, i.e. distal, or proximal reference point will give stenosis figures very similar to angiograms in life. Such data then allows the wealth of information on life expectancy which is available from clinical studies to be used.

Histological methods based on comparing the lumen size to the vessel size at the same site are often made in the belief that they have greater validity than visual assessment. They are more reproducible but have the same limitation in that remodelling is ignored. Pathologists should always remember that the information which is needed is the lumen size relative to the lumen size of the normal vessel either proximally or distally. A pragmatic approach is to cut the artery into 1 cm segments, examine them to exclude thrombus, and then pass a soft malleable probe 2 mm in diameter down the major coronary arteries. If this passes easily there is no significant stenosis present even if many plaques are present. This technique is particularly useful for eccentric plaques in which the lumen is slit or oval in shape.

MYOCARDIAL ISCHAEMIA AND INFARCTION

Myocardial infarction is defined as death of myocardial tissue caused by ischaemia which is a reduction or cessation of blood flow to myocytes to a degree that oxygen delivery is not adequate to meet the metabolic demands of the cells. Ischaemia is initially reversible. Patients with stable angina on exercise have ischaemia which is reversed on rest when oxygen demand falls. Persistent ischaemia is usually due to more severe reduction or cessation of blood flow and leads to structural changes and then death of the myocytes.

Regional infarction

The term infarction is used for a number of entities which have very different pathophysiology (Fig. 2.36). The most common form of infarction recognised clinically and pathologically is an area of regional necrosis which is anterior or lateral or posteroseptal etc and clearly lies in the territory supplied by one major epicar-

dial coronary artery. The clinician recognises such necrosis and localises it anatomically from the ECG appearance. Regional infarction may be transmural or confined to the subendocardial zone. More diffuse ischaemic myocardial necrosis that is unrelated to the area supplied by one coronary artery also occurs. The best recognised form is circumferential subendocardial necrosis due to an overall failure of myocardial perfusion. There are many causes including shock, prolonged hypotension, prolonged hypoxia and use of high doses of inotropic drugs. The condition is always more likely to occur in ventricles with hypertrophy and may be seen after prolonged cardiac bypass for aortic valve stenosis. Diffuse non-regional focal areas of necrosis, identifiable by histology only, are an early form of this type of infarction.

Much of the knowledge about the events which immediately precede regional infarction is derived from a dog model in which a major coronary artery is ligated. Much of this knowledge can be directly applied to man. The dog model (Reimer et al. 1985; Jennings et al. 1995) is simple in that the artery is occluded instantly at a known point in time in a heart without prior collateral flow. Flow can be re-established in the artery at a known time interval. Human infarction is more complex in that the exact time of onset of occlusion is not known, because occlusion often has a stuttering and intermittent onset and collateral flow may or may not have been previously present.

Experimental infarction in the dog

Ligation of a major coronary artery in the dog (usually the left anterior descending artery, but left circumflex occlusion is also used) leads to a regional zone of infarction. A proportion of the animals die within minutes of

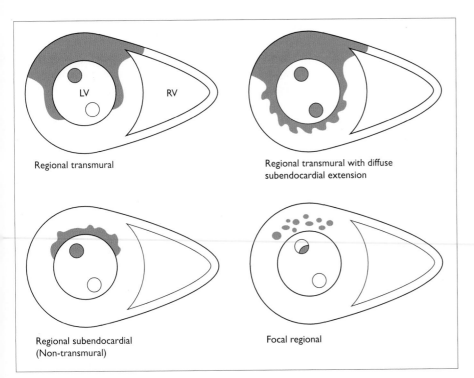

Regional transmural

Regional transmural with diffuse subendocardial extension

Regional subendocardial (Non-transmural)

Focal regional

Figure 2.36
Diagrammatic representation of different forms of regional myocardial infarction. Each type of regional infarction has a different pathophysiology. Regional transmural infarction is due to persistent occlusion of the subtending artery. Regional non-transmural infarction is due to occlusion which spontaneously reopens or has pre-existing collaterals. Focal regional infarction is due to platelet microemboli from a more proximal thrombus. In patients who go into cardiogenic shock diffuse subendocardial necrosis may develop in the rest of the ventricle.

arterial ligation from ventricular fibrillation but in those who survive for a period of over 8 hours the area of necrosis can be recognised at autopsy. The only method of producing such a regional infarct is to occlude the regional artery. The lateral margins of the area of necrosis are defined by the anatomy of the arterial tree and thus are established at the moment of ligation by the site of the occlusion and the coronary anatomy. In the dog model it is possible to reperfuse the area of ischaemia by removing the ligature on the coronary artery. This establishes that the subendocardial myocardium is most susceptible and dies within 20–40 minutes; the infarction then spreads through the wall to reach the epicardial surface in 6 hours. Thus, there are two forms of regional infarction. One is transmural implying that no reperfusion occurred; the other extends only for a part of the wall thickness (non-transmural infarction) implying that reperfusion occurred.

Biochemical and structural changes in experimental infarction

When oxygen supply ceases, within seconds the aerobic mitochondrial respiratory system ceases to function and myocytes stop contracting, but maintain their viability by a switch to anaerobic glycolysis. Myocyte creatinine phosphate falls rapidly followed by a decline in ATP. Anaerobic glycolysis using glycogen as a substrate continues, but leads to lactate accumulation and a rise in intracellular pH. After about 40 minutes, ATP levels fall to zero and the myocytes are effectively dead. They will not recover on reperfusion, i.e. the changes are irreversible. The initial structural changes are a loss of glycogen and an increase in sarcoplasmic spaces due to fluid entering the cells. The major use of energy by ischaemic myocytes which have long ceased contracting is to maintain membrane integrity. Irreversible cell damage is marked by the appearance of breaks in the cell membrane. Blebs of oedema appear beneath the sarcolemma which is lifted away from the underlying sarcomeres and then structural breaks appear. Contiguous with these signs of cell membrane disruption, mitochondrial cristae begin to be disorganised and small dense lipid granules appear. The electron microscopic changes are easy to identify within a few hours and long before light microscopy changes appear. The light microscopy identification of ischaemic necrosis depends on changes in the myofibrils. Loss of myofibrillary architecture and cross-striations and the formation of rather amorphous hypereosinophilic material inside the cell does not occur until 12 hours. An interstitial acute inflammatory cell infiltrate develops by 8 hours before identifiable changes in myofibrils appear by light microscopy. Macrophages appear by Day 3–5, and fibroblasts and new capillary vessels invade the dead area from the margins by 7 days onwards.

Myocytes which are irreversibly damaged but not yet totally dead develop a rather different pattern of histological change if the area of necrosis is reperfused. The myofibrils undergo intense hypercontraction and shunt together leading to the appearance of brightly eosinophilic cross-banding within the myocyte. When present the histological change is striking and appears by 30 minutes, long before other structural criteria of necrosis.

The process of replacing dead myocytes by a collagenous scar may take up to 8 weeks and fibrosis then continues for a further 3–6 months. The area of infarction has to be organised from the margins where there are viable interstitial cells. The process may never be completed and it is possible for mummified myocytes without nuclei to exist within a thick fibrous capsule for many months.

Human myocardial infarction

All the mechanisms and morphological changes in the dog model apply to human disease, but there is considerable added complexity due to the variables of the initiating occlusion being intermittent and the presence or absence of pre-existing collaterals.

Use of macroscopic methods which demonstrate the loss of enzyme activity in the myocardium at autopsy allow the demonstration of the morphology of infarcts more precisely than simple naked eye examination of a fresh tissue slice (Derias and Adams 1978; Anderson *et al.* 1979). Human infarcts can be divided into several forms which have rather different pathophysiological origins (Figs 2.36–2.39). Simple regional transmural infarcts in which the necrosis appears histologically to be all of approximately the same age may occur. All the histological parameters of infarction defined in the dog model are found in human disease (Figs 2.40–2.48). The frequency of the different regions involved is anteroseptal, posteroseptal and lateral by ratios of 3.2.1 reflecting the relative frequency of left anterior descending, right and left circumflex coronary artery thrombi.

The non-transmural form of regional infarction is now common and characteristically appears to have formed by the coalescence of smaller areas of necrosis of differing age. Even within the area of infarction islands of surviving myocytes can be found. A very complex histological picture is produced in which different fields show different stages of necrosis. Survival of interstitial cells within the infarct zone allows very rapid fibroblastic responses.

Determination of duration of infarction

Pathologists may be asked to assess the age of an infarct in order to determine if it pre or post dated an event such as a surgical operation or an accident. Such an exercise is far from easy. The published data (Lodge-Patch 1951) on this matter date to the era when many human infarcts were single regional areas with a uniform age. Today most infarcts have been built up by the coalescence of foci of necrosis occurring over a period of time. All that can be done is to age the oldest foci working on the basis that collagen deposition begins at 5–6 days. The focus of necrosis does not,

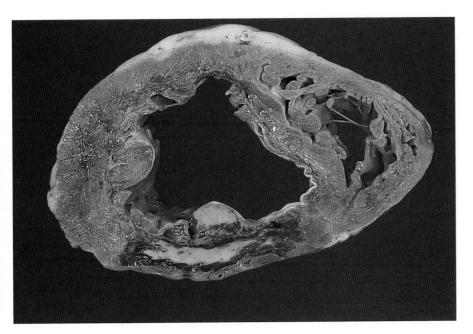

Figure 2.37
Human regional myocardial infarction. In this untreated unfixed slice of myocardium there is an infarct which was between 5 and 7 days in duration by clinical history. By this stage the centre of the infarct is yellow and there is a red rim where vessels are beginning to invade the infarcted tissue to initiate organisation. The infarct is full thickness and involves the posteromedial papillary muscle. The infarct is in the region supplied by the right coronary artery which was occluded by thrombus.

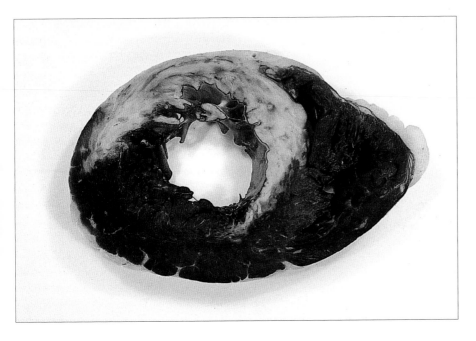

Figure 2.38
Human regional infarction. The transverse slice of tissue taken through the ventricles at the papillary muscle level has been incubated with nitro BT to demonstrate dehydrogenase activity as a deep blue colour. A regional anteroseptal infarction is shown as an absence of enzyme activity. The infarct is full thickness and involves the anterolateral papillary muscle. In the septum there is a segment of the infarct which is not transmural. Left anterior descending coronary artery thrombotic occlusion.

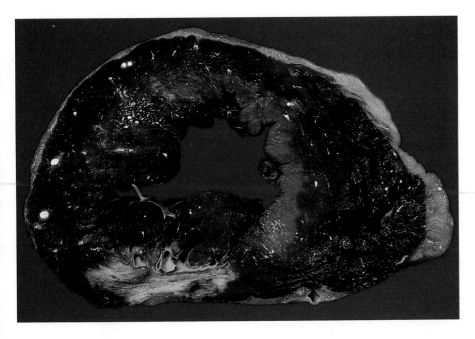

Figure 2.39
Human regional infarction. The transverse slice of ventricular myocardium stained with nitro BT shows enzyme loss in the inner subendocardial zone of anteroseptal area. The infarction is not full thickness at any point. There is an old posterior full thickness infarct scar showing as dense white fibrous tissue. Left anterior descending coronary artery thrombosis with extensive collateral flow due to old right coronary occlusion.

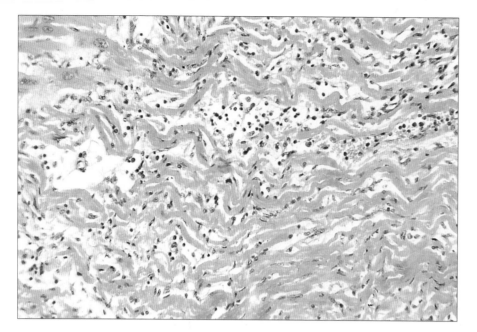

Figure 2.40
Human infarction – histology. There is a diffuse infiltrate of polymorphonuclear cells in the interstitial tissues. This change appears within 8 hours and is often seen before recognisable change within the myocytes themselves (H&E ×56).

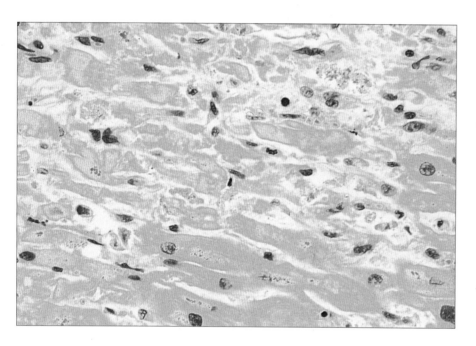

Figure 2.41
Human infarction – histology. The myocytes in the centre of the field have undergone necrosis and the cytoplasm contains irregular clumps of eosinophilic material compared to adjacent cells. Membrane breakdown has begun with release of lipofuscin and macrophages are just beginning to appear. The absence of fibroblastic activity indicates a lesion of 2–3 days in age (H&E ×87.5).

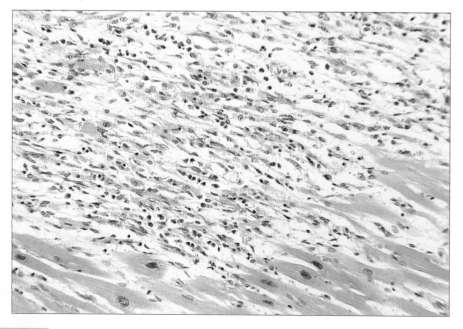

Figure 2.42
Human infarction – histology. In the area of necrosis the majority of the myocyte cytoplasm has vanished and there is an intense macrophage infiltrate, but fibrosis has not begun. This would correspond to 4–5 days of duration of the infarct (H&E ×87.5).

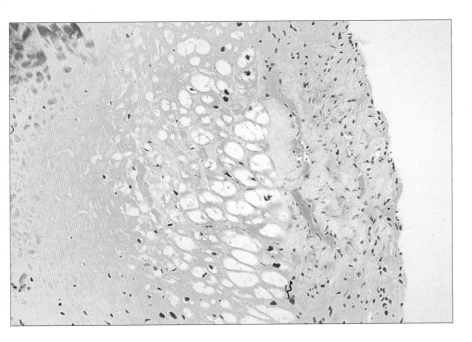

Figure 2.43
Human infarction – histology. In the layer of myocytes just beneath the endocardium the cells remain viable but subject to chronic ischaemia. The myofibrils are lost giving the appearance of vacuolated or empty cells but the nuclei remain intact. The deeper myocardium shows total necrosis. The viable but non-contractile myocytes are the basis of hibernation and can recover function with time if the area is reperfused (H&E ×56).

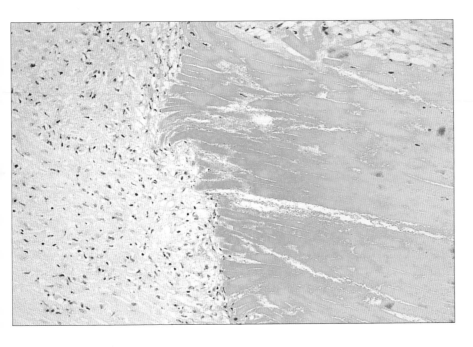

Figure 2.44
Human infarction – histology. There is an area of infarction in which the myocytes remain easily recognised but no nuclei are present. At the margin of the area of necrosis there are some macrophages but there is no evidence of active organisation. Such areas of mummified necrotic myocardium walled in by fibrous tissue may persist for months or even years.

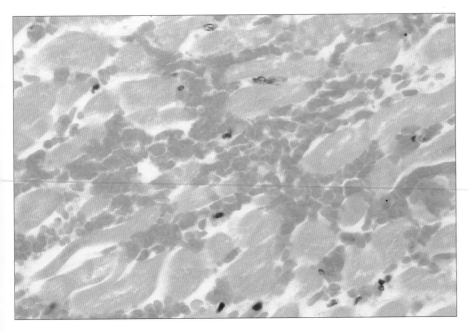

Figure 2.45
Human infarction – histology. Reperfusion of an area of dead myocardium leads to extravasation of red cells into the interstitial spaces and an infarct which to the naked eye appears red and haemorrhagic (H&E ×140).

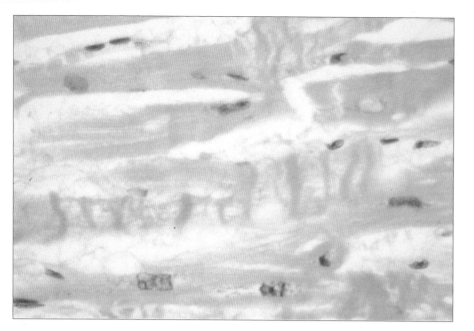

Figure 2.46
Human infarction – contraction band necrosis. In this form of necrosis the myofibrils hypercontract within the cell and form brightly eosinophilic cross-bands at irregular intervals within the cell. It indicates reperfusion of an area of infarction when the myocytes are just viable. Calcium ions enter the cell through the damaged wall membrane and react with myosin ATPase to cause hypercontraction (H&E ×140).

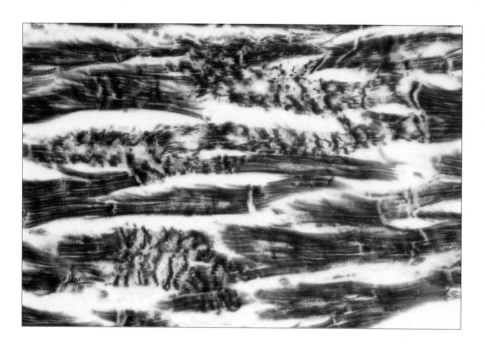

Figure 2.47
Human infarction – contraction band necrosis. In sections stained to highlight the myofibrillary structure such as a PTAH the contraction bands can be more readily observed than in haematoxylin and eosin stained sections (PTAH ×140).

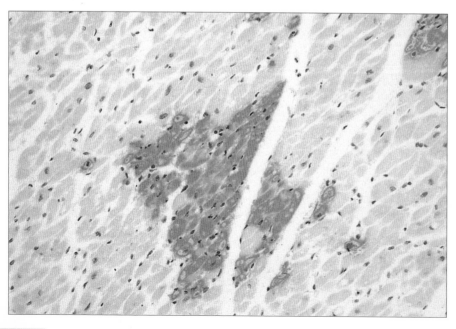

Figure 2.48
Human infarction – complement binding. Foci of myocytes which have undergone recent necrosis stain by immunohistochemistry for the C9 component of complement.

however, necessarily undergo histological changes at the same rate. In foci where the connective tissue stroma survives but the myocytes alone die, collagen deposition may begin within 2–3 days.

Early detection of infarction

Ligation of a coronary artery in the dog consistently produces a regional infarction which can be recognised by macroscopic and microscopic changes from 12 hours after the operation. In animals sacrificed before 12 hours the infarct cannot be recognised. It is therefore apparent that, although the heart muscle in the region begins to die within 10 minutes and is transmural by 6 hours when the necrosis reaches the epicardium, the changes which enable a pathologist to recognise cell death evolve with time (Jennings *et al.* 1995). The same phenomenon must occur in human disease – pathologists regularly encounter human cases with an acute coronary thrombotic occlusion, documented acute ECG changes but no detectable infarct at autopsy. These phenomena lead to a search for more sensitive means of detecting early infarction by histology (Figs 2.46–2.48).

A range of acid or basic fuchsin stains as well as some of the trichrome staining methods will detect changes in the binding of the dyes to the myofibrils of dead myocytes. The loss or reduction of dehydrogenase activity in frozen histological sections has been used to identify dead myocytes. All of these methods involve a subjective analysis by the observer and cannot be used routinely. In all the staining methods judgement is required to carry out differentiation – in effect the observer decides what answer is correct before starting. The C9 component of complement is bound to ischaemic dying myocytes and can also be used to demonstrate early focal necrosis (Fig. 2.48).

Contraction band necrosis (Figs 2.46–2.47) occurs very early after the onset of cell death provided that reperfusion has occurred (Karch and Billingham 1986). The phenomenon is due to restoration of calcium ions to the interstitial tissues; calcium then enters the dying myocyte and invokes intense hyper-contraction of the myofibrils. Contraction banding is easily recognised in haematoxylin and eosin (H&E) sections, but can be accentuated by stains such as phosphotungstic acid haematoxylin (PTAH) (Fig. 2.47). In any heart which has gone into ventricular fibrillation (VF) prior to death some contraction bands will be found. If, however, they are present in large numbers and in particular if they are found in one region only, i.e. anteroseptal but not posteroseptal, they are a reliable means of identifying early infarction. Even when reperfusion had not occurred some contraction band necrosis is usually found at the edge of an infarct which predominantly shows the colliquative pattern of necrosis. Contraction band necrosis has also been called coagulative myocytolysis (Baroldi *et al.* 1979) but this name leads to confusion with other forms of myocyte death such as that occurring in cardiac rejection.

Complications of regional myocardial infarction

Ventricular tachycardia degenerating into ventricular fibrillation is the cause of sudden death in the first 24 hours of myocardial infarction and is responsible for early deaths before the patient reaches intensive care. The risk of VF is not directly related to infarct size and is present even with small infarcts. Cardiogenic shock is responsible for the majority of deaths in patients who have reached intensive care and is a complication directly related to infarct size (Alonso *et al.* 1973). Infarcts which involve more than 40–50% of the total left ventricular mass are rarely survived. Most such

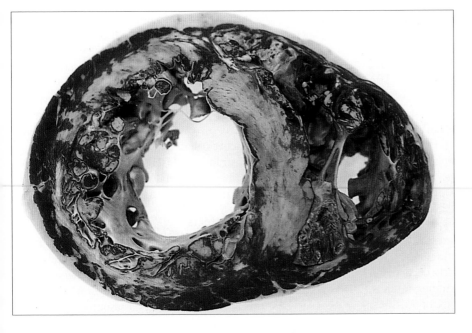

Figure 2.49
Cardiogenic shock from acute infarction. In this cross-section of the ventricles there is a transmural septal regional acute infarction shown by lack of dehydrogenase staining. There is widespread focal areas of necrosis in the subendocardial zone throughout the rest of the ventricles. Old ischaemic scarring is also present on the posterolateral wall.

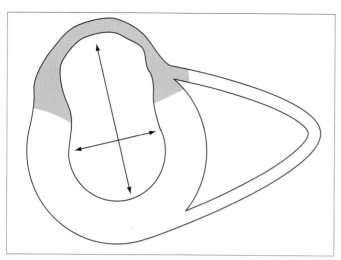

Figure 2.50
Infarct expansion. In infarct expansion the left ventricular wall in the necrotic zone bulges outward and begins to become thinner. The left ventricular cavity becomes asymmetric with one diameter greater than the other. No further necrosis is involved.

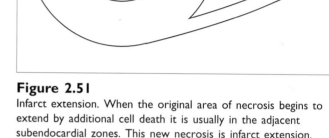

Figure 2.51
Infarct extension. When the original area of necrosis begins to extend by additional cell death it is usually in the adjacent subendocardial zones. This new necrosis is infarct extension.

large infarcts are due to very proximal thrombotic occlusions of the left anterior descending coronary artery. Superimposed subendocardial circumferential necrosis often develops leading to a downward spiral of more necrosis – further decline in left ventricle function – further myocardial hypoperfusion and further necrosis (Fig. 2.49).

Infarct expansion

Infarct expansion (Pirolo *et al.* 1986) is a stretching and thinning of the necrotic region producing an outward bulge (Fig. 2.50). No further necrosis is involved and the process is distinct from infarct extension (Fig. 2.51). Infarct expansion is a complication which develops during the first week in large transmural infarcts. Since it is directly related to infarct size, it is most common in anteroseptal infarcts. Expansion is important because it is a prelude to one form of cardiac rupture (see below) and in its most extreme leads to left ventricular aneurysms. Expansion is also important because when fibrous repair occurs the shape of the expanded acute infarct is retained (Fig. 2.50–2.52). The left ventricle is left with a permanent enlargement of the cavity with a detrimental effect or function (Gaudron *et al.* 1993).

Cardiac rupture

Cardiac rupture leading to tamponade falls into two groups (Becker and van Mantgem 1975). Rupture may occur within 24 hours of the onset of necrosis. Externally there is a slit-like tear in the left ventricle (Fig. 2.53). On cross-sections it is often difficult to see the infarction due to its early state (Fig. 2.53). The tear appears to be at the junction of viable and non-viable tissue and is presumably due to shear stresses between the non-contractile muscle and contracting viable muscle. Left ventricular rupture more rarely occurs later (5–7 days) and is a complication of expanding infarcts. The hole in the left ventricle is at the apex of a distinct

bulge (Fig. 2.54) and there is often overlying acute pericarditis. Cardiac rupture is more common in elderly women than men (Dellborg *et al.* 1985).

Ischaemic left ventricular aneurysms

The commonest form of ventricular aneurysm is the end result of infarct expansion and produces an aneurysmal sac with a relatively wide neck. The wall is fibrous and contains no residual myocardium. The endocardium is white and this white thickening often extends out from the sac itself over the rim into adjacent myocardium. The sac may (Fig. 2.55) or may not contain laminated thrombus. Calcification of the deepest layers of thrombus is common. A much rarer type of aneurysm has a very narrow neck leading to a large external sac. This type is thought to arise from partial tear of the infarct in the acute stage in which a subpericardial haematoma is contained by fibrosis developing in the pericardium. These aneurysms are sometimes called 'pseudo' due to the wall being predominantly formed from the pericardium (van Tassel and Edwards 1972). In fact there is a complete spectrum and histology shows some residual myocardial tissue in the wall of virtually all left ventricular aneurysms. All these aneurysms have a risk of rupture, of systemic emboli and cause abnormal left ventricular function. A striking feature of left ventricular aneurysms is also a marked tendency to episodic ventricular tachycardia. These tachycardias arise in anastomosing strands and islands of surviving myocytes embedded in the endocardial thickening that occurs on the rim of the aneurysmal sac.

Ventricular septal defects

These usually arise from expansion of either an anteroseptal or a posteroseptal infarct (Visser *et al.* 1986; Mann and Roberts 1988). In the acute stage the tear has a ragged edge and in the rare case who survives, this ultimately becomes a smooth-edged defect

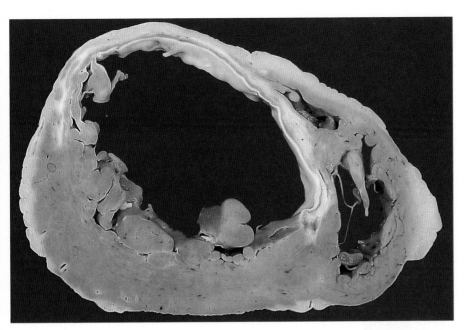

Figure 2.52
Infarct expansion – ventricular remodelling. The cross-section of the ventricles shows a healed expanded anteroseptal infarct. The left ventricular wall is thinned in the scar and the cavity is enlarged. The residual segment of surviving myocardium has undergone hypertrophy and the wall is thick.

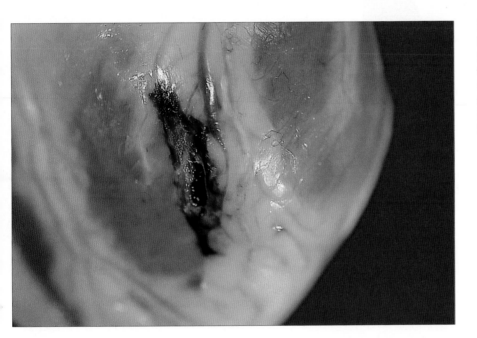

Figure 2.53 a,b
Early ventricular rupture in myocardial infarction. Viewed from the external surface there is a ragged tear in the left ventricle. On the cut surface a slit-like tear traverses the ventricular wall. There is no associated bulge in the contour of the ventricle and infarct expansion has not occurred.

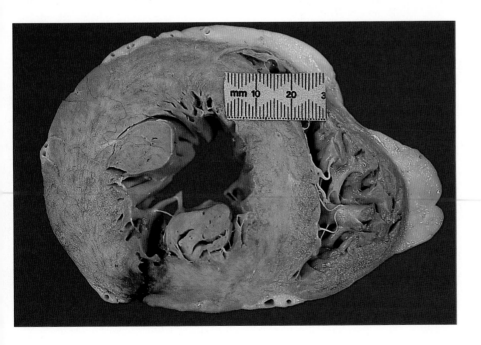

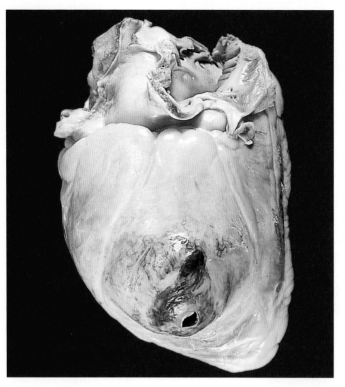

Figure 2.54
Late ventricular rupture in myocardial infarction. Viewed from the epicardial surface there is a localised external bulge with a rupture point at its apex.

(Fig. 2.56). The mortality rate in the acute stage is high and surgical repair is high risk. These risks largely relate to the fact that the infarct size is large.

Papillary muscle rupture

The majority of the complications listed so far are directly related to transmural large infarcts. Papillary muscle rupture (Nashimura *et al.* 1983; Barbour and Roberts 1986) is an exception in that the infarcts can

be small and may not be transmural. Either papillary muscle can rupture. The anterolateral papillary muscle is supplied by the left marginal branch of the left circumflex artery and a distinct entity exists of left marginal artery thrombosis producing papillary rupture without significant infarction of the rest of the left ventricle. The posterior medial artery is supplied from the right coronary artery. Rupture may involve either one subhead or the whole papillary muscle across the base. The stump of the papillary muscle passes back and forward across the mitral valve in life and the chordae become twisted and tangled. The stump is found in the left atrium at autopsy (Fig. 2.57).

NON-ATHEROSCLEROTIC CORONARY ARTERY DISEASE: CONGENITAL ANOMALIES

Non-atherosclerotic coronary artery disease is rare as a cause of significant clinical problems. Congenital anomalies of the origins of the coronary arteries come in a myriad of forms (Fig. 2.58) some of which are dangerous in respect of sudden death (*see* Chapter 8); others are simple anatomical variants without an effect on coronary blood flow (Roberts 1986; Taylor *et al.* 1992). Dangerous anomalies are one artery taking origin from the pulmonary trunk or both arteries taking origin in one aortic sinus with an artery crossing between the aorta and pulmonary trunk. Arteries in the pulmonary trunk create a left to right shunt and often become very large and tortuous. Arteries crossing between the aorta and pulmonary trunk tend initially to have spasm on exercise, then undergo slow obliteration with intimal fibrosis. Both of these dangerous anomalies may present as myocardial infarction or angina in infancy or early adult life and there is always a risk of sudden death. Many cases, however, have good exercise tolerance and only present as sudden

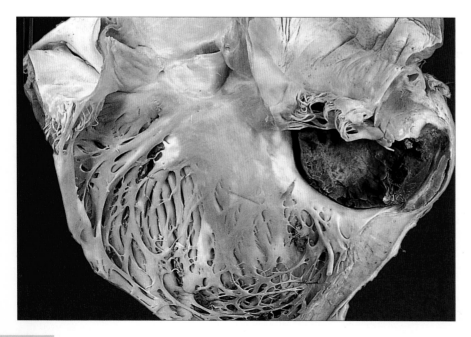

Figure 2.55
Left ventricular ischaemic aneurysm. The aneurysm is a discrete bulge on the posterior wall of the left ventricle with a well defined rim with endocardial thickening. The aneurysm sac contains thrombus which obliterates its cavity.

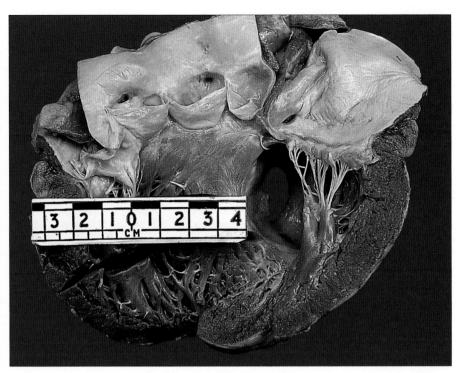

Figure 2.56
Post-infarction ventricular septal defect. There is an acquired ventricular septal defect behind the posteromedial papillary muscle. The defect is smooth edged showing that it occurred at least some weeks previously.

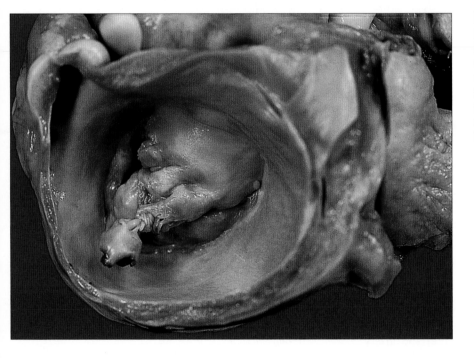

Figure 2.57
Ruptured papillary muscle due to infarction. It is good autopsy practice always to inspect the mitral valve from the left atrium before cutting the valve ring or the ventricle. If this is done papillary muscle rupture will not be missed because the stump of the muscle attached to a tangled mass of chordae is found in the left ventricle.

death. In some infants myocardial ischaemia develops in the area supplied by the anomalous artery and fibrosis develops which may calcify. In infants regional myocardial fibrosis and calcification may be related to segmental aplasia of a short segment of a proximal coronary artery. In such cases large collaterals from the conus branch of the right coronary artery supply the distal left anterior descending artery.

Coronary artery dissection

In adults isolated coronary artery dissection may precipitate acute infarction and sudden death (Basso *et al.*

1996) (*see* Chapter 8). The process is distinct from aortic dissection and starts as a subadventitial haematoma which compresses the vessel lumen from outside. This haematoma may rupture into the lumen and a dissection track is created. The pathogenesis is not clear, but many reports stress that an adventitial inflammatory process is present with eosinophils and basophils. The process is not, however, an arteritis and medial inflammation is absent. Case series collected from individual reports in the literature suggest the process is more common in women and may occur during pregnancy. In subjects who survive, the angiogram can return to close to normal as the

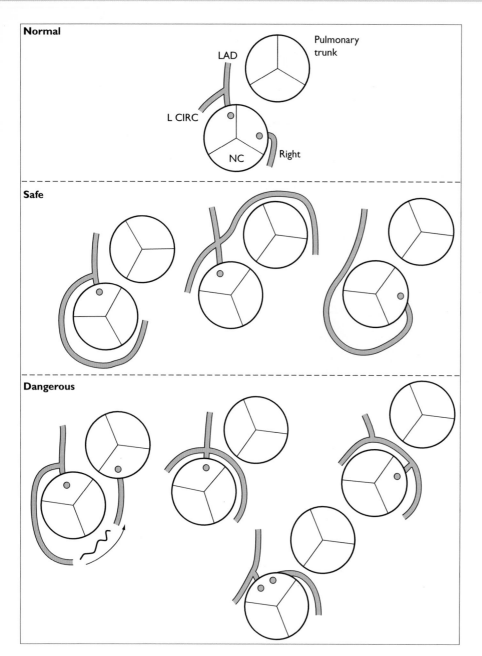

Figure 2.58
Coronary artery anomalies. The dangerous anomalies are when a major arterial branch crosses from right to left or vice versa between the pulmonary trunk and the aorta. Single coronary artery orifices are not inherently dangerous unless they are associated with such crossing. An artery in the pulmonary trunk leads to a left to right shunt through enlarged collaterals.

haematoma is organised and becomes smaller. The lesion can however be recognised as an organised mass of thrombus just below the adventitia in the artery supplying healed infarcts even years after the event. There is no link to Marfan's disease or other connective tissue gene defects in the vast majority of cases.

Ostial stenosis

Ostial stenosis is a traditional feature of syphilitic aortitis but may occur as an isolated phenomenon. The test of ostial stenosis is whether it is easy to pass a 2 mm probe. Isolated ostial stenosis (Fig. 2.59) is more common in women with risk factors for atherosclerosis and lipid-filled foam cells are often present in the intimal thickening suggesting that this is a rare diffuse variant of atherosclerosis rather than a discrete separate entity (Stewart *et al.* 1987; Thompson 1986).

Coronary emboli

Major coronary emboli as distinct from microemboli from exposed mural thrombi over an atherosclerotic plaque in the coronary arteries themselves are rare. The rarity reflects the fact that in systole blood flow is central and rapid through the open aortic valve carrying emboli beyond the coronary orifices. The exception is bacterial endocarditis on the aortic valve where fragments of thrombus lie close to the coronary orifices. Any other cause of thrombus on native or prosthetic aortic valves has a similar risk.

Coronary arteritis and aneurysms

Coronary arteritis is rare. It may occur as part of diseases such as polyarteritis nodosa or Wegener's granulomatosis, but in isolation is an indicator of Kawasaki's disease. This condition follows a few weeks

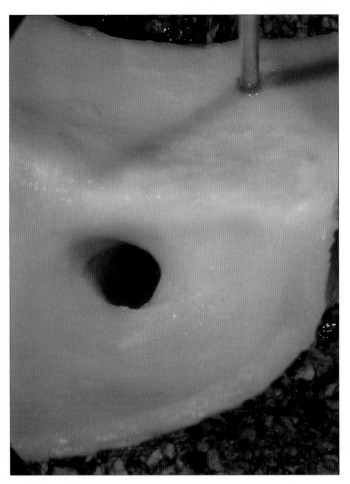
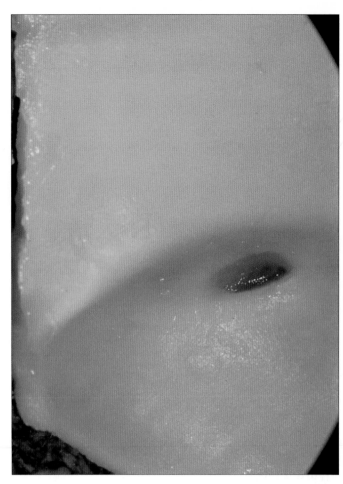

Figure 2.59
Coronary ostial stenosis. The woman of 56 had known risk factors for atherosclerosis and developed stable angina. Angiography showed localised stenosis of the main left coronary artery at its ostia with minimal disease elsewhere. The left ostium is small due to white intimal thickening when compared to the normal right coronary ostium.

after a febrile disease in infants or young children in which there is lymphadenopathy, mouth ulcers and a rash which resembles that of rubella. Cases often present as sudden death. At autopsy the striking feature is massive aneurysmal dilatation of either a localised segment or long lengths of the proximal coronary arteries with occluding thrombus (Fig. 2.60) leading to myocardial infarction. The arteries show an intense transmural arteritis which is indistinguishable from that of polyarteritis nodosa. In Kawasaki's disease, however, arteritis in other organs is absent. The disease is strikingly more common in Japan (Yanagawa *et al.* 1986; Seiguchi *et al.* 1985) although sporadic cases occur world-wide. The pathogenesis is uncertain although all the hallmarks of an immune response to a viral infection are present. There is however as yet no definitive isolation of a particular virus. Cases who survive the acute phase are left with either local (Fig. 2.61) or diffuse aneurysmal dilatation of a coronary artery which may undergo thrombosis some years later (Kato *et al.* 1992). It is being increasingly recognised that the acute phase disease may be misdiagnosed as rubella or be sufficiently mild not to be noticed. Coronary aneurysms may however form and only come to light

when thrombosis occurs years later (Brecker *et al.* 1987).

The finding at autopsy of an aneurysmal dilation of a long segment of one or more coronary arteries needs careful consideration of a number of causes. When one artery opens from the pulmonary artery it often becomes large and tortuous because a left to right shunt develops within the myocardium. If the coronary ostia are normally situated there may be a shunt between the dilated artery and either a chamber or the coronary sinus. The openings are usually easily located. If no fistula is present the case may be a long-term survivor of Kawasaki's disease.

The terms coronary artery aneurysm, aneurysmal dilatation and coronary ectasia are all used to described different points in a continuum which runs from very localised saccular aneurysms to an artery in which stenosis alternates with widely dilated segments. Localised aneurysms may be traumatic, congenital or post-Kawasaki's disease and it is often impossible to determine which process is responsible (Daoud *et al.* 1963). Pathologists are most likely to encounter coronary

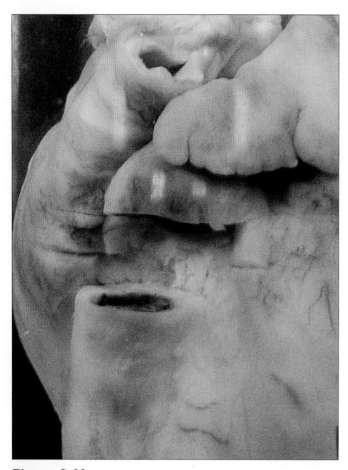 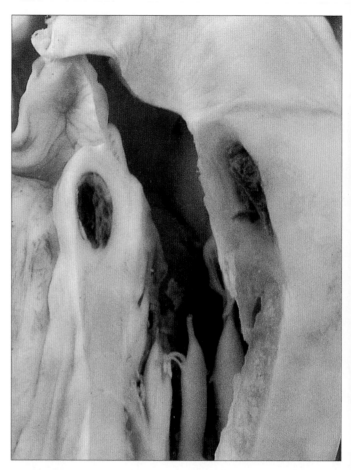

Figure 2.60
Kawasaki's disease. In this case, sudden death occurred within a few weeks of a febrile illness with a rash. The coronary arteries were widely dilated and filled with thrombus.

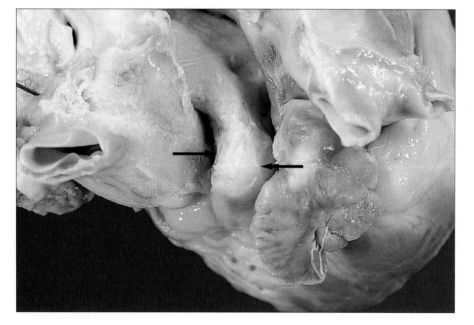

Figure 2.61
Late aneurysm formation – Kawasaki's disease. A male aged 20 died suddenly without previous symptoms. There is a localised aneurysm (arrows) in the main left coronary artery which had undergone recent thrombosis. A similar aneurysm in the right coronary was filled with old thrombus.

ectasia which is relatively common in elderly subjects. In this condition some segments of the artery dilate and have a large lumen despite diffuse intimal atherosclerosis and calcification. Adjacent segments of artery are not dilated and may show stenosis. The condition is usually regarded as a variant of atherosclerosis occurring in older subjects (Swanton *et al.* 1978).

References

Alonso D, Scheidr S, Post M, Killip T. Pathophysiology of cardiogenic shock, quantifications of myocardial necrosis, clinical pathologic and electrocardiographic correlations. *Circulation* 1973;**48**:588–96.

Anderson K, Popple A, Parker D, Sayer R, Trickey R,

Davies M. An experimental assessment of macroscopic enzyme techniques for the autopsy demonstration of myocardial infarction. *J Pathol* 1979; **127**:93–8.

Annex B, Denning S, Channon K, *et al.* Differential expression of tissue factor protein in directional atherectomy specimens from patients with stable and unstable coronary syndromes. *Circulation* 1995; **91**: 619–22.

Ball R, Stowers E, Burton J, Cary N. Evidence that the death of macrophage foam cells contributes to the lipid core of atheroma. *Atherosclerosis* 1995;**114**: 45–54.

Barbour D, Roberts W. Rupture of a left ventricular papillary muscle during acute myocardial infarction. Analysis of 22 necropsy patients. *J Am Coll Cardiol* 1986;**8**:548–65.

Baroldi G, Falzi G, Mariani F. Sudden coronary death: a post mortem study in 298 selected cases compared to 97 'control' subjects. *Am Heart J* 1979;**98**:20–31.

Basso C, Morgagni GL, Thiene G. Spontaneous coronary artery dissection: a neglected cause of acute myocardial ischaemia and sudden death. *Heart* 1996;**75**:451–4.

Becker A, van Mantgem J. Cardiac tamponade: a study of 50 hearts. *Eur J Cardiol* 1975;**3**:349–58.

Bini A, Fenoglio J, Mesa-Tejada R, Kudryk B, Kaplan K. Identification and distribution of fibrinogen, fibrin and fibrin(ogen) degradation products in atherosclerosis. Use of monoclonal antibodies. *Arteriosclerosis* 1989;**9**:109–21.

Brecker S, Gray H, Oldershaw P. Coronary artery aneurysm and myocardial infarction; adult sequelae of Kawasaki disease? *Br Heart J* 1987;**59**:509–12.

Burrig K. The endothelium of advanced arteriosclerotic plaques in humans. *Arteriosl Thromb* 1991;**11**: 1678–89.

Crawford T, Levene C. Medial thinning in atheroma. *J Pathol Bact* 1953;**66**:19–23.

Daoud A, Pankin D, Tulgan H, Florentin R. Aneurysms of the coronary artery: Report of 10 cases and review of the literature. *Am J Cardiol* 1963;**11**: 228–37.

Davies M, Thomas A. Plaque fissuring – the cause of acute myocardial infarction, sudden ischaemic death and crescendo angina. *Br Heart J* 1985;**53**:363–73.

Davies MJ, Thomas AC, Knapman PA, Hangartner JR (1986) Intramyocardial platelet aggregation in patients with unstable angina suffering sudden ischaemic cardiac death. *Circulation* **73**:418–27.

Davies M, Woolf N., Rowles P, Pepper J. Morphology of the endothelium over atherosclerotic plaques in human coronary arteries. *Br Heart J* 1988;**60**: 459–64.

Davies M. Stability and Instability: Two Faces of Coronary Atherosclerosis: The Paul Dudley White Lecture 1995 *Circulation* 1996;**94**:2013–20.

Dellborg M, Held P, Swedberg K, Vedin O. Rupture of the myocardium: occurrence and risk factors. *Br Heart J* 1985;**54**:11–17.

Derias N, Adams C. Nitro blue tetrazolium test: Early gross detection of human myocardial infarcts. *Br J Exp Pathol* 1978;**59**:254–8.

Faggiotto A, Ross R, Harker L. Studies of hypercholesterolaemia in the non-human primate. I Changes that lead to fatty streak formation. *Arteriosclerosis* 1984;**4**:323–40.

Faggiotto A, Ross R. Studies of hypercholesterolaemia in non-human primates. II Fatty streak conversion to fibrous plaque. *Arteriosclerosis* 1984;**4**:341–56.

Falk E. Unstable angina with fatal outcome: dynamic coronary thrombosis leading to infarction and/or sudden death. *Circulation* 1985;**71**:699–708.

Galis Z, Sukhova G, Lark M, Libby P. Increased expression of matrix metalloproteinases and matrix degrading activity in vulnerable regions of human atherosclerotic plaques. *J Clin Invest* 1994;**94**: 2493–503.

Gaudron P, Eilles C, Kugler I, Ertl G. Progressive left ventricular dysfunction and remodelling after myocardial infarction. *Circulation* 1993;**87**:755–63.

Glagov S, Zarins C, Giddens D, Ku D. Mechanical factors in the pathogenesis, localization and evolution of atherosclerotic plaques. In: Camilleri J-P, Berry C, Fiessinger J-N, Bariety J (eds). *Diseases of the arterial wall*. Paris: Springer-Verlag, 1987; 217–39.

Ge J, Erbel R, Zamorano J *et al.* Coronary artery remodeling in atherosclerotic disease: an intravascular ultrasonic study *in vivo. Coronary Artery Disease* 1993;**4**:981–6.

Geng Y, Libby P. Evidence for apoptosis in advanced human atheroma. Colocalization with interleukin-1 beta-converting enzyme. *Am J Pathol* 1995;**147**: 151–266.

Guyton J, Klemp K. Transitional features in human atherosclerosis: intimal thickening, cholesterol clefts and cell loss in human aortic fatty streaks. *Am J Pathol* 1993;**143**:1444–57.

Hangartner J, Charleston A, Davies M, Thomas A. Morphological characteristics of clinically significant coronary artery stenosis in stable angina. *Br Heart J* 1986;**56**:501–8.

Hegyi L, Skepper JN, Cary NRB, Mitchinson MJ. Foam cell apoptosis and the development of the lipid core of human atherosclerosis. *J Pathol* 1996;**179**: 294–302.

Jennings R, Steenbergen CJ, Reimer K. Myocardial ischemia and reperfusion. In: Schoen F, Gimbrone MJ (eds). *Cardiovascular pathology clinicopathologic correlations and pathogenetic mechanisms.* Baltimore: Williams and Wilkins, 1995: 47–80.

Kaplan J, Manuck S, Adams M, Williams J, Register T, Clarkson T. Plaque changes and arterial enlargement in atherosclerotic monkeys after manipulation of diet and social environment. *Arterioscler Thromb* 1993; **13**:254–63.

Karch SB. Billingham ME. Myocardial contraction bands revisited. *Hum Pathol* 1986;**17**:9–13.

Kato H, Inove O, Kawasaki T, Fujiwarr H, Watanabe T, Toshima H. Adult coronary artery disease probably due to childhood Kawasaki disease. *Lancet* 1992;**340**:1127–9.

Libby P. Molecular bases of the acute coronary syndromes. *Circulation* 1995;**91**:2844–50.

Lodge-Patch I. The ageing of cardiac infarcts and its influence on cardiac rupture. *Br Heart J* 1951;**13**:37.

LoSordo DW, Rosenfield K, Kaufman J, Pieczek A, Isner JM. Focal compensatory enlargement of human arteries in response to progressive atherosclerosis. *Circulation* 1994;**89**:2570–7.

Mann JM, Davies MJ. Vulnerable plaque: relation of characteristics to degree of stenosis in human coronary arteries. *Circulation* 1996;**94**:928–31.

Mann J, Roberts W. Acquired ventricular septal defect during acute myocardial infarction: analysis of 38 unoperated necropsy patients and comparison with 50 unoperated necropsy patients without rupture. *Am J Cardiol* 1988;**62**:8–19.

Mintz G, Painter J, Pichard A, *et al*. Atherosclerosis in angiographically 'normal' coronary artery reference segments: an intravascular ultrasound study with clinical correlations. *J Am Coll Cardiol* 1995;**25**: 1479–85.

Nashimura R, Schaff H, Shub C, Gersh B, Edwards W, Takik A. Papillary muscle rupture complicating acute myocardial infarction – analysis of 17 patients. *Am J Cardiol* 1983;**51**:373–7.

Pirolo S, Hutchins M, Moore W. Infarct expansion: pathologic analysis of 204 patients with a single myocardial infarct. *J Am Coll Cardiol* 1986;**7**: 349–54.

Raines E, Ross R. Smooth muscle cells and the pathogenesis of the lesions of atherosclerosis. *Br Heart J* 1993;**69**:S30–S37.

Reimer K, Jennings R, Cobb F. Animal models for protecting myocardium – results of the NHLBI cooperative study. *Circ Res* 1985;**56**:651–65.

Restrepo C, Tracy R. Variation in human aortic fatty streaks among geographic locations. *Atherosclerosis* 1975;**21**:179–93.

Roberts W. Major anomalies of coronary arterial origin seen in adulthood. *Am Heart J* 1986;**111**:941–62.

Roberts W, Virmani R. Formation of new coronary arteries within a previously obstructed epicardial coronary artery (intra-arterial arteries). A mechanism for occurrence of angiographically normal coronary arteries after healing of acute myocardial infarction. *Am J Cardiol* 1984;**54**:1361–2.

Ross R. The pathogenesis of atherosclerosis – a perspective for the 1990's. *Nature* 1993;**362**:801–9.

Seiguchi M, Takao A, Endo M, Asai T, Kawasaki I. On the mucocutaneous lymph node syndrome or Kawasaki disease. In: Yu P, Goodwin J (eds). *Progress in cardiology*. Philadelphia: Lee and Febiger, 1985; 97.

Shiomi M, Tsukaka T, Yata T *et al*. Reduction of serum cholesterol levels alters lesional composition of atherosclerotic plaques. Effect of pravastatin sodium on atherosclerosis in mature WHHL rabbits. *Arteriosc Thromb Vasc Biol* 1995;**15**:1938–995.

Small D, Bond M, Waugh D, Prack M, Sawyer J. Physicochemical and histological changes in the arterial wall of non-human primates during progression and regression of atherosclerosis. *J Clin Invest* 1984;**73**:1590–605.

Stary H, Chandler A, Glagov S, Guyton S, Guyton J, Insull WJ. A definition of initial, fatty streak, and intermediate lesions of atherosclerosis: a report from the Committee on Vascular Lesions of the Council on Atherosclerosis, American Heart Association. Special Report. *Arterioscler Thromb* 1994;**14**: 840–56.

Stary H, Chandler A, Dinsmore R *et al*. A definition of advanced types of atherosclerotic lesions and a histological classification of atherosclerosis. A report from the Committee on Vascular Lesions of the Council on Atherosclerosis, American Heart Association. *Circulation* 1995;**92**:1355–74.

Steinberg D, Parthasarathy S, Carew T, Khoo J, Witztum J. Beyond cholesterol. Modifications of low-density lipoprotein that increases its atherogenicity. *N Engl J Med* 1989;**320**:915–24.

Stewart J, Ward D, Davies M, Pepper J. Isolated coronary ostial stenosis: observations on the pathology. *Eur Heart J* 1987;**8**:917–20.

Strong J. Atherosclerotic lesions. Natural history, risk factors and topography. *Arch Pathol Lab Med* 1992;**116**:1268–75.

Swanton R, Lea-Thomas M, Coltart D, Jenkins B, Webb-Peploe M, Williams B. Coronary artery ectasia – a variant of occlusive coronary arteriosclerosis. *Br Heart J* 1978;**40**:393–400.

Taylor AJ, Rogan KM, Virmani R. Sudden cardiac death associated with isolated congenital coronary artery anomalies. *J Am Coll Cardiol* 1992;**20**:640–7.

Tejada C, Strong J, Montenegro M, Restrep C, Solberg L. Distribution of aortic and coronary atherosclerosis by geographic location, race and sex. *Lab Invest* 1968;**18**:509–26.

Thompson R. Isolated coronary ostial stenosis in women. *J Am Coll Cardiol* 1986;**7**:997–1003.

Tuzcu E, Hobbs R, Rincon G *et al*. Occult and frequent transmission of atherosclerotic coronary disease with cardiac transplantation. Insights from intravascular ultrasound. *Circulation* 1995;**91**:1706–13.

van der Wal A, Becker A, van der Loos C, Das P. Site of intimal rupture or erosion of thrombosed coronary atherosclerotic plaques is characterized by an inflammatory process irrespective of the dominant plaque morphology. *Circulation* 1994;**89**:36–44.

van Tassel R, Edwards J. Rupture of the heart complicating myocardial infarction. Analysis of 40 cases including nine examples of left ventricular false aneurysm. *Chest* 1972;**61**:104–6.

Visser C, Kan G, Meltzer G, Koolan J, Dunning A. Incidence, timing and prognostic value of left ventricular aneurysm formation after infarction. *Am J Cardiol* 1986;**57**:729–32.

Wissler RW. An overview of the quantitative influence of several risk factors on progression of atherosclerosis in young people in the United States. *Am J Med Sci* 1995;**310**:S29–S36.

Yanagawa H, Nakamura Y, Kawasaki T, Shigematsu I. Nation-wide epidemic of Kawasaki disease in Japan during the winter of 1985–1986. *Lancet* 1986;**ii**:1138–9.

THREE

VALVE DISEASE

An understanding of the anatomy of normal cardiac valves is essential for studying the alterations in function produced by pathological processes. The structure and function of the two semi-lunar valves (aortic and pulmonary) is very different from that of the atrioventricular valves (mitral and tricuspid). Most pathological processes mainly affect the mitral and aortic valves because they are subjected to higher haemodynamic pressures compared with the tricuspid and pulmonary valves.

ANATOMY OF CARDIAC VALVES

Aortic valve

The three aortic leaflets have the shape of half moons (semi-lunar) (Figs 3.1,3.2) and are similar but usually not exactly equal in size (Vollebergh and Becker 1977). Viewed from the aorta in the open position, the aortic cusps fold back into their respective sinuses. A white ridge, the linea alba marks the cusp apposition line on the ventricular aspect of each leaflet. The shape of the cusps is one factor which prevents them being forced back into the ventricle when aortic pressure exceeds left ventricular pressure. Another factor is that the total aortic cusp area exceeds that of the aortic orifice by some 50%; this excess allows the ventricular faces of the cusps to abut and mutually support each other in the closed position (Silver and Roberts 1985; Davies 1980). The region of each cusp between its free edge

and the apposition line is called the lunula and in the middle of the free edge of each cusp is a fibrous nodule (of Arantius) (Fig. 3.3). The lunular zone often has small fenestrations which increase in frequency and size with age but have no functional significance. These fenestrations are above the cusp apposition line and thus allow communication between two adjacent aortic sinuses rather than the sinus to the left ventricle. Cusp mobility and flexibility along with lack of adhesion between the cusps right up to their insertion into the aorta are essential for normal opening and closing of the valve. The aortic annulus is a fibromuscular structure (Fig. 3.4) that is shaped like a triradiate crown rather than a simple ring and is 5.7–7.9 cm in circumference in women and 6.0–8.5 cm in men at the level of the supra-aortic ridge. The diameter of the aortic root is determined by the structure of the aortic media just above the supra-aortic ridge. The three commissures occupy the three points of the crown and represents the site of separation of one cusp from its adjacent cusp. The ventriculo-arterial junction is characterised by three sinuses (sinuses of Valsalva) (Fig. 3.2) which support the semi-lunar attachments of the aortic valve. Each sinus bulges outward in the area of the aorta above the attachment of the semi-lunar leaflets, extending up to a distinct ridge encircling the aorta at the commissures, known as the supra-aortic, sinotubular junction or annulo-aortic ridge (Fig. 3.2). The sinus portion of the aorta is 1.5 times wider than the proximal aorta which is appreciated more easily during life with angiography than at autopsy. Two of the sinuses

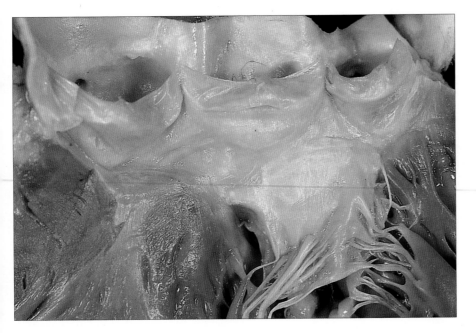

Figure 3.1

Normal aortic valve. The aortic valve has been opened to display the three semi-lunar cusps enface. Each cusp has ridges extending downward and laterally from the central nodule of Arantius. The direct continuity of the aortic valve with the anterior cusp of the mitral valve is seen. On the ventricular face of the anterior cusp of the mitral valve yellow lipid deposits are very common with advancing age. They are of no pathological consequence. The coronary artery orifices open from behind the right and left aortic valve cusps usually close to the sinotubular junction.

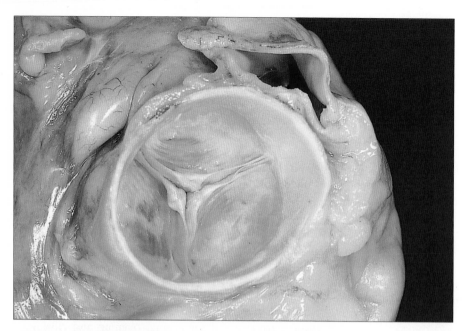

Figure 3.2
Normal closed aortic valve. The valve is viewed from the aorta and has been fixed by perfusion in the closed position. The three aortic cusps meet very precisely and are approximately equal in size. At the central point of the valve aperture each cusp has a small fibrous nodule. The commissures where the cusps are attached to the aortic wall at the junction of the sinus with the aortic root lie on a circumferential ridge (supra-aortic ridge or sinotubular junction). The edges of the adjacent cusps at the commissures are very close together and not separated. Behind each cusp is a sinus of Valsalva.

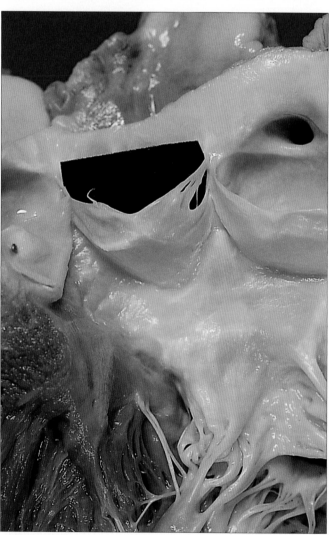

Figure 3.3
Normal aortic valve cusps. The centre of the free edge of the aortic cusps contains a small fibrous nodule from which two ridges extend downward and laterally. The ridges mark the line along which the aortic cusps abut in the closed position. The portion of cusp above the apposition line is the lunula and with increasing age develops small fenestrations. These join adjacent sinuses to each other and are of no functional significance.

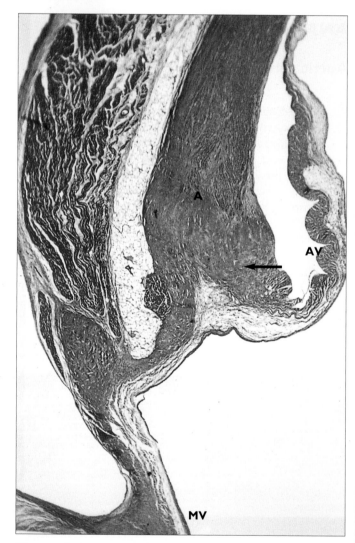

Figure 3.4
Normal aortic root – histology. The plane of the section passes through the non-coronary cusp of the aortic valve (AV) and the anterior cusp of the mitral valve (MV). The base of the sinus (arrow) is made up purely of blue staining collagen; this collagen is continuous with the fibrosa of both the aortic valve cusp and the anterior cusp of the mitral valve. At the upper edge of the fibrous annulus collagen interdigitates with the smooth muscle cells in the media of the ascending aorta (A) (Trichrome ×18.75).

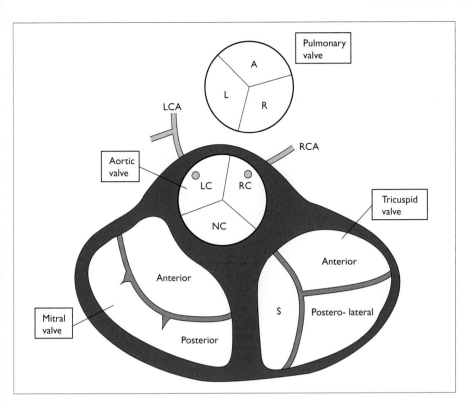

Figure 3.5
Nomenclature of valve cusps. Pulmonary valve: right (R), left (L), anterior (A); Tricuspid valve: septal (S), anterior, postero-lateral; Aortic valve: left coronary (LC) right coronary (RC), and non-coronary (NC); Mitral valve: anterior and posterior.

give rise to the coronary artery ostia which lie just above, on, or just below the supra-aortic ridge. These are the sinuses facing the pulmonary trunk, irrespective of the origin and relationship of the aorta to the pulmonary trunk (Fig. 3.5) (*see* Chapter 1).

Histology of aortic valve

The zona fibrosa forms the structural backbone of each cusp (Fig. 3.4) and is composed of dense collagen which is continuous with the aortic annulus at the sinus attachments. Both sides of the cusp possess subendothelial fibroelastic layers (zona ventricularis and zona aortalis) which are thickest along the closing edge and the ventricular aspect of the valve. The valve cusp is devoid of blood vessels.

Mitral valve

The mitral valve has two leaflets of markedly dissimilar shape and circumferential length (Figs 3.6, 3.7) and when fully open has a large orifice of 4–8 cm² which allows high volume flow at the relatively low pressure differential that exists between the left atrium and ventricle in diastole. The annular circumference is 5–10 cm. In the closed position the valve forms a flat floor to the left atrium, most of which is formed by the most anteriorly located leaflet which is square in shape

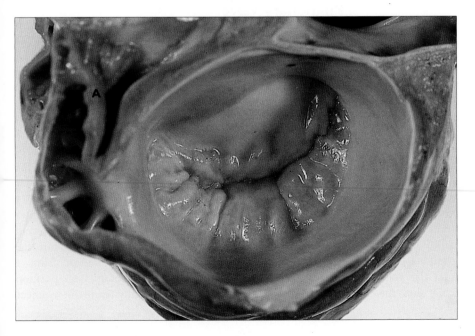

Figure 3.6
Normal mitral valve. The mitral valve is closed and viewed from the left atrium. The left atrial appendage (A) is long and thin and points anteriorly. The line of cusp apposition is concave. The anterior cusp is a flat rather featureless structure viewed from the atrial aspect. The curved posterior cusp is often subdivided as here into a number of scallops. In this normal valve there is no projection upward of any portion of either cusp which lie at the same level making a flat floor to the left atrium.

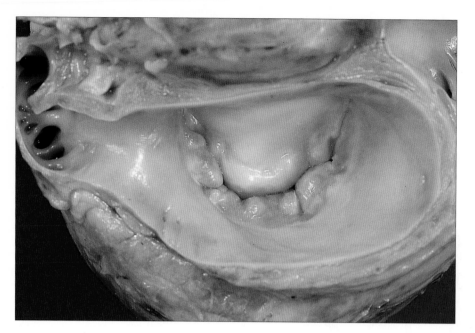

Figure 3.7
Normal mitral valve – hooding. The valve is viewed from the left atrium and is fully competent without any residual defect in this closed position. Along the posterior cusp a series of small upward projections of cusp tissue have occurred between chordal insertions. This process known as hooding is a common age-related change of no functional significance usually seen in people over 60 years of age. Also note the thickening of the edge of the anterior cusp.

and takes up one third of the annular circumference (Fig. 3.6). During systole the two leaflets of the closed valve do not bulge into the left atrium. A ridge on the atrial aspect of the anterior leaflet situated 0.5 cm from the free edge of the cusp defines the line of cusp apposition. It increases in prominence with age (Fig. 3.7) and should not be mistaken for pathological fibrous thickening of the leaflet. The anterior leaflet hangs down like a veil into the left ventricle during diastole, separating the inflow and outflow tract of the left ventricle (Fig. 3.8 a,b). The crescentic shaped posterior leaflet is long and thin making up two thirds of the annular circumference. It is often divided into three smaller scallops by small clefts. Examination of the valve from below (Figs 3.9, 3.10) show that numerous fan-shaped chordae are attached to both cusps on the ventricular aspect in an area described as the rough zone of the cusp. The chordae originate from two prominent papillary muscles (anterolateral and posteromedial) which have their origins very close together in the apical trabecular muscle of the left ventricle.

Histology of mitral valves

Each cusp has a dense fibrous core (zona fibrosa) which is continuous with the valve ring or annulus at its edge and is also continuous with the chordae tendineae. There is a layer of loose connective tissue on the atrial aspect of the valve (zona spongiosa) within which layers of fine irregular elastic fibrils form with age. The ventricular aspect of the valve has a narrow fibroelastic layer covered by endothelium. The line of closure on the atrial aspect of each leaflet has localised plaques of fibroelastic tissue. Blood vessels, lymphatics and nerves lie at the base of the valve. On the ventricular aspect of the anterior cusp myocardial muscle cells and a thin layer of smooth muscle cells, accompanied by blood vessels, may extend into the cusp for half its length. Lipid-filled foam cells in this layer cause flat yellow patches to become visible macroscopically and these increase with age.

Tricuspid valve

The tricuspid valve has three leaflets – anterosuperior, septal and inferior – which are separated from each other by the anteroseptal, supero-inferior and inferoseptal commissures, respectively (see Chapter 1). Like the mitral valve all three leaflets are supported by chordae tendineae with papillary muscle attachment. The anterior muscle is the largest and usually springs directly from the body of the septum. Chordae supporting the anteroseptal commissure are attached to the medial papillary muscle (of Lancisi), a relatively small muscle which springs either as a single band or as a small sprig of cords from the posterior part of the interventricular septum. The inferior muscle is usually the smallest and may be represented by several small muscles. The inferior leaflet takes its origin exclusively from the diaphragmatic wall of the ventricle and is often called the mural leaflet.

Pulmonary valve

The major feature of the pulmonary outlet from the right ventricle is that it is a complete muscular structure (conus muscle) and the pulmonary valve lies 1.5 cm above the level of the aortic valve. The structure of the valve is very similar to that of the aortic valve with three semi-lunar leaflets. These three leaflets are named the anterior, right and left (Fig. 3.5). The annulus is 5–8 cm in circumference. Each cusp is similar to that in the aortic valve but is often more delicate and the nodules of Arantius are more prominent. The muscular band which separates the tricuspid and pulmonary valves is called the supraventricular crest (see Chapter 1). The pulmonary valve is thus easy to remove during life and is often used as an autograft to insert into the aortic position while an aortic homograft from a cadaver donor is inserted into the pulmonary position (Ross procedure). This is especially useful in younger patients to avoid the use of mechanical valves.

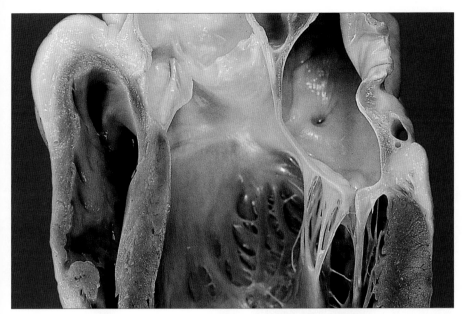

Figure 3.8 a,b

Long axis view of heart. (a) The left atrium, left ventricular outflow tract, aortic and mitral valves are shown in a long axis transection in the same plane as used in clinical echocardiography. The anterior cusp of the mitral valve forms one border of the left ventricular outflow tract, the other border being the interventricular septum. The anterior cusp of the mitral valve is in direct continuity with the aortic valve. Both mitral cusps abut and are held at exactly the same level by chordae which insert into the ventricular aspects of the cusps. (b) Diagram of structures shown in Fig. 3.8a.

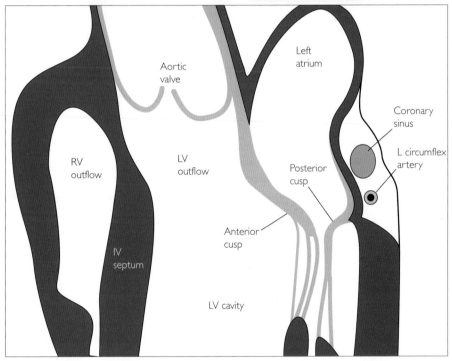

Figure 3.9

Normal mitral valve. The picture is taken looking directly up the left ventricular outflow tract to the aortic valve. The ventricular aspect of the anterior cusp of the mitral valve forms one boundary of the outflow tract. Chordae from the papillary muscles insert into the two rough zones of the cusp leaving a smooth central zone (C) without chordal attachments. The ventricular aspect of the mitral cusp shows some lipid deposition.

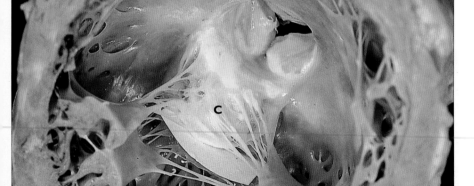

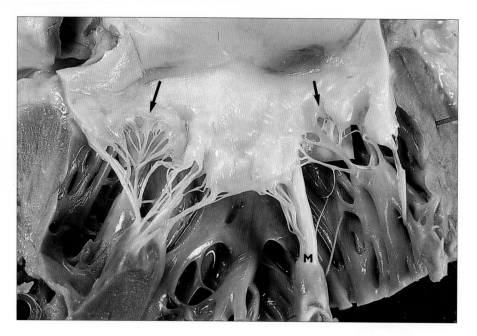

Figure 3.10
Normal mitral valve. The valve ring was divided through the posterior cusp and the heart opened to show the atrial aspect of the cusps. The commissures (arrows) are marked by two fan-shaped chordae. One of the papillary muscles gives rise to a very thick chorda with a thick endocardial coat. This chorda inserts into the anterior cusp. The structure is a muscular chorda (M), so called because it has a core of myocardial tissue contiguous with the papillary muscle, and is a minor anatomical variant of no consequence. This should not be mistaken for mild rheumatic disease.

AGE-RELATED CHANGES IN CARDIAC VALVES

Age-related degenerative changes may appreciably alter the aortic valve and should be taken into account in any morphological evaluation. With increasing age there is a progressive increase in the diameter of the aortic root at the level of the supra-aortic ridge such that by the age of 80 years, the aortic and mitral annuli have similar dimensions. This dilatation is due to the loss of smooth muscle cells from the aortic media with fragmentation of the elastic laminae and a shift to a more fibrous rather than an elastic structure. The cusps appear to have the capacity to remodel and expand in area with age to maintain the normal relation between the root and cusp area which is essential for valve competence (Davies 1980; Silver and Roberts 1985).

Age-related degenerative wear and tear lesions of the valve cusps (Kitzman *et al.* 1988) include focal fibrosis, lipidosis and calcification. One principle governing the pathology of cardiac valves is that mechanical trauma will invoke fibrous thickening in the zona ventricularis. Thus, with age the apposition lines on the faces of the aortic cusp steadily become more prominent. Mild fibrosis and lipoidosis starting in early middle age lead to an increase in cusp thickness at the base of each cusp. After the age of 65 years the aortic and mitral annuli thicken with acquired calcific deposits. It is this calcification at the base of each aortic valve cusp that is known as aortic sclerosis. Minor degrees of calcification are also common in the connective tissue in the angle between the base of the posterior cusp of the mitral valve and the posterior ventricular wall. Fibrous whisker-like projections may form along the closing edge, free edge and nodule of Arantius which are known as Lambl's excrescences.

EXAMINATION OF THE HEART VALVES WITHIN THE HEART

At autopsy the valves are best studied intact and both aspects of each valve should be examined. The tricuspid valve is exposed by a lateral incision through the right atrium from the superior vena cava 1 cm above the valve annulus into the atrial appendage. Similarly, the mitral valve can be studied by opening the left atrium via an incision extending from one of the left pulmonary veins to one of the right pulmonary veins. Mitral stenosis is usually obvious and can be assessed by inserting one, two or three fingers through the orifice. By gently squeezing the left ventricle after washing out blood clot, an impression can be formed of whether the cusps are mobile and whether there is any prolapse into the atrium. The ventricular aspects of the atrioventricular valves may be viewed following transverse sectioning of the ventricle. The semi-lunar valves are best examined after removal of the aorta and main pulmonary artery about 3 cm above the origin of both great vessels. Stenosis of the aortic valve can be assessed by passing a finger through the valve. More sophisticated techniques such as perfuse fixation for 24 hours with formalin give very exact appreciations of the presence or absence of regurgitation in the aortic and mitral valve but are time-consuming and require a pressure pump. Once the valves have been examined intact they can be opened but any chance of convincing a sceptical clinician of functional abnormality may be lost. Very good exposure of the aortic and mitral valves can be made by a cut which passes from the left atrium down the lateral margin of the heart through the mitral valve followed by a left ventricular long-axis cut passing from apex through the outflow tract through the aortic valve. Similarly the pulmonary valve and infundibulum may be visualised with a long-axis cut to the right ventricle. Measurements of the circumference of the mitral and tricuspid valve

Table 3.1

Measurements of the mitral, tricuspid and aortic valves

	Mitral valve		Tricuspid valve		Aortic valve	
	Male	Female	Male	Female	Male	Female
Mean circumference (cm)	7.8	7.7	11.4	11.0	7.1	7.1
95% Population range (cm)	5.3–10.3	5.3–10.2	8.5–14.3	8.1–13.9	5.2–9.5	5.3–9.3

annuli can be made in the opened valves (Table 3.1). The value of this practice is discussed below.

Procedures for evaluation of resected valves

After the surgical specimen is received the clinical details should be obtained before (Dare *et al.* 1993) gross morphological observations are recorded. Macroscopic examination is by far the more reliable way of determining the nature of valve disease rather than histological examination. Features to be recorded include the number of cusps, fibrous thickening, calcific deposits, perforation, indentation of valve edge, tissue excess, commissural fusion, vegetations, chordae tendineae (fused, elongated, shortened, ruptured), and abnormal papillary muscles. The cardiac valves may be radiographed for calcific deposits. Clinical information from catheterisation studies and echocardiography as well as operative descriptions are necessary to arrive at a proper diagnosis in many cases, especially if the resected valve is received in a fragmented state. It is not possible to define the cause of aortic regurgitation without knowledge of the aortic diameter either by echocardiography or from the operation notes. Histology can be used to confirm the macroscopic features but taken in isolation microscopy findings can be very misleading owing to the very limited tissue responses in the valve.

STRUCTURE/FUNCTION CORRELATIONS IN VALVES

The cardiac valves are simple tissues and their response to pathological insults are limited.

Mechanical trauma

Mechanical trauma to an endocardial surface, whether this is by impact with adjacent structures or other cusps or by a regurgitant jet hitting the surface, causes division of fibroblastic cells in the superficial zones of the cusp and leads to surface fibrous thickening. This secondary non-specific fibrous response is seen in almost every abnormal valve and should not be confused with the primary disease process.

Chronic rheumatic valve disease

Acute rheumatic fever is discussed in detail in Chapter 5. The valvulitis of the acute phase is neither functionally important nor macroscopically striking. The microscopy, however, shows that the cusp is inflamed with a mixture of acute and chronic inflammatory cells and that blood vessels begin to extend into the cusp from the base by 6 to 8 weeks after the acute phase. What are known as valvar interstitial cells increase in number and size (MacManus and Davies 1996). These cells, which appear phenotypically somewhere between fibroblasts and smooth muscle cells, and could be equally well called myofibroblasts, begin to synthesise collagen. The changes involve all three layers of the cusp, and the trilaminar architecture is finally obliterated by dense collagen thickening the valve. The cusps also are often retracted, i.e. reduced in area. The synthesis of collagen within the valve appears to continue over long periods, although why it is not self-limiting is unclear. Some of the myofibroblasts will stain with antibodies to streptococcal wall antigens. Fragments of excised rheumatic valves, many years after the acute disease, still show high rates of collagen synthesis when compared with normal valve tissue. In addition to cusp fibrosis, another hallmark of chronic rheumatic valve disease is fusion of adjacent valve cusps at their commissures. The characteristic pathology of chronic rheumatic valve disease is therefore to produce any combination of stenosis due to commissural fusion, with regurgitation due to cusp retraction in the mitral and aortic valves (Table 3.2).

The long latent periods which occur between acute rheumatic fever and chronic rheumatic valve disease

Table 3.2

Structural–functional correlates in valve disease

Mechanisms of stenosis	
Commissure fusion	
Calcification	
Mechanisms of regurgitation	
Annulus dilatation	
Cusp retraction Chordal shortening	Fibrosis
Cusp expansion Chordal lengthening	Myxoid change
Cusp perforation/destruction	Infective endocarditis

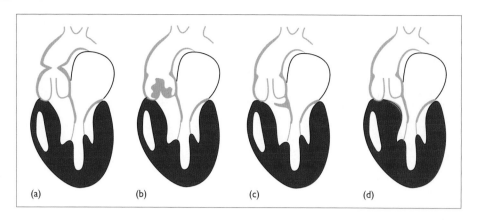

Figure 3.11
Left ventricular outflow obstruction. Left ventricular outflow obstruction occurs at supra-aortic, (a) valvar (b) and sub-valvar. Subvalvar outflow obstruction is either membranous (c) or muscular (d).

imply that a low-grade stimulus to collagen production must be continuing. One view is that repeated subclinical attacks of streptococcal infection occur; another is that once a valve is damaged abnormal mechanical force will operate to continue the fibrotic process. It is also recognised that some other diseases will produce a valvulitis which has very similar valve pathology, an example being systemic lupus. Many cases of what are regarded as chronic rheumatic valve disease on morphological grounds do not give a history of acute rheumatic fever in childhood. This absence of a previous history is particularly a feature of rheumatic valve disease in older subjects in developed countries. These considerations have led to a view that chronic rheumatic type valves with no Aschoff bodies in an atrial appendage, and no history of acute rheumatic fever, should be designated as post-inflammatory valvulitis. The suggestion has not gained much acceptance because no other cause than post-rheumatic fever has been established.

Calcification

Calcification is a very common age-related change in the aortic valve cusps, just below the insertion of the mitral valve cusp into the mitral annulus. It is thought to reflect mechanical stress exerted on collagen. Calcification is also a feature of bicuspid aortic valves and of all rheumatic valves. The calcification appears to develop within mature collagen, but has also been linked to rather specific mechanisms involving a phenotypic change in the fibroblastic cells to a more osteoblastic-like cell expressing osteopontin. Calcium induces cusp rigidity and therefore valve stenosis.

Mucoid/myxomatous change

The central fibrous core of valve cusps is normally made up of dense collagen arranged in a regular lamellar pattern. In the mitral valve especially around the chordal insertions, focal areas of a more loosely organised connective tissue (valve spongiosa) are found normally. In some conditions, notably the floppy mitral valve, the fibrosa breaks down into very loosely arranged connective tissue with fragmented elastic fibrils and large pools of connective tissue mucin. Inflammatory cells and vascularisation are absent, although mast cells may be prominent. The

mucopolysaccharides are not abnormal in structure. The basis of the change which is often confined to the mitral valve cusps is uncertain. It is an observed pathology in patients with Marfan's disease due to genetic abnormalities of fibrillin and in other genetic disorders of collagen synthesis.

AORTIC VALVE PATHOLOGY

Aortic outflow obstruction

Obstruction of the left ventricular outflow tract occurs at several levels (Fig. 3.11). The functional effect of all these dissimilar processes on the left ventricle is identical.

Valvar stenosis

There are three common causes of valvar stenosis and some rarer ones (Table 3.3). The different forms are usually easily recognisable by viewing the valve from the aortic aspect (Fig. 3.12).

Table 3.3
Causes of isolated aortic valve stenosis

Common
Bicuspid calcific aortic stenosis
Tricuspid calcific aortic valve stenosis
Chronic rheumatic disease
Rare
Congenital aortic valve stenosis
Myxoid dysplasia of aortic valve
Very rare
Familial hypercholesterolaemia
Ochronosis
Fabry's disease
Radiation
Rheumatoid
Systemic lupus erythematosus (SLE)
Mucopolysaccharidosis

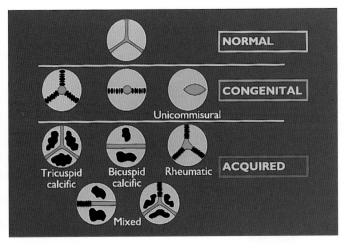

Figure 3.12
Types of valvar aortic stenosis. By viewing the valve from the aortic aspect and noting the variables of the number of cusps, calcification, orifice shape and commissural fusion, the aetiology can usually be established.

The bicuspid aortic valve and stenosis

Bicuspid aortic valves (Edwards 1961) occur in 1–2% of the general population and affect men three or four times more frequently than women. 40–50% of patients with aortic coarctation have bicuspid valves (Becker *et al.* 1970). The valve has two cusps, which may be equal in size (Fig. 3.13) or more commonly one cusp is larger than the other. In over 80% of cases, the larger cusp contains a shallow ridge or raphe which is the site of congenital fusion of the original commissures (the conjoined cusp) (Fig. 3.14).

Two types of bicuspid aortic valve occur with unequal frequency: anteroposterior (AP) and right–left. The AP type (75% of cases) arises as a result of fusion of the right and left cusps and have both coronary artery ostia arising from behind the anterior cusp. The right–left type of bicuspid aortic valve has a coronary ostium arising from each of the sinuses and when present, the raphe is always located in the right cusp. It is unclear

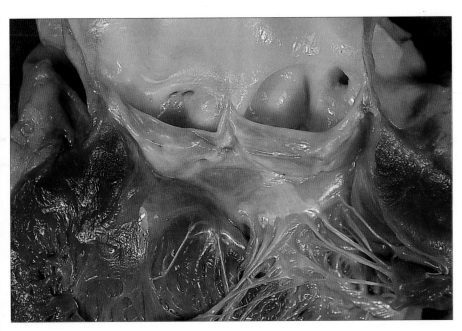

Figure 3.13
Coincidental bicuspid aortic valve. This valve has two almost morphologically normal cusps of equal size with a coronary artery arising from each sinus. This is the rarest form of a congenital bicuspid valve and was causing no functional abnormality. It may be a true congenital lesion since there is no indication of an abortive attempt to form a commissure *in utero*.

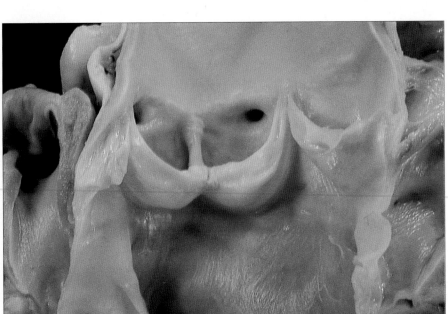

Figure 3.14
Coincidental bicuspid aortic valve. This is the far more common variety of a bicuspid aortic valve with one cusp very much larger than the other. This larger cusp has a ridge or raphe running across the sinus up to the free edge of the cusp. Both coronary arteries arise from the sinus related to the cusp with a raphe.

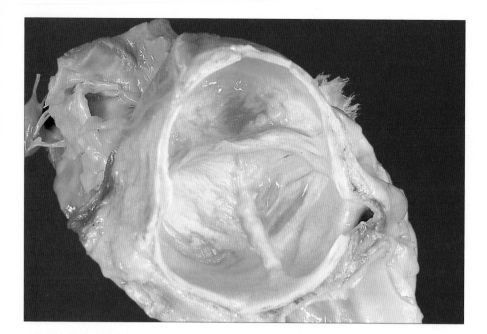

Figure 3.15
Mild aortic calcific biscuspid valve stenosis.
The closed valve is viewed from the aorta.
The larger cusp has a calcified raphe
running across the base of the sinus. Mild
aortic valve stenosis in life.

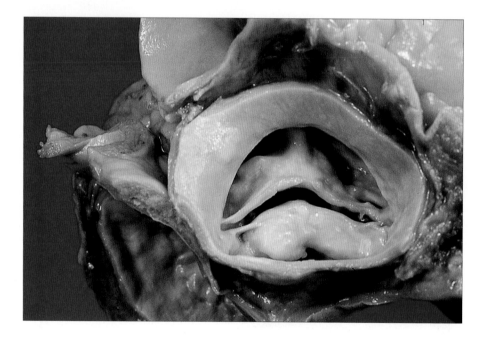

Figure 3.16
Bicuspid calcific aortic stenosis. Both cusps
contain nodules of calcification and there is
a raphe. The orifice is a transverse slit.

why the commissure between the right and left cusps is more prone to congenital fusion. The majority of bicuspid valves have three interleaflet triangles suggesting the commissures formed *in utero*, but then fused. The cause of this acquired defect *in utero* is not known. A minority of bicuspid valves have two sinuses, two equal sized cusps two interleaflet triangles (Fig. 3.13) suggesting a true genetic defect (Angelini *et al.* 1989).

Patients with bicuspid aortic valves are usually asymptomatic in the first 2–3 decades of life although the valve abnormality can be detected by auscultation as a systolic click and by echocardiography. Only a proportion of patients will develop functional abnormalities. In most cases the bicuspid valve undergoes calcification leading to stenosis (Roberts 1970). The exact proportion of subjects with bicuspid valves who develop steno-

sis is unclear, but cannot be anything like 100%; a non-calcified bicuspid aortic valve should not be over-interpreted as an autopsy finding. Bicuspid valves, provided they are not stenotic, do not cause sudden death. The gradient of pressure across the stenotic aortic valve in systole that is the difference between left ventricular pressure and the pressure in the aorta may be as great as 100 mm Hg. In a normal valve the gradient is usually zero. Calcification characteristically first occurs along the raphe and forms an immobile strut that hinders the motion of the conjoined cusp (Fig. 3.15). An arch of calcification also commonly forms along the aortic aspect of the non-conjoined cusp and further contributes to cusp rigidity as does secondary valvar fibrosis. All these features contribute to the development of progressive stenosis and the resulting valvar orifice assumes the shape of an irregular transverse

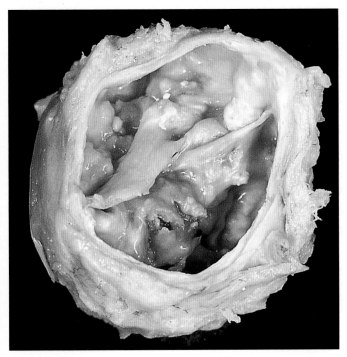

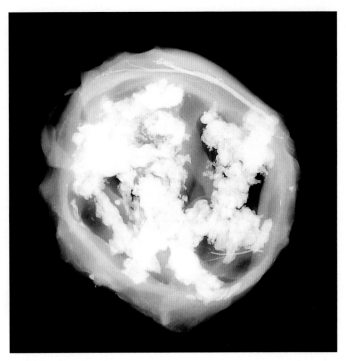

Figure 3.17
Bicuspid calcific aortic stenosis. The cusps are almost totally replaced by nodules of calcification although it is just possible to make out that the orifice was a transverse slit. Radiography shows an extreme degree of calcification. The severity of the gradient in life across bicuspid valves is directly related to the degree of calcification. In this woman it was over 100 mm Hg; sudden death prior to surgery.

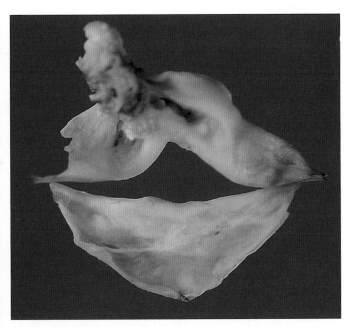

Figure 3.18
Bicuspid calcific aortic stenosis. In surgical specimens the valve cusps are usually removed separately allowing recognition it was bicuspid. Here one cusp has a calcified raphe with a notch in the free edge of the cusp. The other is remarkably normal.

material the original pathological process cannot be identified.

Degenerative or tricuspid calcific valve stenosis

The majority of stenotic aortic valves of this type are found in patients over 65 years of age. The valve is characterised by having three cusps without commissural fusion and with nodular calcific deposits in all three cusps (Figs 3.19, 3.20). On the aortic aspect of each cusp, the calcium forms nodular arch-like deposits that are anchored to the annulus. This effectively hinders the normal hinge-like motion of the cusp leading to stenosis. Commissural fusion is minimal or absent, and the valvar orifice assumes a triangular shape with inward bowing. These features serve to differentiate the degenerative form of aortic valve disease from other causes, particularly post-inflammatory cases. Minor degrees of aortic calcification are very common over 70 years of age, and account for the short mid-systolic aortic sclerotic murmur which is frequently heard in elderly people. It is very difficult clinically to decide when a patient has passed from aortic sclerosis to aortic stenosis because the two conditions are a continuum. The pressure gradient across the valve rises slowly as more calcification occurs. The same problem faces pathologists carrying out autopsies in deciding whether aortic calcification was clinically significant. If a finger can be passed through the valve without undue force being exerted and no left ventricular hypertrophy is present stenosis was not severe. Very severe aortic stenosis is, however, sometimes encountered in old age without ventricular hypertrophy, probably reflecting total lack of physical exercise in an immobile old person.

slit-like opening (Figs 3.16, 3.17). In surgical valve excisions by counting the cusps and analysing the morphology, a large proportion of calcified bicuspid valves can be recognised (Fig. 3.18). When valves are removed piecemeal in multiple fragments of calcified

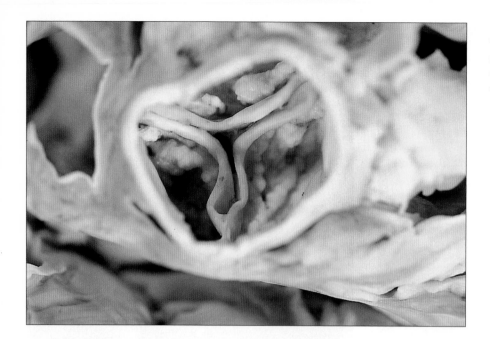

Figure 3.19
Tricuspid calcific aortic stenosis. Viewed from above the valve is seen to have three cusps without commissural fusion. In each cusp there are large calcified nodules.

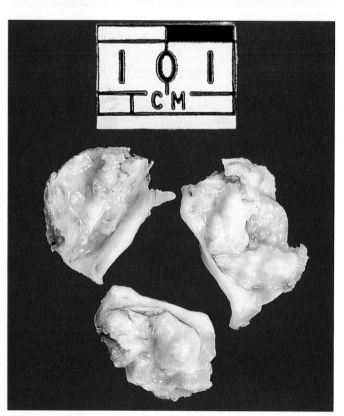

Figure 3.20
Tricuspid calcific aortic valve stenosis. In surgical excision specimens the lack of commissural fusion allows the three cusps to be removed separately. The cusps contain C-shaped calcific nodules.

Pathogenesis of tricuspid calcific aortic valve stenosis

The exact pathogenesis of the calcification that occurs in the three aortic cusps with increasing age is currently a subject of considerable interest. Epidemiological studies of age-related valve calcification using echocardiography do not support the concept that everyone will develop calcification of their aortic valve if they live long enough (Lindroos *et al.* 1993). One view is that calcification may simply be a wear and tear phenomenon that occurs in collagen which is mechanically stressed. Others have proposed that it is a more active process related to inflammatory activation in the cusp (Olsson *et al.* 1994). In a high proportion of the population, some lipid is laid down within macrophages on the aortic aspect of the cusps deep in the sinuses. Some inflammatory activation occurs with the expression of class II MHC molecules on smooth muscle cells and macrophages and with osteopontin expression. The mechanism of calcification therefore has some affinity with that which occurs in atherosclerosis.

In familial hypercholesterolaemia in which the plasma cholesterol is very high, a great deal of lipid is laid down at the base of the sinuses and leads to the development of aortic stenosis at a young age. In subjects who undergo valve replacement for tricuspid aortic calcific stenosis, the frequency of inserting vein grafts for coronary artery disease is higher than that in bicuspid aortic stenosis. This suggests that risk factors for atherosclerosis play a part in the pathogenesis of tricuspid calcific aortic valve stenosis (Davies *et al.* 1996). When bicuspid and tricuspid calcified cusps are compared, there are differences in the distribution of the nodules of calcium. In the former they are in the fibrosa; in the latter they are far more superficial and protrude onto the aortic face into the sinus (Isner *et al.* 1990). The evidence linking calcification of aortic valves with hyperlipidaemia is, however, inconsistent; one study found that when patients with bicuspid and tricuspid calcific aortic stenosis were compared, the latter were linked in a logistic regression model with elevated plasma cholesterol (Mautner *et al.* 1993). In contrast, in another study which also compared similar groups of patients, it was found that only females were associated with tricuspid calcific aortic stenosis (Mohler *et al.* 1991). Yet another study which looked at all causes of aortic valve calci-

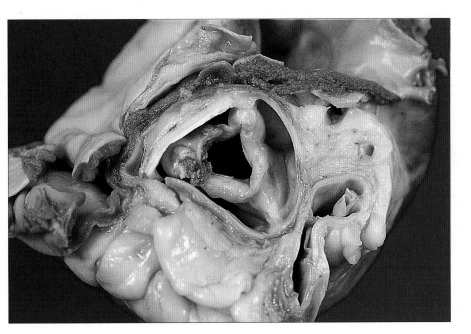

Figure 3.21
Aortic valve stenosis due to chronic rheumatic disease. The valve orifice is triangular in shape due to fusion of all three commissures. The cusps are thick and fibrous. Although the dominant haemodynamic abnormality was stenosis, such fixed small orifices also allow some regurgitation. The mixed haemodynamic picture is typical of chronic rheumatic disease.

fication identified by echocardiography found no relation to hyperlipidaemia (Lindroos *et al.* 1994).

A third potential risk factor for developing calcification in tricuspid aortic valves is the individual propensity to calcify soft tissue. Paget's disease of bone (Strikberger *et al.* 1987), chronic renal failure (Maher *et al.* 1987) and hyperparathyroidism (Niederle *et al.* 1990) all lead to valve cusp calcification and potentially aortic stenosis. It is postulated that other diseases such as osteoporosis which also mobilise calcium from the bones may potentiate aortic valve calcification, explaining the excess risk in women (Ouchi *et al.* 1993).

Quadricuspid aortic valves are far more rare than bicuspid valves, being found in less than one in a thousand individuals. The use of echocardiography to give an enface view of the aortic valve in life is, however, identifying more cases. Quadricuspid valves are very variable in the shape and morphology of the cusps, and liable to become stenotic as calcification develops. The natural history is not different from that of bicuspid valves (Hurwitz and Roberts 1973).

Rheumatic aortic stenosis

Stenotic aortic valves of rheumatic origin are characterised by fusion of at least one and usually two or three commissures in the presence of an anatomically abnormal valve with fibrous thickening (Fig. 3.21). Extensive fusion of all three commissures produces a characteristic central triangular orifice. The cusp fibrosis is associated with the commissural fusion and rigidity and thereby adds to the valvar stenosis. Secondary calcification often develops on the aortic and ventricular aspects of the cusps and may further hinder cusp motion.

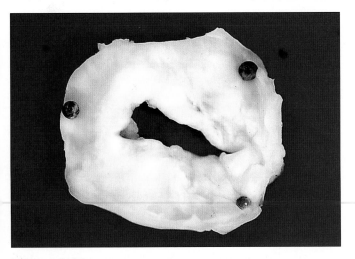

Figure 3.22
Congenital aortic valve stenosis. Stenotic valve removed from female aged 17 showing a fibrous diaphragm without separate cusps and having a central aperture.

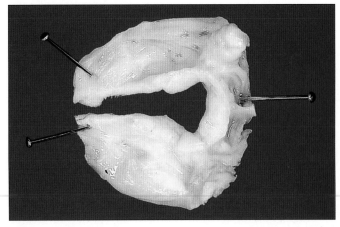

Figure 3.23
Unicommissural aortic valve stenosis. The surgically excised valve shows an eccentric tear drop shaped orifice with one commissure which is not fused. A raphe marks the site of another abortive attempt to form a commissure. Male aged 31 – murmur since birth.

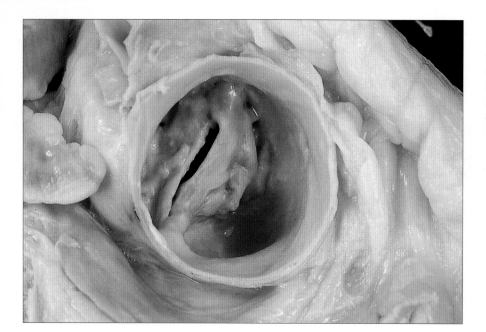

Figure 3.24
Mixed aortic valve disease. The orifice is a transverse slit, but there is fusion of both commissures and the valve is clearly bicuspid. Mitral valve disease was also present suggesting that this is a bicuspid aortic valve with concomitant chronic rheumatic disease.

Congenital aortic stenosis

The term congenital aortic stenosis is applied to valves in which a significant pressure gradient exists across the valve from infancy. The aortic bicuspid valves discussed above, while being congenital anomalies, do not develop a gradient until calcification supervenes in the fourth decade of life onward. Congenital aortic valve stenosis comes in several forms. There may be a dome-shaped diaphragm with a central hole (Fig. 3.22) with three ridges representing rudimentary commissures. There may be an eccentric tear drop or keyhole-shaped orifice. This arises when the valve is unicommissural, i.e. a single leaflet takes origin from the aortic wall and swings around to be inserted close to its point of departure. The single cusp may have two ridges marking the site of failed commissural formation. Most congenitally stenotic aortic valves need to be replaced surgically in the first or second decade of life but the unicommissural form (Fig. 3.23) may last until the third decade (Falcone *et al.* 1971). In some cases, the valve does not appear to have organised cusps which are represented only by nodular masses of myxoid tissue without a trilamellar structure. These valves are referred to as myxoid dysplasia and are typical of Noonan's syndrome, but also can occur in isolation.

Mixed forms of aortic valve stenosis

A number of morphological types of aortic stenosis do not fit into the patterns described so far. Bicuspid aortic valves undergoing calcification do not usually develop commissural fusion; the exceptions are if there has been concomitant chronic rheumatic valve disease (Sadee *et al.* 1994) or if there has been an episode of treated bacterial endocarditis in the past.

Valves are encountered in which there is acquired fusion of one commissure (Fig. 3.24) only. Such valves highlight the difficulty in laying down criteria for distinguishing failure to form a commissure leaving just a

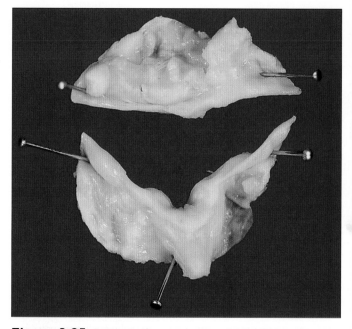

Figure 3.25
Rheumatic aortic valve stenosis. This excised valve is a fibrous diaphragm with a central aperture. There are ridges marking the commissural sites. This could be interpreted as a congenital stenotic valve or a rheumatic type valve. The presence of mitral disease favoured a rheumatic origin.

raphe from commissural fusion acquired in adult life. There are some valves which will always be categorised differently, even by experienced cardiovascular pathologists (Figs 3.25–3.27).

The spectrum of morphological forms of bicuspid aortic valves is very wide. At the end of the spectrum which is easily recognised are valves with two sinuses of equal size and cusps with normal morphology. In the centre of the spectrum there are two sinuses of unequal size. In the cusp relating to this larger sinus, there is a raphe

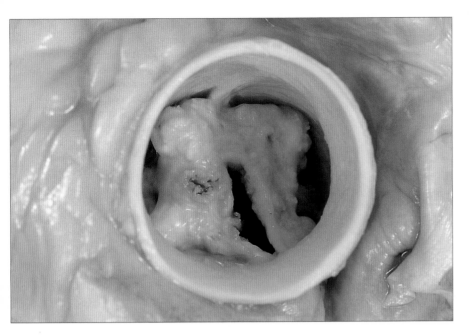

Figure 3.26
Aortic valve stenosis – undetermined type. The orifice is eccentric and elliptical and this could be a unicommissural valve with calcification – it could equally be a bicuspid aortic valve with acquired fusion of one commissure. The age (37) and absence of mitral disease somewhat favours a unicommissural valve.

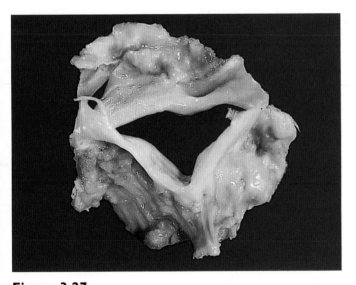

Figure 3.27
Aortic valve stenosis – undetermined type. The challenge here is to decide whether this is a bicuspid valve with a very pronounced notch and raphe acquired fusion of one commissure in a tricuspid aortic valve. The adjacent cusp edges on histology went up to the aortic wall favouring an acquired fusion. However, there was no mitral disease or history of rheumatic fever to confirm a rheumatic pathogenesis.

and this means taking a thick histological block and cutting levels. The effort is rarely worth while and most pathologists make a decision on the macroscopic appearances alone.

Acquired fusion of one commissure in adult life does however clearly occur. If there is concomitant fibrosis in the mitral valve cusps it is reasonable to assume a rheumatic aetiology. If the mitral valve is normal the pathogenesis of the aortic valve abnormality is unknown.

Relative frequencies of causes of aortic valve stenosis

The relative proportion of the different forms of isolated aortic valve stenosis depends on the geographic population and age of the subjects being analysed and is reported in many series (Subramanian *et al.* 1984; Dare *et al.* 1993). A recent surgical series of 465 adult patients (Davies *et al.* 1996) showed that 63.7% had bicuspid calcified valves, 26.9% tricuspid calcific valves, 5.4% rheumatic, 2.6% mixed pathology and 1.5% unicommissural valves. The average age of patients undergoing aortic valve replacement for bicuspid and tricuspid calcific aortic stenosis overlaps but differ by a decade (Fig. 3.29).

There are marked changes in the frequency of the different causes of aortic valve stenosis over the last three decades. These can be best appreciated in the results reported by the Mayo Clinic over the last few decades (Tazelaar 1995) where tricuspid calcified valves have overtaken bicuspid valves as the major cause of isolated aortic stenosis. Tricuspid calcific aortic valve stenosis, which predominates in the older age groups, is under-represented in surgical series due to age bias. In Saudi Arabia, South America and India, rheumatic aortic stenosis remains common due to the persistence of acute rheumatic fever in childhood.

which forms a ridge at the base of the cusp. The other extreme of the bicuspid spectrum has two very unequal sinuses, and the cusp related to the larger has a deeply notched free edge and a raphe that reaches the supra-aortic ridge. It is this extreme that cannot easily be distinguished from acquired fusion of one commissure in adult life. The usual criteria which are applied are whether two cusp edges can be found in the 'raphe' and whether they can be traced up to the supra-aortic ridge. The two edges may be seen by the naked eye (Fig. 3.28) or histologically in sections taken in the transverse plane. The plane of section has to be exactly aligned

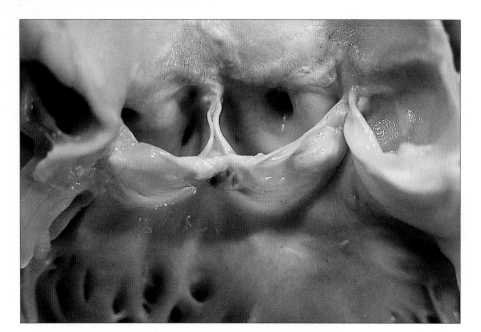

Figure 3.28
Acquired fusion of aortic valve commissure. One commissure is fused but the free edge of each cusp can be traced as separate entities up to the aortic wall. This indicates that the fusion occurred after infancy. Aetiology unknown. Functionally the valve had no abnormality in life but has become, in effect, a bicuspid aortic valve. Such valves are sometimes called acquired pseudo-congenital bicuspid aortic valves.

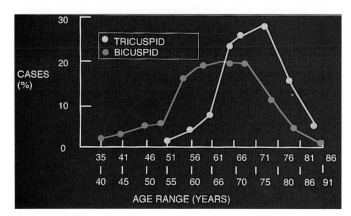

Figure 3.29
Age distribution of bicuspid and tricuspid aortic valve stenosis at time of surgery. The age ranges overlap to a very large extent but the median for tricuspid aortic valve is about a decade later in life.

Supravalvar aortic stenosis

Supra-aortic stenosis may take one of three forms. The lesion may be present as a discrete shelf, as a so-called hour-glass deformity, or as a tubular variety in which most of the aortic arch and its branches are also involved. The tubular type is probably the rarest. The other varieties show an underlying disordered mosaic architecture in the elastic tissue of the aortic media. When a supravalvar lesion obstructs the outlet from the left ventricle, the ascending aorta becomes divided into segments at high and lower pressures. The coronary arteries arise from the segment under high pressure, this feature accounting for their dilated and tortuous course and probable early onset of atherosclerosis. This, in combination with left ventricular hypertrophy, is responsible for sudden deaths in this condition. Whatever the nature of the supravalvar stenosis, the abnormality of the wall involves the commissural attachments of the leaflets. The abnormal commissural attachments predispose to early degeneration of the

leaflets. Supravalvar aortic stenosis is the least common type of left ventricular outflow obstruction, and most patients with this condition either have Williams' syndrome or a positive family history. William's syndrome is also referred to as idiopathic infantile hypercalcaemia and patients go on to develop renal calcification. Virtually all cases have mental retardation with characteristic elfin type faces. Deletions in a gene controlling elastin production on chromosome 7 are responsible (Ewart *et al*. 1993). Cases of supra-aortic stenosis which are familial, with or without the characteristic facial appearance, and without other manifestations, are also common. It is not clear at the moment whether these are different mutations or different genes. Progression with time has been demonstrated. Mortality is highest in patients with multi-level obstruction, and this indicates the serious nature of this particular condition.

Subvalvar aortic stenosis

A fibrous shelf which extends from the ventricular septum beneath the aortic valve onto the facing surface of the mitral valve is a cause of congenital aortic stenosis (Fig. 3.30). Only rarely is the lesion a completely circular obstruction and partial membranes are sometimes found as coincidental findings at autopsy. Muscular hypertrophy of the interventricular septum in hypertrophic cardiomyopathy may also be a cause of subaortic obstruction (Chapter 5).

Rare causes of aortic valve stenosis

Infiltration of the valve cusps by histiocytic cells can lead to stiffening and obstruction to flow. This phenomenon is seen in all the six varieties of mucopolysaccharidosis, in ochronosis, Fabry's disease and Whipple's disease. The histiocytic cells contain an abnormal storage product. Very rarely rheumatoid granulomas are large enough to cause obstruction, but more commonly cause valve incompetence (see below).

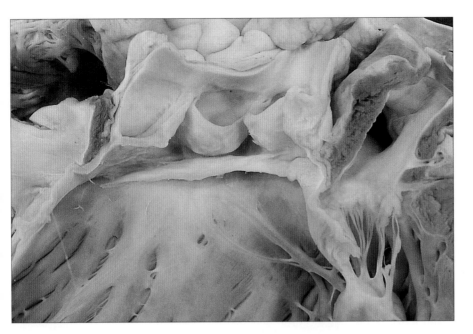

Figure 3.30
Membranous subaortic stenosis. A discrete fibrous shelf extends from the anterior cusp of the mitral valve to pass along the ventricular septum just below the aortic valve cusps.

Familial hypercholesterolaemia leads to abundant lipid-filled histiocytes within the cusps, in the sinuses and in the intima of the ascending aorta. Calcification leads to obstruction, both at valve level and at the level of the supra-aortic ridge.

Mixed aortic valve stenosis and regurgitation

The pathological processes described so far largely produce isolated aortic valve stenosis. Combined aortic stenosis and regurgitation is characteristic of chronic rheumatic disease in which the central triangular orifice is a fixed aperture which neither opens wider nor closes. Some bicuspid valves which calcify also have an element of regurgitation. Series which report the different diseases responsible for surgical replacement of the aortic valve often differ in whether they include or exclude cases in which the mitral valve is abnormal; this is another reason alongside geographic and age selection factors that make series difficult to compare.

Gastrointestinal bleeding in aortic stenosis

Recurrent gastrointestinal bleeding is a feature of a small proportion of patients with aortic valve stenosis. The cause is thought to be small arteriovenous malformations in the submucosa of the gastrointestinal tract, particularly the stomach. The association has been the subject of considerable controversy and how the vascular lesions arise is unknown, but the bleeding diminishes after valve replacement (Scheffer and Leatherman 1986; Mehta *et al.* 1989).

AORTIC REGURGITATION

Pure aortic regurgitation is less common than aortic valve stenosis. The aetiology of aortic regurgitation can be subgrouped into those conditions primarily affecting

Table 3.4
Aortic regurgitation – mechanisms

Cusp disease	
Perforated	Bacterial endocarditis
Retracted	Chronic rheumatic, rheumatoid, SLE
Notched	Bicuspid valve
Root enlarged/distorted	
Aortitis	Syphilis, ankylosing spondylitis, rheumatoid
Aortopathy	Idiopathic
	Marfan's
Lack of cusp support	
Above	Dissection of aorta
Below	Ventricular septal defect

the aortic valve cusps and those primarily affecting the aortic root (Table 3.4). In the normal aortic valve, total cusp area exceeds root area and disturbance of this relationship, either by decreasing cusp area by fibrosis or increasing root area by dilatation or distortion, leads to regurgitation. The cusps also need to be structurally intact, i.e. without tears or perforations. The causes of regurgitation are multiple and vary between surgical series due to selection bias (Table 3.5).

As in the case of aortic stenosis, appreciable changes have taken place in the relative frequency of the various causes of aortic regurgitation (Dare *et al.* 1993; Passik *et al.* 1987). The most common aetiologies were rheumatic disease followed by endocarditis and aortic root dilatation but these studies are from the 1980s. A more recent study from Italy shows that aortic root dilatation is the most frequent in their series, as it is in the most recent Mayo Clinic data (Dare *et al.* 1993).

Table 3.5

Causes of isolated aortic regurgitation

Common
Idiopathic aortic root dilatation (non-inflammatory)
Chronic rheumatic valve disease
Aortitis (all types)
Post-bacterial endocarditis
Bicuspid aortic valves

Rare
Ehlers–Danlos syndrome – osteogenesis imperfecta, Marfan's disease
Systemic lupus erythematosus (SLE)
Rheumatoid
Ankylosing spondylitis/Reiter's syndrome
Behçet's syndrome
Whipple's disease

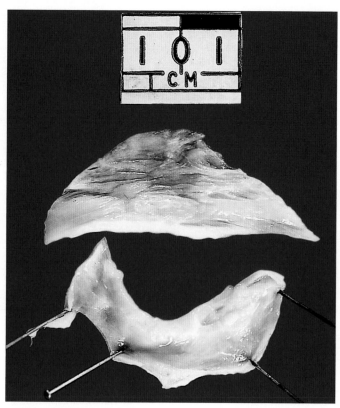

Figure 3.31
Aortic regurgitation – bicuspid valve. The valve has two cusps one of which has a concave free edge. The other cusp has a slight nodular thickening along its free edge as a result of regurgitant flow. Neither cusp is thickened or calcified. Pure aortic regurgitation necessitated valve replacement.

Aortic regurgitation – cusp disease

Congenital bicuspid valve

As already stated, 1–2% of the population have bicuspid aortic valves from birth. These can develop pure regurgitation (Sadee *et al.* 1992; Roberts *et al.* 1981) but this outcome is much rarer than stenosis. Regurgitation is particularly likely to occur with cusps which are unequal in size, or in which one cusp has a deep notch in the free edge (Fig. 3.31). In such cases, one cusp slips under the edge of the other causing regurgitation. In rare cases the larger cusp is supported by a strand of tissue joining its free edge to the aortic wall. If this cord breaks regurgitation occurs. Finally (see below) there is an undue association of bicuspid valves with idiopathic dilatation of the aortic root.

Rheumatic and post-inflammatory aortic valve disease

In some patients fibrosis primarily produces scar retraction of the cusps without appreciable commissural fusion, thereby resulting in valvar incompetence. When pure incompetence occurs, calcification tends to be mild or absent. It is unclear why chronic rheumatic disease produces stenotic commissural fusion in one patient and regurgitant flow due to cusp retraction in another. Regardless of the functional state, however, annular dilatation is not a feature of post-inflammatory valve disease. Regurgitation is due to a reduction in total cusp area relative to a normal root area. In surgical specimens the cusps are thick and fibrous and noticeably reduced in area.

Post-bacterial endocarditis

In the healed stage of endocarditis with virulent organisms, perforations are present through the body of the cusp which allow free communication between the aortic and left ventricle when the valve is closed. Both bicuspid and tricuspid valves may be involved. Aneurysms of the cusp may also occur (Chapter 4).

The floppy aortic cusp syndrome and aortic cusp prolapse

In aortic root dilatation (see below) the degree of cusp overlap is reduced and this will ultimately lead to one cusp slipping down beneath the edge of the others in the closed position leading to regurgitation. Some authors have described an entity in which the cusps become expanded and so soft that even when there is a normal degree of overlap, prolapse occurs despite the root being normal in size. The condition is described as being analogous to the floppy mitral valve and myxoid change is present in the valve cusps (Tonnemacher *et al.* 1987; Allen *et al.* 1985). To substantiate such a condition there has to be certainty that the aortic root size at the level of the supra-aortic ridge is normal in size and the aortic root is normal in structure. We have only seen one such case; the most recent Mayo Clinic series of aortic regurgitation undergoing surgical replacement has none (Dare *et al.* 1993).

Aortic root disease

Aortic root disease may be inflammatory (aortitis) or non-inflammatory (Chapter 7). Both processes can cause aortic root dilatation or distortion which disturbs the normal cusp/root relation. Macroscopic examination can often distinguish the two forms of root disease, although there can be considerable overlap in the

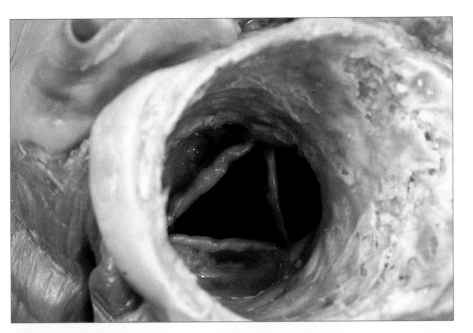

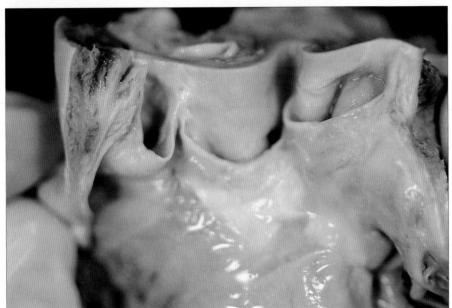

Figure 3.32a,b
Inflammatory aortic valve disease. (a) In syphilitic disease the involvement is predominantly in the root of the aorta with tree-bark scarring of the intima and widening of the commissural attachments. The free edges of the cusps are abnormal but this is secondary to regurgitant flow over the cusp. (b) In rheumatoid disease granulomas have developed in the base of the cusps and sinuses causing the cusps to retract and become thick. The whole area of the base of the anterior cusp of the mitral valve where it is contiguous with the aortic valve and the membranous septum is replaced by white fibrous tissue.

features. Aortitis often distorts the root as well as causing dilatation, and the aortic wall is thick. In non-inflammatory disease, the wall is thin and the degree of dilatation greater. A wrinkled intima with stellate depressions (tree-barking) is common to all forms of root disease.

Inflammatory aortitis

In syphilis (Chapter 7) the condition maximally affects the first 3 cm of the ascending aortic wall and the commissural region. The sinuses are not involved. The characteristic feature is a thickened, wrinkled intimal surface, with widening of the commissural attachments (Fig. 3.32). There may be coronary ostial stenosis. Diffuse calcification develops in the aortic wall. The cusps are normal apart from pronounced linear thickening of the free edges of the cusps. In rheumatoid arthritis (Roberts *et al*. 1968) granulomas cause a filling in of the base of the sinuses and the cusps retract (Fig.

3.32). In ankylosing spondylitis and other HLAB27-related conditions such as Reiter's disease, the aortitis extends outside the aortic root to involve the valve cusps which become distorted with fibrosis and retraction (Fig. 3.33). This fibrosis extends down onto the anterior cusp of the mitral valve and outward into the atrial septum to destroy the AV node and cause complete heart block (Bulkley and Roberts 1973; Liu and Alexander 1969; Paulus *et al*. 1972; Reid *et al*. 1979).

The histology of the root of the aorta in the various forms of aortitis causing regurgitation is less discriminatory than the macroscopic findings, apart from rheumatoid arthritis which has the characteristic palisaded granulomas (Fig. 3.34). Serology for syphilis, rheumatoid arthritis and the HLA status are needed to distinguish the cause with certainty. In all these conditions there is focal destruction of the media with an adventitial infiltrate of lymphocytes and plasma cells,

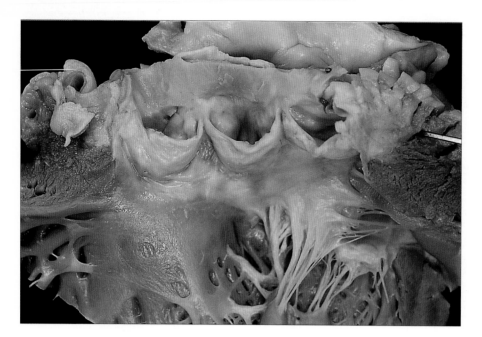

Figure 3.33
Aortic regurgitation in anklyosing spondylitis. The cusps are thickened, distorted and retracted from the base. Fibrosis extends into the base of the mitral valve and has obliterated the area of the membranous septum. The macroscopic appearances are often very similar to rheumatoid disease but are easily distinguished by histology.

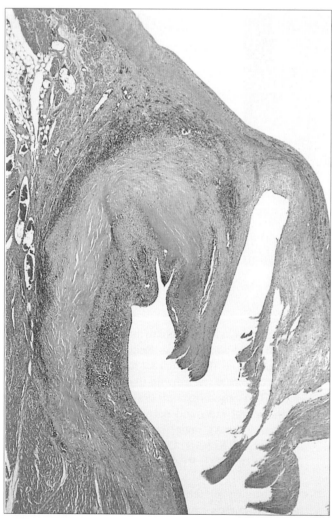

Figure 3.34
Rheumatoid arthritis – mitral valve. The characteristic site for rheumatoid granuloma is the base of the aortic cusps and in the angle between the mitral cusp and the ventricular wall from where the inflammatory mass extends into the underlying myocardium (H&E ×9.375). Note the cuff of lymphocytes around the rheumatoid nodule.

which extend into the media along the vasa vasorum. The adventitia thickens and small vessels show marked endarteritis obliterans. The intima also thickens and may develop diffuse atherosclerosis.

In ankylosing spondylitis, fibrous tissue with heavy inflammatory cell infiltration extends into the atrial septum adjacent to the aortic root and may destroy the AV node, causing heart block. Syphilis will only extend if there is localised gumma formation, in which case small giant cell granulomas related to necrosis develop. The granulomas of rheumatoid arthritis also can extend into the AV nodal area. In ankylosing spondylitis, the cardiac manifestations may occur before the disease appears in the joints. Idiopathic giant cell aortitis (see Chapter 7) may also involve the aorta just above the aortic valve and cause dilatation and regurgitation.

In non-inflammatory disease, the aortic wall is thinner and tree-barking is far less pronounced, although intimal wrinkling may occur due to intimal fibrosis associated with patchy medial destruction. Viewed from above, the aortic root is widened and the supra-aortic ridge is effaced in one or more sinuses (Figs 3.35, 3.36). The reduction in the degree of overlap of the cusps leads either to one prolapsing under its neighbours or a central defect. Nodular thickening along the free edge as a result of regurgitation occurs as in other causes of aortic regurgitation (Fig. 3.37). The dilatation of the aortic root is due to medial destruction of the aorta. The medial destruction in non-inflammatory disease takes various forms. At one extreme it is simply a loss of medial smooth muscle, and there may be large areas in which the media is acellular but the elastic laminae are intact. At the other extreme, typical of Marfan's disease, there are large areas of cystic change with fragmentation of the elastic laminae. The most extreme degrees of aortic root dilatation are usually seen in Marfan's disease

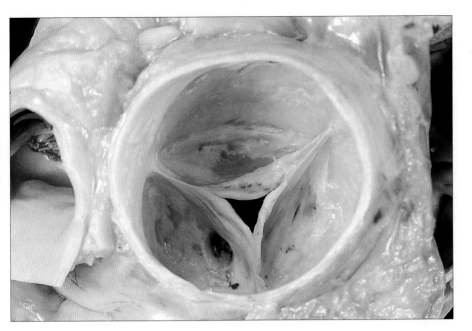

Figure 3.35
Aortic regurgitation due to non-inflammatory root dilatation. The aortic valve has been fixed by perfusion under pressure in the closed position. There is a residual central defect between the cusps. The root area is increased and the supra-aortic ridge marking the boundary between the sinus and the aorta has been smoothed out.

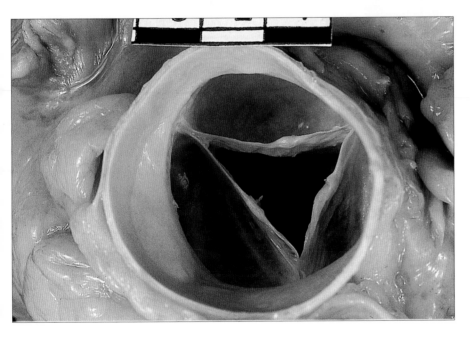

Figure 3.36
Aortic regurgitation due to non-inflammatory root dilatation. There is a much larger central triangular deficit due to the cusps not meeting than in Fig. 3.35. The supra-aortic ridge is more preserved although the whole root is dilated.

(Fig. 3.38). The aortic medial changes are discussed in more detail in Chapter 7.

Due to the decline in rheumatic disease, non-inflammatory aortic root dilatation is becoming a more common cause of aortic regurgitation. It has a variety of names, including idiopathic aortic root dilatation and annulo-aortic ectasia. Some familial cases are now being recognised which are due to abnormalities of the fibrillin gene without the other skeletal manifestations of Marfan's syndrome.

It is very easy to appreciate aortic regurgitation due to root dilatation in hearts which have been perfuse-fixed to close the valve under systemic pressure. It is less easy in specimens dissected in the routine way, particularly if the valve ring has been cut. The essence of this form of aortic regurgitation is that the aortic root is dilated and

measurements of the circumference of the aorta at the level of the valve commissures on the supra-aortic ridge are increased. The valve cusps are however not static structures, and will increase in area to compensate for the enlarging root. Only when this compensatory mechanism is overcome by either the rate or degree of root enlargement does regurgitation occur. Valves of the root circumference between 9 and 11.0 cm may or may not be associated with mild regurgitation. Confirmatory evidence for regurgitation in the form of the nodular thickening of the cusp edge, jet lesions or a dilated left ventricle is needed (Fig. 3.39). Above a circumference of 11.0 cm regurgitation will occur.

Aortic regurgitation due to loss of commissural support

An aortic dissection tear immediately above the commissures will allow one or more cusps to prolapse

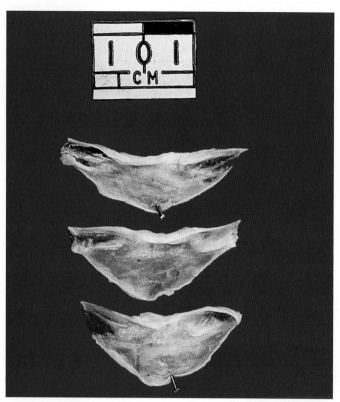

Figure 3.37
Aortic regurgitation due to non-inflammatory root dilatation. The excised cusps are large and are of normal thickness. There is no fibrosis in the body of the cusp although along the free edges there is a very discrete linear thickening. This is the result of regurgitant jets passing over the cusp edge and not a primary cause of the regurgitation.

Table 3.6
Causes of mitral valve stenosis

Common
Chronic rheumatic valve disease
Rare
Congenital
Ring calcification
Very rare
Carcinoid
Rheumatoid arthritis
Systemic lupus erythematosus
Amyloid
Methysergide therapy
Fabry's disease
Mucopolysaccharidosis
Radiation

MITRAL VALVE DISEASE

Mitral stenosis

The aetiology of mitral stenosis is virtually limited to chronic rheumatic type disease. There are other causes of mitral stenosis (Table 3.6) but these are very rare.

Rheumatic mitral valve disease

In its simplest form, there is a fibrous diaphragm with a central oval aperture due to fusion of both commissures (Fig. 3.40). In these cases, a simple valvotomy with splitting of the commissures can be highly successful without recourse to cardiac bypass and valve replacement. Such cases occur in younger individuals and are far more common in geographical areas where rheumatic fever is still endemic such as Egypt and India.

downwards. In ventricular septal defects which come right up to the base of the cusp without an intervening strip of septal muscle, prolapse of a cusp down into the ventricle can also occur.

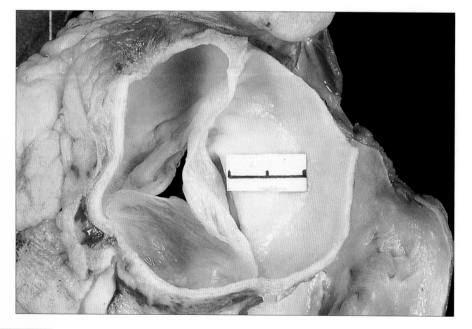

Figure 3.38
Aortic regurgitation in Marfan's disease. The aortic root is very large measuring 15.7 cm in circumference. The aortic root has been opened out with complete loss of the supra-aortic ridge. Two cusps have prolapsed under the edge of the cusp related to the sinus with the greatest dilatation.

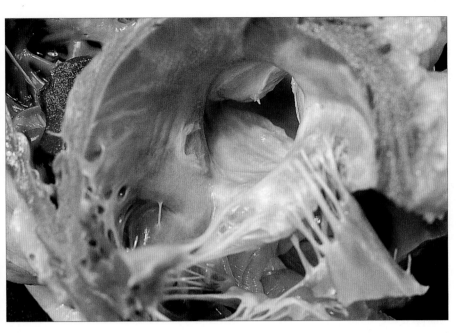

Figure 3.39
Aortic regurgitation due to root dilatation.
The left ventricular outflow is viewed
looking up toward the aortic valve which
although it was fixed closed has a central
defect. On the endocardium of the
interventricular septum there is a crescentic
patch of endocardial thickening due to the
impact of the regurgitant jet. Such jet
lesions may also occur on the ventricular
face of the anterior cusp of the mitral valve.
The left ventricular cavity is dilated and the
wall thickness reduced due to volume
overload.

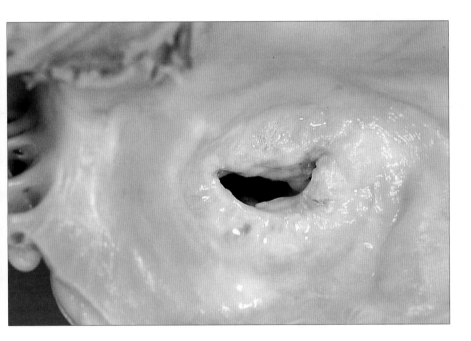

Figure 3.40
Rheumatic mitral stenosis. Both
commissures have fused leaving a small oval
aperture in a fibrous valve. The atrium is
moderately enlarged but there is no
thrombus present in the appendage.

In areas where rheumatic fever has declined, symptomatic patients with mitral stenosis are older and there is usually advanced cusp calcification. Diffuse thickening of each leaflet is seen with calcified deposits particularly at the edges of the leaflets and at both commissures (Fig. 3.41). In some cases, cusp calcification and fibrosis causes stenosis in the absence of commissural fusion. Calcific masses often ulcerate onto the atrial surface of the cusp (Fig. 3.41). Below the level of the cusps, the chordae tendineae are also thickened, shortened and fused, giving an element of subvalvar stenosis. Such valves have to be replaced with a prosthesis to relieve obstruction and requires cardiac bypass.

In countries such as the UK, many cases of mitral stenosis occur in patients over the age of 50 years. Often there is no history of rheumatic fever. This may indicate

that the history is unreliable after such a time lapse, or the acute phase was subclinical, or that there are other causes of an acute valvulitis leading to chronic stenosis. Atrial appendages removed during mitral valve surgery, when examined histologically may contain Aschoff bodies in the absence of any sign of acute rheumatic activity. The frequency falls with increasing age of the patient suggesting that Aschoff bodies are long-lived granulomas that persist long after acute rheumatic fever has resolved (Davies 1980).

There is often a dilated left atrium in association with mitral stenosis and thrombus may be present, but this can be variable. The dilatation may be related to the myocarditis found in the acute phase, or be a result of the stenosis combined with regurgitation, or follow the onset of atrial fibrillation. Thrombus usually starts in

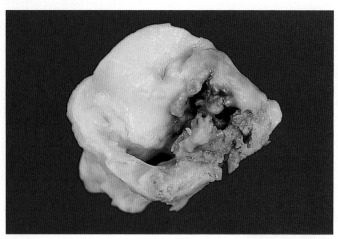 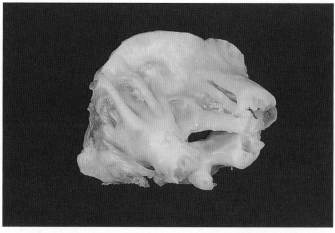

Figure 3.41
Rheumatic mitral stenosis. The excision specimen is viewed from the atrial aspect in (a). The orifice is very small due to commissural fusion and in addition the formation of large nodules of calcification, some of which have undergone ulceration. In (b) the valve is viewed from the ventricle. The chordae are fused together to form solid pillars of fibrous tissue causing additional sub-valvar stenosis.

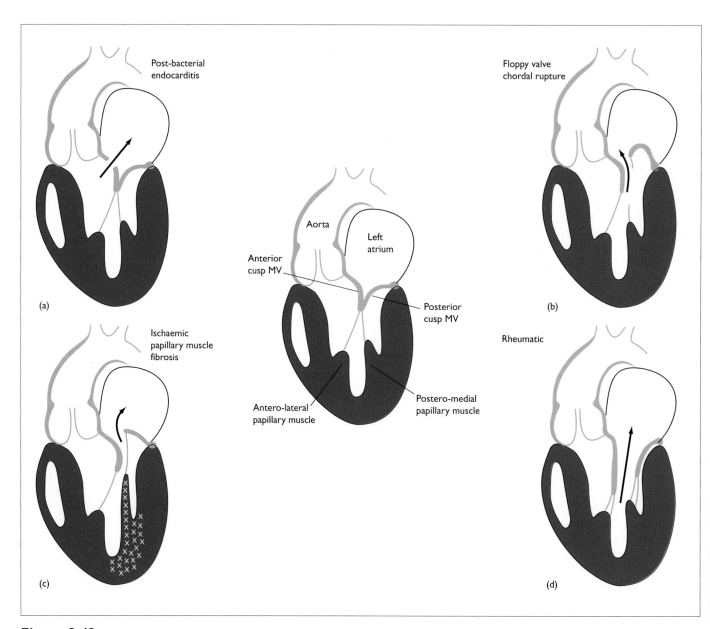

Figure 3.42
Mechanisms in mitral regurgitation. The main mechanisms responsible for mitral regurgitation are cusp perforation: bacterial endocarditis – (a); cusp prolapse, floppy valve – (b); ischaemic papillary muscle damage – (c); chordal shortening (rheumatic) – (d).

Table 3.7

Mechanisms of pure mitral regurgitation

Cusps	
Perforated	Bacterial endocarditis
Retracted	Chronic rheumatic disease, SLE
Expanded	Floppy valve
Chordae	
Short	Chronic rheumatic disease
Long/broken	Floppy valve
Papillary muscle	
Rupture	IHD
Fibrosed	IHD, Cardiomyopathy
Ring dilated	Marfan's disease
Ring rigid	Mitral ring calcification
Ventricle dilated	Functional mitral regurgitation

Table 3.8

Causes of mitral valve prolapse

Physiological	Normal structure valve
Structural abnormality of cusps/chordae	Floppy valve, Marfan's disease
Papillary muscle disease	Ischaemic heart disease Dilated cardiomyopathy

the left atrial appendage, and can extend over the surface of the whole chamber and undergo calcification.

Mitral incompetence

In contrast to stenosis, the causes for this are multiple (Table 3.7) (Fig. 3.42). These can be approached by whether the abnormality lies in the cusps, chordae, papillary muscle or annulus.

The floppy mitral valve and cusp prolapse

The advent of echocardiography allowed clinicians to gain a far deeper insight into valve function than was previously possible. It was realised that prolapse of a part of a mitral cusp into the left atrium during ventricular systole was a very common phenomenon. Prolapse is a strange word for what is an upward movement, but it is the one used. In a proportion of subjects with mitral cusp prolapse regurgitation develops at the end of systole. The auscultatory findings are very characteristic with an audible click as the upward movement of the cusp is halted, associated with a late systolic murmur as regurgitation occurs.

There are several causes of mitral valve prolapse (Table 3.8). Large scale surveys of fit young individuals show that minor degrees of cusp prolapse without regurgitation are commonplace, and can be regarded as minor physiological anomalies. Subjects who develop mild late systolic mitral regurgitation, however, have anatomical abnormalities of the valve. The majority of these abnormalities involve expansion of the cusp area and elongation of the chordae, to which the name floppy mitral valve has been given. Papillary muscle fibrosis can however also cause cusp prolapse.

The name floppy valve was given to the condition by surgeons who were replacing mitral valves for what was initially diagnosed as a rheumatic valve. It was recognised at surgery that the cusps were large and voluminous and soft to feel, quite unlike the typical retracted hard cusps of rheumatic disease.

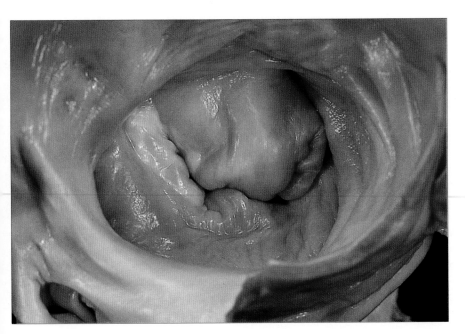

Figure 3.43

Floppy mitral valve. In the mildest forms of the floppy valve viewed from the left atrium the cusps are dome shaped and project upward into the atrium but their edges still coapt and there is no significant degree of regurgitation. This is the minimal macroscopic appearance required for a floppy valve.

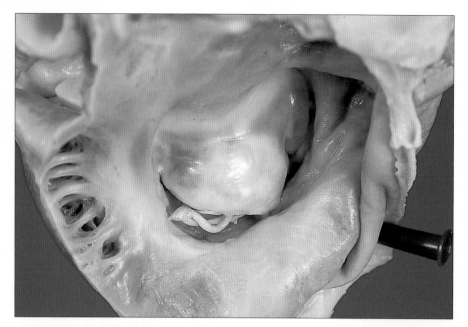

Figure 3.44
Floppy mitral valve with regurgitation. In this heart the anterior cusp is dome-shaped and projects upward into the atrium, having risen above the edge of the posterior cusp. The stumps of ruptured chordae can be seen. Severe mitral regurgitation was present.

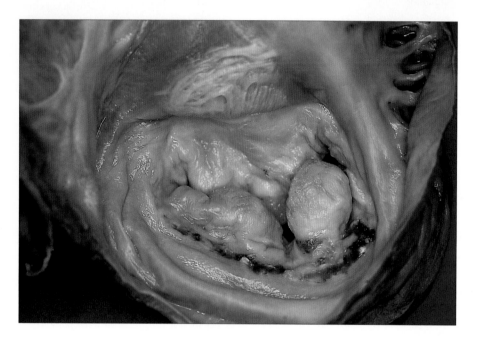

Figure 3.45
Floppy mitral valve with severe regurgitation. The posterior cusp shows two dome-shaped segments which protrude up into the atrium and have prolapsed far above the level of the edge of the anterior cusp. On the wall of the atrium where the regurgitant jet from under the edge of the posterior cusp hits the endocardium there is a very pronounced jet lesion. Small foci of flat thrombus are noted along the base of the posterior cusp. Large thrombi (vegetations) do not develop unless there is superimposed bacterial endocarditis.

The striking macroscopic feature of the floppy mitral valve is expansion of the cusps which adopt a dome shape. Viewed from the left atrium at autopsy one or both cusps bulge up into the atria (Figs 3.43–3.45). The cusp involvement may be very local and occur in one or more segment of the posterior cusp or involve both cusps. Along with the cusp expansion the chordae elongate. The soft rather gelatinous feel of the cusps is characteristic. By the time subjects with floppy valves come to autopsy or surgical replacement (Figs 3.46–48) many of the cases show advanced surface fibrosis over the cusps making them thick and white. This is probably the reason why the condition was not clearly distinguished from chronic rheumatic disease in the past. The cusp area expansion and the soft feel, however, remain distinguishing features even in late cases. The surface fibrosis is a result of thickening of the superficial layer

of the cusp, due to mechanical trauma as the hypermobile cusp hits the ventricular wall and the other cusp.

The histological appearances of the floppy valve (Fig. 3.48) are replacement of the solid fibrosa of the cusp with loosely arranged myxomatous tissue. These myxoid areas are cellular with many spindle-shaped fibroblastic cells and collagen and elastin fibrils are fragmented. There is a high content of acid mucopolysaccharide and an increased number of mast cells, but the cusp is not vascularised or inflamed. The surface of the cusp is often covered by a well-organised new layer of fibrous tissue containing elastic laminae. Small platelet thrombi are common on the surface of the cusp due to mechanical trauma to the hypermobile cusps. Histological examination of cusp tissue in floppy valves requires care in taking the histological blocks, so

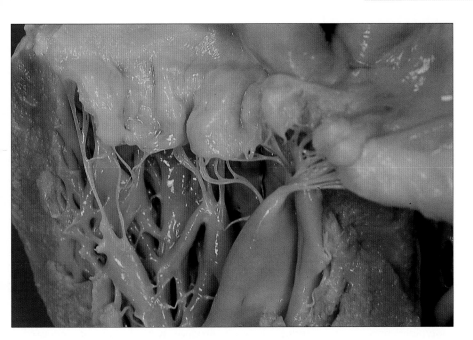

Figure 3.46
Floppy mitral valve. In this specimen in which the valve ring has been opened it is possible to recognise the enlarged dome-shaped cusps which are white and opaque. The chordae are long but not ruptured.

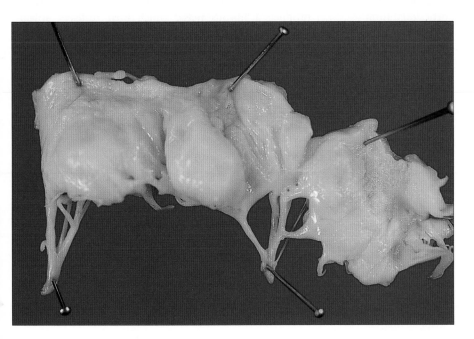

Figure 3.47
Surgically excised floppy valve. The dome-shaped thick and opaque cusps can be recognised easily if the valve is pinned out flat. The size of the cusps and the fact that they feel soft when handled distinguishes the condition from rheumatic disease.

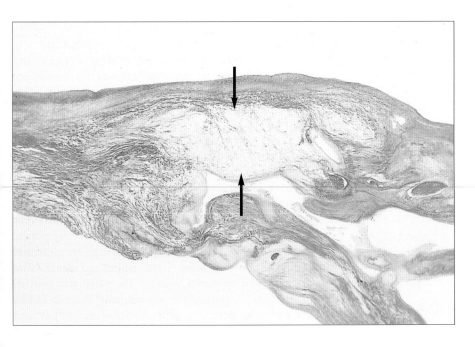

Figure 3.48
Floppy mitral valve histology. The cusp is thick with surface fibrosis but within the centre are large pale areas devoid of collagen (arrows) (EVG ×17.5).

as to demonstrate the cusp architecture. Floppy valves are not easily recognised by taking random blocks which may easily pass through the normal spongiform areas of the cusp. Blocks should be taken in the long axis of the cusp at right angles to the atrioventricular insertion of the valve.

Floppy mitral valves are common. Their frequency appears to rise steadily with age. They are becoming the commonest cause of isolated mitral regurgitation in patients undergoing valve replacement in populations in the developed world, where chronic rheumatic disease has declined.

The pathogenesis of the floppy mitral valve is contentious. There is no doubt that floppy valves are a complication of all the genetic disorders of connective tissue synthesis including Marfan's disease, osteogenesis imperfecta and Ehlers–Danlos syndrome. There is also increasing recognition that partial phenotypic expressions of these genetic diseases occur. For example the the mitral valve prolapse and mild aortic dilatation syndrome (MAAS) (Chapter 7) with mild aortic root dilatation and a floppy mitral valve is now recognised to be due to mutations of the fibrillin gene in which the amount of mutant type product is below 10% and no skeletal manifestations occur. A familial trend is well-recognised in floppy valves without any other systemic abnormality. Floppy valves are however so common that genetic abnormalities can only explain a proportion of cases. Other theories include an ageing wear and

tear phenomenon acting on a valve which was congenitally abnormal, perhaps lacking chordal support to certain parts of the cusp.

The natural history of a floppy mitral valve is probably to remain a mild condition with trivial regurgitation unless complications develop (Table 3.9).

Chordal rupture in floppy mitral valves is due to excessive mechanical stress operating on the thinned and elongated chordae; a proportion of cases also develop mitral ring dilatation. This is particularly true of floppy valves associated with gene disorders of connective tissue such as Marfan's disease. Bacterial endocarditis is a risk in any floppy valve which has even mild regurgitation. The most contentious and least understood risk is that of sudden death (see Chapter 8). A rare complication is fusion of the chordae onto the posterior wall of the left ventricle (Fig. 3.49). The hypermobile chordae hit the endocardium to produce vertical lines of endocardial fibrosis, which occasionally fuse with the chordae to produce a fibrous mass, which now restricts upward movement of the cusp and alters the mechanism of regurgitation (Salazar and Edwards 1970). Up until 10 years ago the mitral valve was usually replaced surgically, but more recently surgical repair has been introduced. The aim is to excise the most dome-shaped portion of the cusp and then stitch the rest of the cusp together, thus reducing its area and ability to prolapse (Fig. 3.50).

Rheumatic mitral incompetence

In pure regurgitation due to chronic rheumatic disease, there is diffuse fibrous thickening of the cusps and chordae without calcific deposits and commissural fusion. The commonest pattern is for the posterior cusp to be immobile and reduced in size. Chordae shorten (Fig. 3.51) and often fuse together preventing the cusps moving to meet in the closed position.

Infective endocarditis (Chapter 4)

The leaflets have a perforated or indented appearance with vegetations or combinations of these changes. This can occur on previously damaged valves, i.e. rheumatic or floppy, or the valve can be normal. Certain conditions such as floppy mitral valve are easily recognisable even with endocarditis, but mild previous inflammatory disease with fibrosis may be masked by healed or healing endocarditis.

Chordal rupture

Rupture of chordae occurs most frequently in the floppy valve and also in infective endocarditis. Ischaemic heart disease does not cause chordal rupture, since these are avascular structures. Severe closed chest trauma may cause chordal rupture in a mitral valve that appears otherwise normal. Such cases may cause considerable medico-legal problems over potential compensation following road traffic accidents. The question will be raised whether the valve was normal or abnormal previously if replacement is needed. The surgical specimen will need careful examination and

Table 3.9

Natural history of a floppy mitral valve

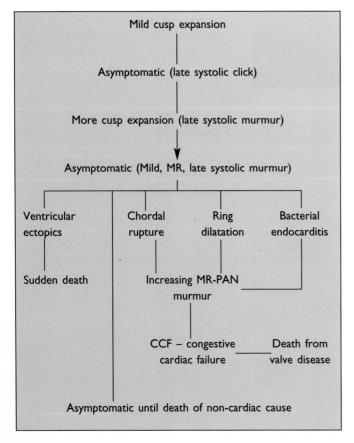

Mild cusp expansion

Asymptomatic (late systolic click)

More cusp expansion (late systolic murmur)

Asymptomatic (Mild, MR, late systolic murmur)

Ventricular ectopics — Chordal rupture — Ring dilatation — Bacterial endocarditis

Sudden death — Increasing MR-PAN murmur

CCF – congestive cardiac failure — Death from valve disease

Asymptomatic until death of non-cardiac cause

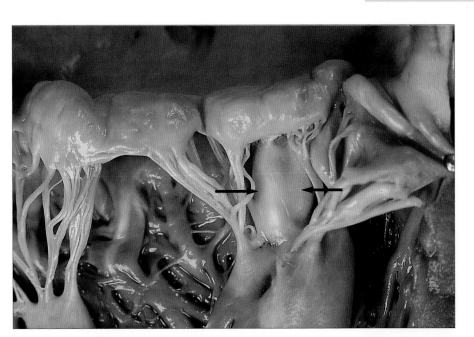

Figure 3.49
Chordal fusion (arrows) in floppy mitral valve. The posterior cusp has the typical dome shape of a floppy mitral valve. The chordae are incorporated into a fibrous mass attached to the endocardial surface of the posterior wall of the left ventricle.

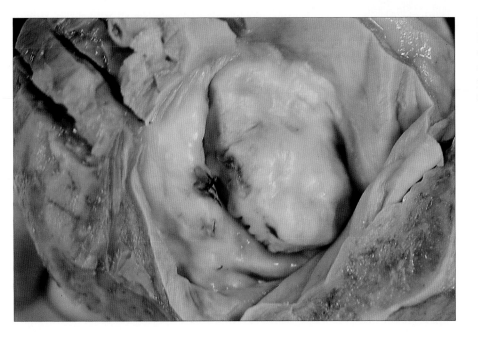

Figure 3.50
Floppy mitral valve – surgical repair. Both cusps are strikingly dome-shaped; the repair of the posterior cusp carried out some years earlier can be recognised by the blue suture material embedded in the cusp.

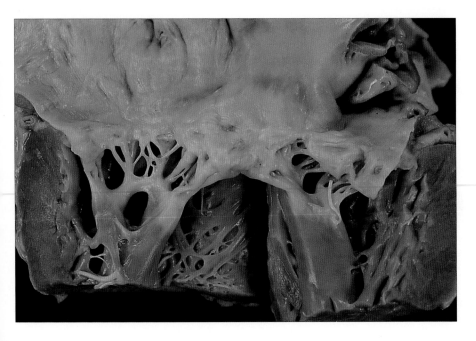

Figure 3.51
Rheumatic mitral regurgitation. The predominant change in this valve is shortening of the chordae which restricts cusp movement. The degree of commissural fusion is minimal and the cusps show only moderate fibrous thickening.

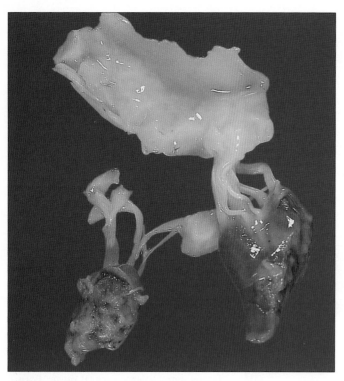

Figure 3.52
Ischaemic mitral regurgitation. The excised valve shows stumps of two heads of a ruptured papillary muscle.

macroscopic photography, as well as correctly orientated histological blocks.

Papillary muscle

Ischaemic papillary muscle damage leads to all degrees of severity of regurgitation. At one extreme there is rupture following acute myocardial infarction when the distal tip or the base of the muscle becomes necrotic (Fig. 3.52). The stump of the papillary muscle crosses the mitral valve *in vivo* and at autopsy the ruptured head is found in the left atrium. At the other extreme, healing of papillary muscle necrosis with fibrosis may either shorten the papillary muscle or allow it to elongate; both processes cause mild regurgitation. Calcification of the fibrotic apex of the elongated papillary muscle often occurs. Fibrosis of the left ventricular wall at the base of the papillary muscle following infarction alters the axis of the pull on the chordae leading to mild regurgitation. Overall ischaemic damage to the papillary muscle complex is probably the commonest cause of very mild regurgitation of the mitral valve in developed countries but only rarely requires valve replacement.

Mitral regurgitation due to annular dilatation

Large and chronic increases in annular circumferences can lead to mitral regurgitation. This can be primary as in Marfan's disease or be associated with severe volume overload due to aortic or mitral regurgitation. When ring dilatation is associated with mitral regurgitation due to a floppy valve, consideration should be given to a generalised connective tissue defect. This cannot be done by histology and has to be by consideration of the family history. The mild MAAS form of fibrillin gene abnormality is the commonest form found.

Functional mitral regurgitation

In patients with severe left ventricular failure where the ventricle becomes globular in shape, mitral regurgitation can occur despite the mitral annular size being normal. The condition is thought to be caused by altering the axis of traction by the papillary muscles on the cusps. Regurgitation ceases if treatment reverses the globular shape of the ventricle. An analogous form of functional tricuspid regurgitation exists.

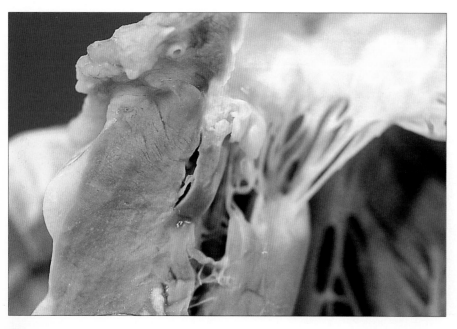

Figure 3.53
Mitral ring calcification. The calcific mass occurs in the angle between the base of the cusp and the left ventricular endocardium. The base of the cusp is pushed up toward the atrium.

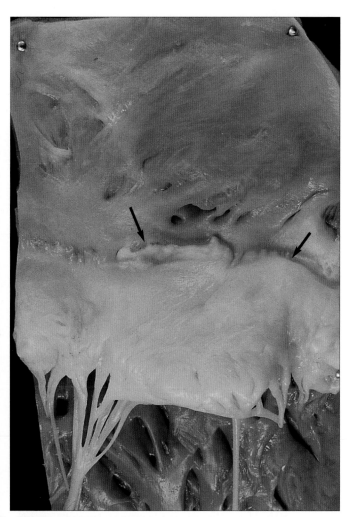

Figure 3.54
Mitral valve calcification in Marfan's disease. There is a very pronounced expansion and doming of the posterior cusp. Calcification which began below the cusp base has now extended and pushed through the atrial endocardium (arrows).

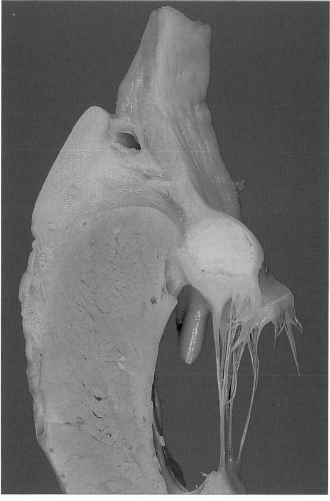

Figure 3.55
Mitral ring calcification. In this case the calcium in the ring has undergone necrosis and breakdown to form soft caseous-like material. The lesion should not be mistaken for TB or rheumatoid. More solid calcification is usually found at other points in the ring.

Mitral valve calcification

Mitral valve calcification just below the insertion of the posterior cusp into the atrioventricular ring becomes increasingly common with age. Figures on frequency are very variable due to the sensitivity of the methods used to identify the calcification, but a figure of 10% of individuals over 50 years of age identifiable by X-ray is credible. Macroscopic calcification at autopsy is rare under 70 years, but increases steadily in frequency thereafter (Pomerance 1970).

Calcification develops just beneath the insertion of the posterior cusp and forms a bar 2–7 cm long (Figs 3.53, 3.54). The base of the cusp is pushed upward, giving it an appearance very like a floppy mitral valve. Both conditions are age-related and often coexist. The calcification is regarded as a wear-and-tear phenomenon, and may therefore be enhanced by the very mobile cusps in the floppy valve. In Marfan's disease where there is an extreme degree of floppy mitral valve, ring calcification (Fig. 3.54) can occur at a young age. In extreme cases, the calcium becomes contiguous with age-related calcification in the aortic valve and completely encircles the mitral orifice. The calcification is rather like that seen in the aortic valve, and occurs in a nodular fashion. Within the centres of the nodules the tissue breaks down and is very eosinophilic in histology sections. The central breakdown may reach the point where the tissue becomes a pultaceous mass which is yellow and soft (Fig. 3.55). Some inflammatory cells and foreign body giant cells often form at the margin and the lesion is often misdiagnosed, and even reported in case reports as a tuberculoma or gumma of the mitral valve.

Mitral ring calcification is rarely symptomatic, most examples being coincidental findings either seen on chest X-rays, or ECHO in life or found at autopsy. The normal mitral valve ring decreases in size when the left ventricle contracts, and this is in part responsible for normal competence. When there is a complete ring of calcium around the valve orifice, it becomes fixed neither able to increase nor decrease. The result is a mild to moderate combination of mitral stenosis and regurgitation, but in inactive elderly subjects this is rarely of

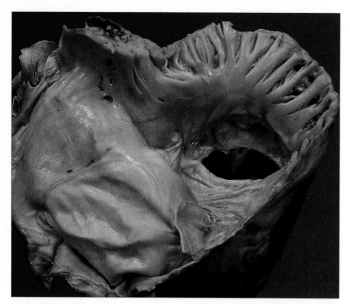

Figure 3.56
Rheumatic tricuspid valve stenosis. There is commissural fusion to produce a fibrous diaphragm with an oval aperture.

clinical significance. When calcification is very heavy it may extend onto the ventricular septum and sever the bundle of His, causing complete heart block. This association is known as Rytand's syndrome (Fulkerson *et al.* 1979; Takamoto and Popp 1983). The calcific deposits in the ring occasionally erode through the base of the mitral valve cusp and become exposed. The valve then becomes vulnerable to bacterial endocarditis. The presence of exuberant mitral ring calcification in association with aortic calcification in subjects under 60 years should also lead to the investigation of possible enhanced soft tissue calcification. This may occur in chronic renal disease, hyperparathyroidism and Paget's disease of bone (Nestico *et al.* 1983).

TRICUSPID AND PULMONARY VALVE DISEASE

These valves are rarely surgically excised. Rheumatic tricuspid disease (Fig. 3.56) occurs with concomitant aortic and mitral disease. Tricuspid stenosis is due to commissural fusion and calcification and marked fibrous thickening of the cusps are very rare. The most common form of rheumatic tricuspid regurgitation is in fact due to severe dilatation of the annulus following right ventricular dilatation in pulmonary hypertension. The valve orifice is too large to be closed by the cusps which are only mildly reduced in size by fibrosis.

Pulmonary atresia or stenosis is seen in the context of congenital stenosis as in tetralogy of Fallot when the valves cusps are often thickened and dysplastic. Bicuspid and quadricuspid pulmonary valves are more common than the equivalent aortic lesions, but are of no consequence. The carcinoid syndrome with release of vasoactive peptides into the circulation from liver

metastases results in fibrosis of the right-sided valve cusps (Roberts and Sjoerdsma 1964) (Fig. 3.57). The cusps become covered by a layer of dense white fibrous tissue which extends in the mitral valve onto the ventricular endocardium and in the pulmonary valve into the sinuses. The extension into the base of the pulmonary trunk leads to a characteristic constriction at commissural level. Balloon dilatation is becoming a standard method to relieve the symptoms, but is not always successful. All combinations of stenosis and regurgitation are produced in both valves. Histological examination shows the pathology to be surface fibrosis which is encasing relatively normal underlying cusp architecture.

Two other relatively unimportant features in terms of function occur in the tricuspid valve but may be noticed at autopsy. In pulmonary hypertension the anterior cusp of the tricuspid valve develops nodular thickening of its surface, facing the right ventricular outflow. This thickening may have yellow ulcerated areas. In old age the tricuspid leaflets and chordae often expand and lengthen giving, in effect, a floppy tricuspid valve (Fig. 3.58). The change may or may not accompany similar changes in the mitral valve. This floppy tricuspid valve is rarely of significance. The haemodynamics in the low pressure right side of the heart are such that the pulmonary or tricuspid cusps can be absent or removed without detriment providing there is no pulmonary hypertension. The septal cusp of the tricuspid valve is often absent or hypoplastic, and is a congenital anomaly of no clinical significance.

PROSTHETIC HEART VALVES

Replacing abnormal heart valves began in the 1950s and there is now a bewildering variety of prosthetic valves. Valve replacement is so common and patient survival so good that every pathologist, even those outside specialised centres, will encounter autopsies in which comments on the function of a prosthetic valve will be required. There are national registers for monitoring prosthetic valve performance and surgeons are always appreciative of follow up autopsy data.

Types of prosthetic valve

Valve prostheses can be divided into mechanical prostheses made of plastics, Teflon or metal and tissue valves. Each type has its vices and virtues; metal prostheses have a high risk of thromboembolism requiring lifetime anticoagulation, but the valves last for years. Tissue valves have a high risk of failing within 10 years and will not last a lifetime, but they have a negligible risk of thromboembolism and anticoagulation is not required.

Mechanical valves

Numerous types exist. All have a ring covered by Teflon which is sewed into the native valve annulus after the

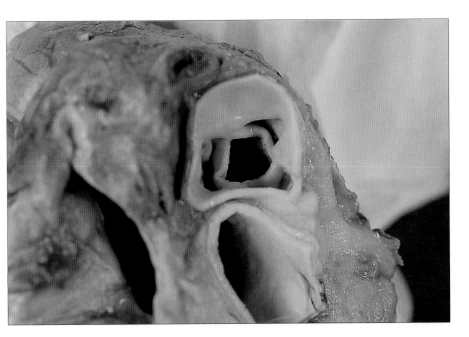

Figure 3.57
Carcinoid valve disease. The pulmonary valve cusps are thickened and the annulus is constricted at the level of the commissures producing a mixture of pulmonary stenosis and regurgitation.

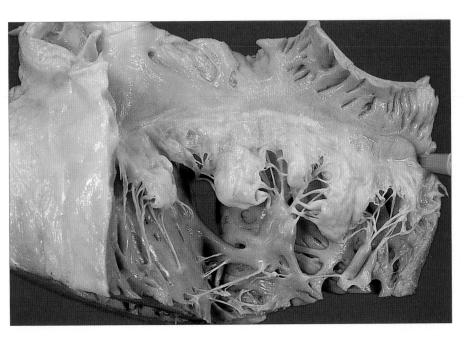

Figure 3.58
Floppy tricuspid valve. The cusps are all enlarged and opaque with a dome shape. This change is the analogue of a floppy mitral valve but is very rarely of any clinical significance.

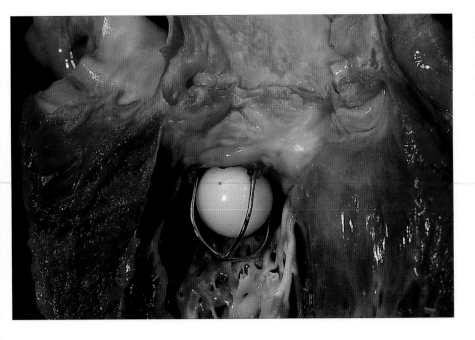

Figure 3.59
Starr type prosthetic valve. There is a prosthetic valve in the mitral position. The cage has metal struts and the ball is Silastic. Other models have metal balls and struts covered by Teflon.

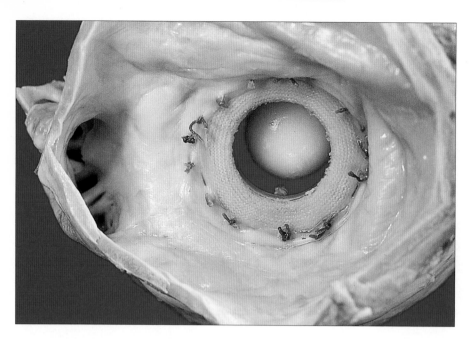

Figure 3.60
Starr type prosthetic valve. Viewed from the left atrium the ring of the prosthetic valve covered by a Teflon weave is seen to be neatly sutured into the original valve ring. All the sutures are intact without a para-prosthetic leak being present. No thrombus hinders the ball seating into the ring.

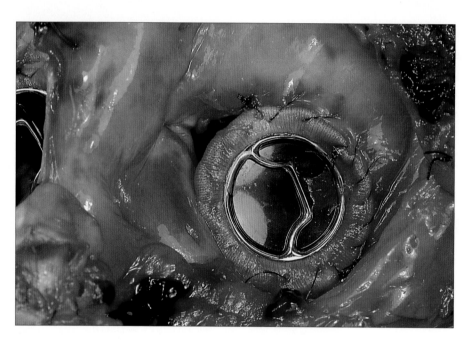

Figure 3.61
Tilting disc prosthesis. A prosthesis with a spring-controlled tilting disc is shown in the mitral position. Some of the sutures into the sewing ring of the prosthetic valve have cut through the atrial wall allowing the prosthetic valve to tilt and creating a para-prosthetic leak.

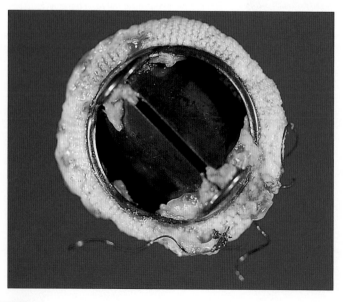

Figure 3.62
Hinged bileaflet prosthesis. This prosthetic valve was excised as an emergency due to thrombus extending from the ring and interfering with the free movement of the flaps.

cusps have been removed. In cage and ball prostheses of the Starr–Edwards type, a ball-shaped poppet moves inside a cage (Figs 3.59, 3.60). There may be three struts (aortic) or four (mitral) and the ball is made of a variety of materials including metal, plastic or Silastic. In order to obtain both a better flow profile and to avoid the necessity of a large cage in the ventricle, low profile valves have been designed. These may have a disc-shaped poppet in a cage, a tilting metal disc controlled by a spring (Fig. 3.61) or two hinged metal flaps (Fig. 3.62).

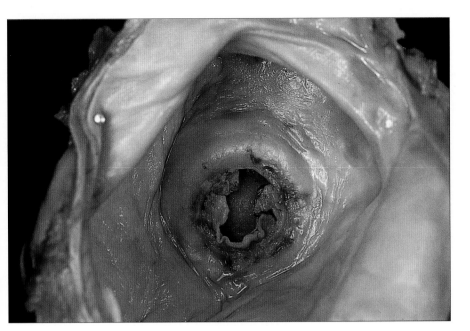

At autopsy it is relatively easy to check the normal functioning of these mechanical prosthetic valves after opening the left atrium and washing out post mortem blood clot, cutting the aorta across just above the supra-aortic ridge and making a short axis cut across the ventricles at mid-ventricular level. Both aspects of mitral and aortic prosthetic valves can then be inspected. Adherent post mortem clot is usually easily washed or picked out of the valve and is deep red in colour. Ante-mortem thrombus is brick red and strongly adherent. It is relatively easy to see if balls move freely in cages or if hinged valves open or shut. Major mechanical disasters are very obvious. The earlier Starr valves had balls which absorbed lipid and swelled becoming jammed in the cage. The later models have steel balls which do not have this problem. Silastic balls may crack or fissure and embolise fragments of the ball or jam in the cage. Strut fractures may occur due to metal fatigue. With hinged and tilting prostheses, thrombus on the ring may prevent the correct movements (Fig. 3.62).

In mitral valve replacements, some surgeons will remove the whole valve including the papillary muscles to give ample room for the prosthetic cage. Other surgeons argue that better left ventricular contraction is preserved when the papillary muscles are left *in situ*. There is, however, a danger that residual valve tissue may impinge on the movement of the prostheses. Perivalvar leaks are usually due to one of the ring sutures cutting through the tissue or breaking (Fig. 3.61). All mechanical valves that have been *in situ* more than a few months develop a layer of white fibrous tissue over the sewing ring through which the ends of the sutures project (Fig. 3.63). This layer is often called neointima and it does appear to diminish thrombus formation. Projection of this layer as a pannus out across the valve orifice may occur, however, obstructing flow (Fig. 3.63). It is very difficult for the pathologist at autopsy to judge the relation between the size of

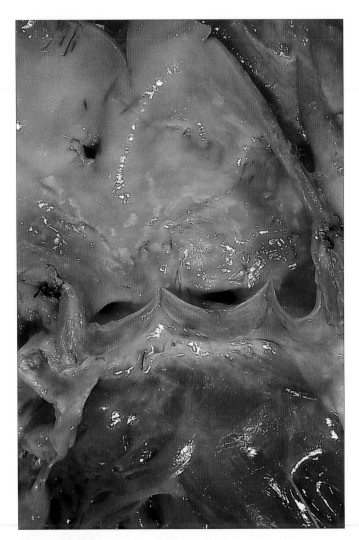

Figure 3.64
Aortic homograft valve. The aortic valve has been replaced with a human cadaver valve. The valve has been *in situ* for 2 years. The cusps appear normal. This has been covered in and is only just recognisable due to some suture material showing through the new intima that has formed. Vein grafts were also inserted into the coronaries and the orifice of one of these is seen in the aorta. Normal aortic valve function.

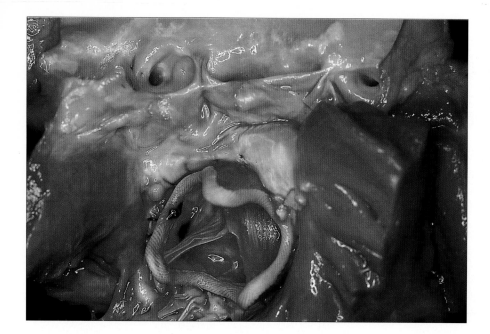

Figure 3.65
Porcine prosthetic valve. This valve has been inserted into the mitral position. It consists of a pig valve sewn into a three-pointed stent.

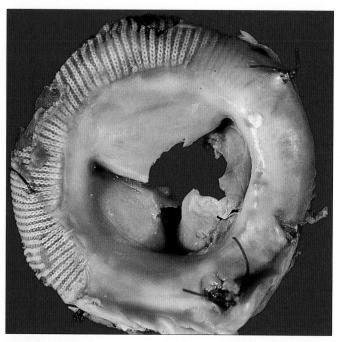

Figure 3.66
Porcine prosthetic valve tear. This Hancock type prosthesis was removed from the mitral position after regurgitation developed some years after implantation. The valve ring shows a covering of neointima. Regurgitation was due to cusp tears.

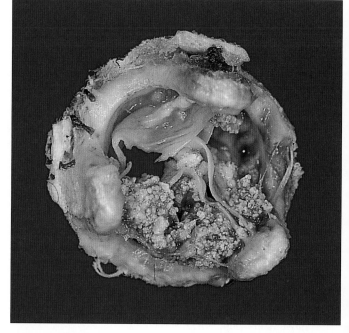

Figure 3.67
Tissue prosthetic valve calcification. This Hancock type prosthesis was removed due to recurrent stenosis. The stenosis is caused by nodular masses of calcium which begin where the cusps are stitched to the stent. Note also the tear in the cusp.

the prosthetic valve used in relation to the original native valve orifice. In aortic regurgitation the aortic root is often dilated and relatively large prostheses can be inserted. In stenosis some of the aortic roots are small and even a small prosthesis seems jammed in very tightly with relatively little space around the cage to allow blood to pass around the ball. In such cases a strut may impinge on the orifice of a coronary artery (Schoen 1995).

Tissue valves

The tissue valves which have been or are in current use include non-stented human aortic homografts (Fig. 3.64) and stented valves within which semi-lunar cusps were either made from pericardium or fascia lata. Aortic valves from pigs (Fig. 3.65) are also used. The animal tissues used are all treated with gluteraldehyde and there is no question of viable tissue being used in a graft situation. The prosthesis depends on the mechanical properties of collagen which has been fixed in gluteraldehyde. The use of human material is rather different. In children one option is to remove the pulmonary valve and instantly insert it into the aortic position. Such valves are viable and appear to grow and remodel in the new position. The pulmonary valve is replaced by a tissue prosthesis. The philosophy is that in the low pressure pulmonary position, a prosthetic valve lasts far longer. In adults the aortic valve may be replaced by human aortic valves removed either from cadavers or from explanted hearts from patients with cardiomyopathy or ischaemic heart disease, undergoing cardiac transplantation. The human valves are treated in a variety of ways depending on the centre involved. They may be simply kept in an antibiotic solution and used fresh or fixed in gluteraldehyde. Centres which use stored fresh valves claim there is a graft element, i.e. fibroblasts in the new valve begin to divide and actively maintain the collagen; others find no evidence that this occurs. Human homograft valves are usually used in the aortic position alone and are unstented.

The Hancock bioprosthesis introduced in the 1970s had a pig aortic valve mounted inside a 3-pronged stent covered by knitted polyester. The whole valve was sewn inside the stent, so that there was some extra-valvar tissue present. This tended both to project into the valve orifice and to calcify. Later Hancock models have the three cusps sewn separately onto a flexible acetal resin stent. The Carpentier–Edwards valve is similar in design, but has a flexible metal frame.

The long-term survival of both aortic homografts and animal tissue valves is limited by primary failure of the cusp tissue which tears (Fig. 3.66) and by heavy calcification (Fig. 3.67) which develops within the cusps. Subjects under 15 years of age calcify tissue valves very rapidly, leading to early failure which is why switching the pulmonary valve to the aortic valve has become established.

References

Allen W, Matloff J, Fishbein M. Myxoid degeneration of the aortic valve and isolated aortic regurgitation. *Am J Cardiol* 1985;55:439–44.

Angelini A, Ho S, Anderson R *et al.* The morphology of the normal aortic valve as compared with the aortic valve having two leaflets. *J Thorac Cardiovasc Surg* 1989;89:363–7.

Becker A, Becker M, Edwards J. Anomalies associated with coarctation of the aorta: particular reference to infancy. *Circulation* 1970;41:1067–75.

Bulkley B, Roberts W. Ankylosing spondylitis and aortic regurgitation – description of the characteristic cardiovascular lesion from study of eight necropsy patients. *Circulation* 1973;68:1914–27.

Davies MJ. *Pathology of cardiac valves*. London: Butterworths, 1980.

Davies M, Treasure T, Parker D. Demographic characteristics of patients undergoing aortic valve replacement for stenosis: relation to valve morphology. *Heart* 1996;75:174–8.

Dare A, Harrity P, Tazelaar H, Edwards W, Mullany C. Evaluation of surgically excised mitral valves: revised recommendations based on changing operative procedures in the 1990s. *Hum Pathol* 1993;24:1286–93.

Edwards J. The congenital bicuspid aortic valve. *Circulation* 1961;23:485–8.

Ewart AK, Morris CA, Atkinson D. Hemizgosity at the elastin locus in a development disorder. Williams' syndrome. *Nature Genet* 1993;5:11–16.

Falcone M, Roberts W, Morrow A, Perloff J. Congenital aortic stenosis resulting from a uncommissural valve. Clinical and anatomic features in 21 adult patients. *Circulation* 1971;44:272–80.

Fulkerson P, Beaver M, Auseon J, Grabler H. Calcification of the mitral annulus. Aetiology clinical association complications and therapy. *Am J Med* 1979;66:967–77.

Hurwitz L, Roberts W. Quadricuspid semilunar valve. *Am J Cardiol* 1973;31:623–6.

Isner J, Chokshi S, DeFranco A, Braimen J, Slovenkai G. Contrasting histoarchitecture of calcified leaflets from stenotic bicuspid versus stenotic tricuspid aortic valves. *J Am Coll Cardiol* 1990;15:1104–8.

Kitzman DW, Scholz DG, Hagen PT, Illstrup DM, Edwards WD. Age-related changes in normal human hearts during the first 10 decades of life. Part II (maturity); a quantitative anatomic study of 765 specimens from subjects 20 to 99 years old. *Mayo Clin Proc* 1988;63:137–46.

Lindroos M, Kupari M, Heikkila J, Tilvis R. Prevalence of aortic valve abnormalities in the elderly: an echocardiographic study of a random population sample. *J Am Coll Cardiol* 1993;21:1220–5.

Lindroos M, Kupari M, Valvanne J, Strandberg T, Heikkila J, Tilvis R. Factors associated with calcific aortic valve degeneration in the elderly. *Eur Heart J* 1994;15:865–70.

Liu S, Alexander C. Complete heart block and aortic insufficiency in rheumatoid spondylitis. *Am J Cardiol* 1969;23:888–92.

McManus BM, Davies MJ. Heart Disease in the Adult. In: Damanjov I, Linder J (eds). *Anderson's pathology*, 10th edn. St.Louis: Mosby, 1996; Chapter 45.

Maher E, Pazianas M, Curtis J. Calcific aortic stenosis: a complication of chronic uraemia. *Nephron* 1987;47:119–22.

Mautner G, Mautner S, O'Connon III R, Hunsberger S, Roberts W. Clinical factors useful in predicting aortic valve structure in patients >40 years of age with isolated valvular aortic stenosis. *Am J Cardiol* 1993;72:194–8.

Mehta P, Heinsimer J, Bryg R. Reassessment of the association between gastrointestinal arteriovenous malformation and aortic stenosis. *Am J Med* 1989;86:275–7.

Mohler E, Sheridan M, Nicholls R, Harvey W, Waller B. Development and progression of aortic valve stenosis: atherosclerosis risk factors – a causal relationship? A clinical morphological study. *Clin Cardiol* 1991;14:995–9.

Nestico P, DePace N, Kotler M, Rose L, Brezin J,

Swartz C. Calcium phosphorus metabolism in dialysis patients with and without mitral annular calcium. Analysis of 30 patients. *Am J Cardiol* 1983;**51**: 497–500.

Niederle B, Stefenelli T, Glogar D, Woloszczuk W, Roka R, Mayer H. Cardiac calcific deposits in patients with primary hyperparathyroidism: preliminary results of a prospective echocardiographic study. *Surgery* 1990;**108**:998–9.

Olsson M, Rosenqvist M, Nilsson J. Expression of HLA-Dr antigen and smooth muscle cell differentiation markers by valvular fibroblasts in degenerative aortic stenosis. *J Am Coll Cardiol* 1994;**24**:1664–71.

Ouchi Y, Akishita M, de Souza A, Nakamura T, Orino H. Age-related loss of bone mass and aortic/aortic valve calcification-revaluation of recommended dietary allowance of calcium in the elderly. *Ann N Y Acad Sci* 1993;**6**:297–307.

Passik C, Ackermann D, Pluth J, Edwards W. Temporal changes in the causes of aortic stenosis: a surgical pathological study of 646 cases. *Mayo Clin Proc* 1987;**62**:119–23.

Paulus H, Pearson C, Pitts W. Aortic insufficiency in five patients with Reiter's syndrome: a detailed clinical and pathological study. *Am J Med* 1972;**53**: 464–72.

Pomerance A. Pathological and clinical study of calcification of the mitral valve ring. *J Clin Pathol* 1970;**23**:354–61.

Reid G, Patterson M, Patterson A, Cooperberg P. Aortic insufficiency in association with juvenile ankylosing spondylitis. *J Pediatr* 1979;**95**:78–80.

Roberts W. The structure of the aortic valve in clinically isolated aortic stenosis. An autopsy study of 162 patients over 15 years of age. *Circulation* 1970;**42**:91–7.

Roberts W, Kehoe J, Carpenter D. Cardiac valvular lesions in rheumatoid arthritis. *Arch Intern Med* 1968;**122**:144–56.

Roberts W, Morrow A, McIntosh C. Congenitally bicuspid aortic valve causing severe, pure aortic regurgitation without superimposed infective endocarditis: analysis of 13 patients requiring aortic valve replacement. *Am J Cardiol* 1981;**47**:206–9.

Roberts W, Sjoerdsma A. The cardiac disease associated with the carcinoid syndrome (carcinoid heart disease). *Am J Med* 1964;**35**:5.

Sadee A, Becker A, Verheul H, Bouma B, Hoedemaker G. Aortic valve regurgitation and the congenitally bicuspid aortic valve: a clinico-pathological correlation. *Br Heart J* 1992;**67**:439–42.

Sadee A, Becker A, Verheul J. The congenital bicuspid aortic valve with post-inflammatory disease – a neglected pathological diagnosis of clinical relevance. *Eur Heart J* 1994;**15**:503–6.

Salazar A, Edwards J. Friction lesions of ventricular endocardium relation to tendineae of mitral valve. *Arch Pathol* 1970;**90**:364–76.

Scheffer S, Leatherman L. Resolution of Heyde's syndrome of aortic stenosis and gastrointestinal bleeding after aortic valve replacement. *Ann Thorac Surg* 1986;**42**:477–80.

Schoen FJ. Pathological considerations in replacement heart valves and other cardiovascular prosthetic devices. In: Schoen FJ, Gimbrone KMA (eds). *Cardiovascular pathology clinicopathologic correlations and pathogenetic mechanisms*. Baltimore: Williams and Wilkins, 1995; 194–222.

Silver MA, Roberts WC. Detailed anatomy of the normally functioning aortic valve in hearts of normal and increased weight. *Am J Cardiol* 1985;**55**: 454–61.

Strikberger S, Schulman S, Hutchins G. Association of Paget's disease of bone with calcific aortic valve disease. *Am J Med* 1987;**82**:953–6.

Subramanian R, Olsen L, Edwards W. Surgical pathology of pure aortic stenosis. A study of 374 cases. *Mayo Clin Proc* 1984;**59**:683–90.

Takamoto T, Popp R. Conduction disturbances related to the site and severity of mitral annular calcification: a 2-dimensional echocardiographic and electrocardiographic correlative study. *Am J Cardiol* 1983;**51**:1644–9.

Tazelaar HD. Surgical pathology of the heart: endomyocardial biopsy, valvular heart disease and cardiac tumors. In: Schoen FJ, Gimbrone KMA (eds). *Cardiovascular pathology clinicopathologic correlations and pathogenetic mechanisms*. Baltimore: Williams and Wilkins,1995; 81–107.

Tonnemacher D, Reid C, Kawanishi D. Frequency of myxomatous degeneration of the aortic valve as a cause of isolated aortic regurgitation severe enough to warrant aortic valve replacement. *Am J Cardiol* 1987;**60**:1194–6.

Vollebergh F, Becker A. Minor congenital variations of cusp size in aortic valves. Possible link with isolated aortic stenosis. *Br Heart J* 1977;**39**:1006–11.

INFECTIVE ENDOCARDITIS

INTRODUCTION

Infective endocarditis occurs when a microorganism (bacterial, fungal or Rickettsial) settles and grows within a mass of thrombus (vegetation) (Figs 4.1, 4.2) on the endocardial surface of a valve. More rarely, infected vegetations occur on the endocardium of a cardiac chamber or on the intimal surface of the aorta.

PATHOGENESIS OF INFECTIVE ENDOCARDITIS

Experimental models of bacterial endocarditis (Baddour *et al.* 1989) show the necessity for two concurrent events in the establishment of infection on the endocardium. One factor is endothelial denudation over the valve cusp associated with platelet deposition; the

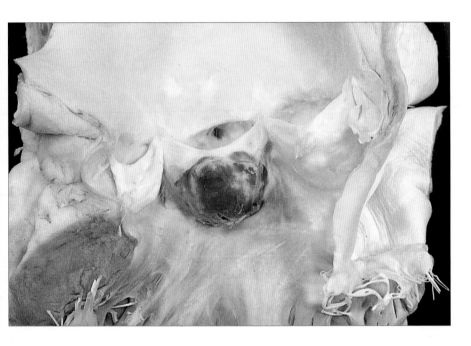

Figure 4.1
Bacterial endocarditis – aortic valve. A single large red vegetation is attached to the ventricular aspect of one aortic cusp. There is no obvious pre-existing valve abnormality. Staphylococcal endocarditis in an elderly subject.

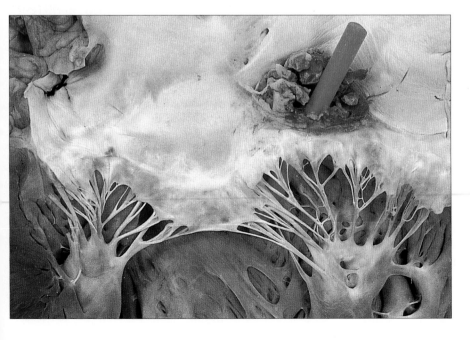

Figure 4.2
Bacterial endocarditis – mitral valve. A large red vegetation is attached to the atrial aspect of the posterior cusp of the mitral valve. The cusp is perforated. The valve does not appear to have been previously abnormal. *Staphylococcus aureus* grown.

other is an episode of bacteraemia. Neither factor alone will establish the infection. The animal models use an indwelling catheter across a cardiac valve to cause endothelial damage, followed by the intravenous injection of known numbers of an organism. Organisms vary widely in their pathogenicity, i.e. the number needed to establish infection. Organisms which can bind via receptors to fibronectin or other subendothelial components or to platelets are the most virulent, i.e establish infection when small numbers are injected. These facts suggest that adhesion of an organism to either platelets or to an exposed subendothelial component of the valve matrix is the primary event. The organism then begins to divide at the site and becomes surrounded by thrombotic material. Within this thrombus, the organism lies in a privileged site remote from polymorphonuclear attack. An acute inflammatory response is generated in the underlying valve with a fibroblastic, neutrophil and monocyte component. This inflammatory reaction does not, however, reach the organism ensconced in the thrombus. The organisms deepest in the thrombus often cease to divide, but remain viable, while bacterial division continues in the more superficial zones of the thrombus. The implication is that prolonged treatment with bactericidal drugs is needed to sterilise the vegetations. The characteristics of the human disease indicate that the principles laid down in animal models also apply to human bacterial endocarditis (Bayliss et al. 1983).

Bacteraemia is not uncommon, both in normal humans and in a wide range of disease states. Bacteria are however rapidly cleared by the reticuloendothelial cells of the liver and spleen. Brushing the teeth, dental irrigation and even chewing hard food invokes bacteraemia in subjects with chronic gingivitis. Dental work increases the frequency of bacteraemia (Freeman and Hall 1996). Any operation on the gastrointestinal or genitourinary tract will invoke transient bacteraemia with faecal streptococci or Gram-negative coliforms. Any direct intravenous instrumentation carries a risk of bacteraemia. Acute pyogenic infections such as staphylococcal boils or pneumococcal pneumonia release bacteria into the circulation. With the plethora of episodes of bacteraemia, it is surprising that infective endocarditis is not more common. This has led to the view that the organisms which commonly cause human endocarditis at the relatively low numbers circulating must have some special characteristics. The explanation is thought to lie in the ability of some organisms to bind to fibronectin or platelet surfaces. Staphylococci and streptococci may bind by receptor mediated mechanisms, but can also produce dextrin-like compounds and ribitol or lipoteichoic acid which readily bind to fibronectin. Organisms which have the ability to break down proteins in the valve also have enhanced capacity to divide once infection has started. Agglutinating antibodies produced to some streptococci also appear to enhance the capacity of the organism to initiate infection on valves.

A wide range of valve abnormalities and all prosthetic valves predispose to human infective endocarditis. The risk is greatest with valve lesions which involve high pressure jets. Thus, mitral regurgitation has a higher risk than mitral valve stenosis. The increased risk with regurgitant jets is due to direct damage to the endocardium by the local haemodynamic forces. It is however becoming more frequent for bacterial infection to become established on valves which are not clinically regarded as being previously abnormal. In this context, however, age-related changes in normal subjects predispose to small platelet thrombi on valve cusps at the lines and points of cusp apposition. Lambl's excrescences are probably the result of organisation of such thrombi. Small thrombi not of a size either to be of any haemodynamic consequence or be barely visible, may act as a nidus on which highly virulent organisms such as Staphylococcus aureus can establish infection.

CLASSIFICATION OF INFECTIVE ENDOCARDITIS

The old classification of infective endocarditis dating back to Osler into acute, subacute or chronic was based on the course of the untreated disease. This course was largely determined by the nature of the organism itself, and today it is more usual to qualify the term endocarditis by the organism, i.e. staphylococcal endocarditis, Streptococcus viridans endocarditis etc. The pattern of the disease has changed radically throughout this century (Uwaydah and Weinberg 1965). In considering infective endocarditis today, distinction is also made between infection on the natural native valve (NVE) and prosthetic valve endocarditis (PVE). The latter is often subdivided into early (< 60 days after insertion) and late. Infective endocarditis in intravenous drug users (IVDU) is another group in which the characteristics of the disease and the range of organisms responsible is somewhat different than that found in infective endocarditis on native valves acquired outside hospital.

Clinical diagnosis of infective endocarditis

The clinical diagnosis of infective endocarditis is often not easy – reviews of clinical practice continue to emphasise that the diagnosis is often made very late.

It has been suggested that the diagnosis can be considered as firmly based when there are two major criteria, one major and three minor criteria or five minor criteria (Table 4.1). Such criteria are not absolute, and merely give an indication of the probability of the disease being infective endocarditis, ranging from definite through probable to possible. The criteria are, however, useful (Durack et al. 1994) in comparing the treatment and survival of cases between different hospitals.

Prior to the antibiotic era, bacterial endocarditis was inevitably fatal. The mortality remains surprisingly high at 15–30%, with late diagnosis being a major factor in

Table 4.1

Criteria for the diagnosis of infective endocarditis in life

Major	Minor
Two positive blood cultures	Systemic emboli
	Fever
Vegetation on valve by ECHO	Ostler's nodes
	Splinter haemorrhages
Cusp destruction on ECHO	Known predisposing cause
	IV Drug user
	Abnormal valve
	Prosthetic valve *in situ*
	Positive serology for organism known to cause infective endocarditis
	Progressive valve dysfunction

Table 4.2

Conditions predisposing to infective endocarditis

Structural cardiac abnormalities
Aortic valve stenosis regurgitation – any cause
Bicuspid aortic valves (particularly with mild regurgitation)
Mitral regurgitation – rheumatic or cusp prolapse (floppy valve)
Mitral stenosis – (only if concomitant regurgitation is present)
Senile mitral ring calcification
Hypertrophic cardiomyopathy – (subaortic mitral impact lesion infection)
Ventricular septal defect
Patent ductus arteriosus
Coarctation of aorta
Atrial septal defect (primum only due to the abnormal mitral valve)

Prostheses and catheters
All mechanical valves
Tissue valves with stents – (very rare on non-stented human homograft valves)
Indwelling vascular catheters
Pacing wires (intravenous)
Shunts for hydrocephalus

Factors causing bacteraemia
Dental work and gingivitis
Drug abuse (intravenous)
Urogenital/gastrointestinal operations
Septic focus elsewhere

Factors altering immunity
Immunosuppression
Diabetes
Chronic alcoholism

the failure to achieve better results (Skehan *et al.* 1988; Bayliss *et al.* 1983; Malquarti *et al.* 1984). A joint survey by the British Cardiac Society and the Royal College of Physicians in 1986 suggested that in Britain, with a population around 50 million, there were 577 patients diagnosed as having infectious endocarditis. This is highly likely to be an underestimate depending as it did on voluntary registration of cases by physicians. In these patients 137 had known pre-existing chronic valve disease thought to be rheumatic in origin (23.7%), 108 had congenital valve lesions (18.8%), 145 (25.3%) had non-rheumatic valve disease including bicuspid aortic valves and mitral valve prolapse, while the remaining 183 (31.9%) had no known predisposing cause. While such data are of some interest, the pattern of the disease is changing rapidly. Rheumatic valve disease is declining and mitral valve prolapse and bicuspid aortic valves are relatively increasing as predisposing causes. Prosthetic valves and the rising incidence of drug abuse are also altering the disease pattern (Uwaydah and Weinberg 1965; Sanabria *et al.* 1990). The factors predisposing to infective endocarditis are shown in Table 4.2. The changing pattern is emphasised by the fact that it is estimated that today one third of all episodes of infective endocarditis occur on prosthetic valves (Freeman and Hall 1996).

MICROORGANISMS CAUSING INFECTIVE ENDOCARDITIS

The relative proportions of cases of infective endocarditis due to different organisms has changed over the last few decades due to the decline in chronic rheumatic valve disease, the use of antibiotics, the advent of cardiac surgery making patients with prosthetic valves common in the community, better oral hygiene in the community, the increasing numbers of intravenous drug abusers and the use of immunosuppressive treatment. It is rarely possible to compare series which describe the types of organisms causing infective endocarditis because the case selection and case mix differs. This variation in case type will influence the relative proportions of different organisms.

Streptococci of the types found in the mouth (viridans group) have declined as a cause of native valve endocarditis (NVE) but are still responsible for about a third to a half of cases acquired in the community. The organisms enter the blood from the mouth, and classically followed dental work. Today only about 15% of cases give a history of recent visits to the dentist (Wahl 1994; Guntheroth *et al.* 1984). The majority of cases are, however, associated with poor oral hygiene and gingivitis. Bacterial taxonomy undergoes very regular changes, but even allowing for this factor the range of β-haemolytic streptococci causing infective endocarditis is far wider than that found 30 years ago. *Streptococcus viridans* is an extremely broad group of organisms producing α-haemolysis on culture media containing red cells. Common strains causing infective endocarditis include *S. sanguis*, *S. mitis*, *S. milleri*, *S. mutans* and *S. salivarius*. The disease produced is subacute in its clinical type. Enterococci are now responsible for many cases of infective endocarditis and are more frequent than the viridans group in infections which follow urogenital and gastrointestinal tract operations, and in drug addicts. Various types of faecal enterococci are recognised as the major contributors. These include *S. bovis*, *S. faecalis*, *S. faecium* and *S. durans*. *S. bovis* infection is particularly linked to gastrointestinal operations for carcinoma of the colon and ulcerative colitis. In general, the disease is subacute in type but on occasion more acute with septic emboli.

Gram-negative bacteria account for up to 10% of cases in some series and are relatively more common in drug addicts and on prosthetic valves (Cohen *et al.* 1980). *Staphylococcus aureus* is the archetypal organism capable of settling on functionally normal valves and causes extensive tissue damage and septic emboli. Most series of native valve endocarditis now record it to be almost as common as *S. viridans* endocarditis.

A vast range of other organisms, many reported as single cases or small series, can cause infective endocarditis. Identification of such a diverse range of organisms requires a wide range of culture conditions (Bouvet and Acar 1984). Pneumococci and gonococci more than 30 years ago accounted for 10% of cases of infective endocarditis. Their frequency has been reduced to sporadic single cases (Wolff *et al.* 1984; Wall *et al.* 1989). Fungal endocarditis is rare as a primary event on native valves with *Candida*, *Histoplasmosis* and *Aspergillus* being the commonest – very large vegetations are produced. The diagnosis is often made first on the histology of vegetations when a valve is surgically replaced (Walsh *et al.* 1980).

Rickettsia and *Chlamydia* (Etienne *et al.* 1992) cause a very chronic and slowly progressive endocarditis with an insidious onset as does *Brucella* endocarditis (Perry *et al.* 1969). Infection usually occurs on previously abnormal valves, and diagnosis is made in life by serology rather than isolation. Cases seen by pathologists have usually been treated extensively and identification by morphology of the organism on the vegetation is very rarely successful. All these very chronic forms of infective endocarditis give rise to valves which are impossible, by morphology alone, to distinguish from treated *S. viridans* endocarditis or even end-stage rheumatic disease. A history of working with agricultural animals is present in more than 50% of cases of *Brucella* and Q fever endocarditis.

Prosthetic valve endocarditis

On prosthetic valves the predominant organisms are staphylococci. Coagulase-positive staphylococci often cause early endocarditis, while coagulase-negative groups of the albus (epidermidis) type often cause the later infections. Albus type organisms are probably introduced at the time of surgery, but produce a slowly progressive disease. It is however now apparent that some coagulase negative staphylococci such as *S. lugdunensis* can behave in a very much more acute and aggressive manner (Vandenesch *et al.* 1993; Etienne and

Eykyn 1990). Native valve infection is now also recognised to occur (Caputo *et al.* 1987).

Infective endocarditis in intravenous drug abusers

Infections in intravenous drug abusers are marked by the diversity and unique nature of the organisms (Banks *et al.* 1973; Dismukes *et al.* 1973; Dressler and Roberts 1989). *Staphylococcus aureus* endocarditis, fungal and enterococcal infections are all common. Fungal isolates make up 10% of cases in drug addicts. *Pseudomonas aeruginosa* and *P. cepacia* make up close to 50% of isolates in drug addicts, being almost unique to this group of patients (Reisberg 1979; Cohen *et al.* 1980).

CULTURE-NEGATIVE ENDOCARDITIS

The cornerstone to the successful clinical treatment of infective endocarditis is the isolation of the organism from blood cultures with antibiotic therapy being specifically matched to the sensitivity of the organism. In up to 10% of cases of infective endocarditis diagnosed by clinical criteria, however, blood cultures remain sterile (Tunkel and Kaye 1993). In many of these cases the clinical diagnosis seems certain and the term culture-negative infective endocarditis is used. The explanation usually lies in either the previous use of sub-therapeutic antibiotic therapy, or that the organism has growth requirements which make its growth *in vitro* difficult. In infections with streptococci of the viridans groups, a single dose of penicillin will prevent blood cultures being positive for some weeks while not sterilising the vegetations. A wide range of organisms are, however, difficult to grow in culture. Some have very complex growth factor requirements, or need culturing under anaerobic conditions. Others such as *Coxiella burnetti*, *Chlamydia* and *Bartonella* are best initially diagnosed by serological investigation.

PATHOLOGY OF INFECTIVE ENDOCARDITIS

Morphology of vegetations

Infective endocarditis is caused by microorganisms with a wide range of capabilities for tissue destruction. These characteristics determine to some extent the morphology of vegetations and of the adjacent heart valves. Marked destructive lesions are noted in *Staph. aureus* infections (Fig. 4.2), whereas less marked destruction plus a reparative fibrotic response are features of streptococci of the viridans group (Fig. 4.3). The vegetations of infective endocarditis are most commonly found attached to the atrial aspect of atrioventricular valves and to the ventricular aspect of semi-lunar valves.

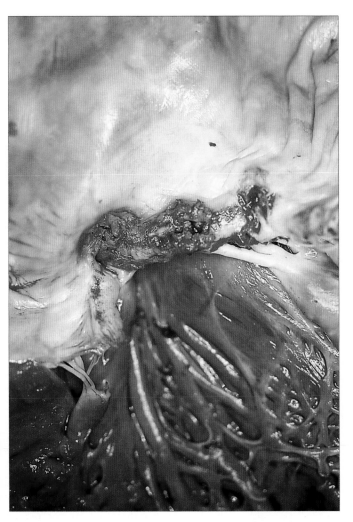

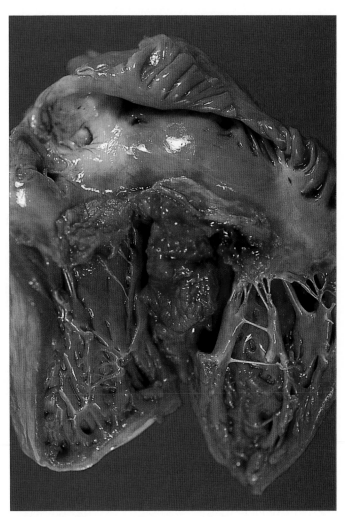

Figure 4.3
Bacterial endocarditis – mitral valve. Flat rather diffuse yellow/red vegetations are present on the anterior cusp of the mitral valve along the apposition line. The chordae are very thickened even remote from the vegetations and the left atrium was dilated, indicative of prior rheumatic mitral regurgitation. *Streptococcus viridans* isolated.

Figure 4.4
Bacterial endocarditis – tricuspid valve. The patient was known to inject drugs intravenously. There is a very large vegetation which has destroyed the anterior cusp and hangs into the ventricular outflow tract. Vegetations have also spread onto the posterior cusp.

Usually they are related to the line of cusp apposition, but if large they may involve adjacent parts of a cusp or leaflet or contiguous structures, e.g. chordae tendineae or the sinus of Valsalva. Vegetations may also arise at a site away from the cusps themselves at the site where a regurgitant jet hits the endocardium.

Vegetations vary in size with fungal infections being the largest. Vegetations can vary in colour from red (Fig. 4.4) through pink to yellow (Fig. 4.5) and may be soft and friable or firm. They can have a smooth surface, but more often are irregular and granular. Vegetations may be single or multiple. Unless the diagnosis has been made live from blood cultures, any vegetation found at autopsy should be swabbed in sterile conditions in order that the organism can be identified. Attempts to isolate the organism, even from the vegetations directly after antibiotic therapy has been instituted, however, are not always successful. Histological examination of a vegetation to identify the presence of an organism should indicate the use of a Gram stain, periodic acid-

Schiff stain, (PAS) and a Gomori methenamine silver stain. This combination is useful because it not only delineates fungal spores and hyphae, but may also reveal cocci that have lost their staining characteristics to the Gram stain, possibly as a result of an alteration in their surface coating or because they are dead. Other stains, e.g. Giemsa or Machiavello's stains, may be used for particular infections such as Rickettsial endocarditis. Electron microscopy may be useful if one is looking for microorganisms that lack a cell wall and which do not stain by the Gram stain method. The vegetations of infective endocarditis will calcify with time after antibiotic treatment, and care must be taken to distinguish between the irregularly sized granules of calcium occurring in vegetations and viable bacteria. Fresh vegetations consist of platelets and fibrin with polymorphonuclear leukocytes abundant in some areas. Colonies of bacteria or fungal hyphae may be demonstrated both at the edge of and within the thrombus and it is often striking that organisms are embedded in relatively acellular fibrin (Fig. 4.6). If the infection is

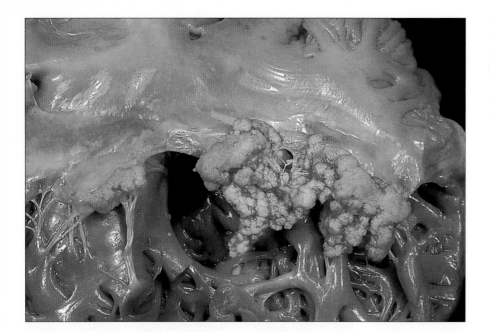

Figure 4.5
Fungal endocarditis – tricuspid valve. The anterior cusp of the tricuspid valve is covered by polyploid yellow vegetations. The patient was a known drug addict. Candida present in vegetation and in blood cultures.

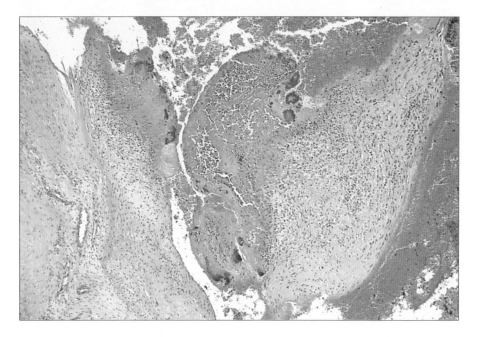

Figure 4.6
Bacterial endocarditis – histology. The valve cusp is covered by a mass of eosinophilic thrombus within which colonies of basophilic bacteria can be seen. These colonies are within the deeper layers of the thrombus. The valve cusp is heavily inflamed, but the inflammatory cells are not in contact with the bacterial colonies. Focal collections of polymorphs are present in the thrombus but these also are not in direct contact with the bacterial colonies (H&E ×56).

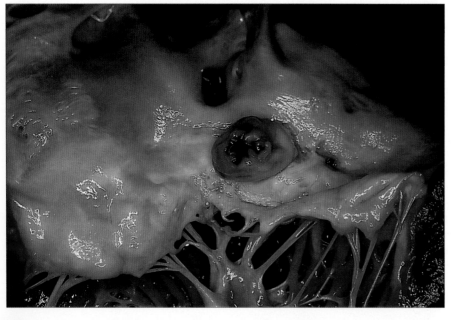

Figure 4.7
Mitral valve – infective endocarditis. There is a mass of vegetations on the atrial aspect with a central hole. The anterior cusp of the mitral valve is dome-shaped indicating a pre-existing floppy valve.

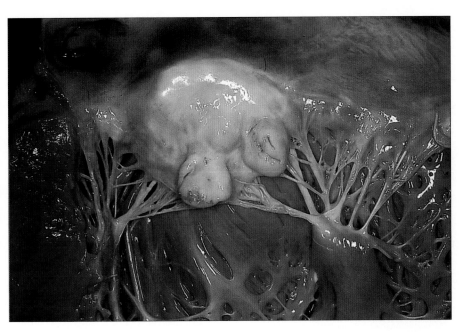

Figure 4.8
Mitral cusp aneurysms – post-infective endocarditis. The anterior cusp shows two aneurysmal bulges at the site of previous vegetations.

chronic, the vegetation often shows a varying degree of organisation and vascularisation from the underlying cusp and/or calcification. Chronic inflammatory cells and a few giant cells may occur. Numerous giant cells are a feature of vegetations in patients with endocarditis caused by *Coxiella burnetii* (Q fever).

With organisms which cause tissue necrosis, the edge of the cusp may ulcerate, chordae rupture or the body of the cusp perforate (Figs 4.2, 4.7) leading to incompetence of the valve. An infection may also weaken the fibrosa of a cusp, leading to aneurysm formation. Aortic valve aneurysms are usually small, 2–3 mm, and bulge towards the left ventricle. Mitral valve aneurysms usually affect the anterior leaflet (Fig. 4.8); they may be 3–4 mm in diameter, have a smooth surface or have a larger orifice and wind sock-like appearance, with the sock being conical and several centimetres long. A cusp aneurysm may cause symptoms of regurgitation immediately or become apparent by echocardiography several months after the infection has been treated. Occasionally a perforation can be found at the apex of such aneurysms.

Vegetations may spread from the aortic valve cusps to the endocardial surface of the interventricular septum or the ventricular face of the anterior cusp of the mitral valve. This spread often follows a regurgitant jet. Vegetations on the posterior mitral valve cusp may extend up onto the endocardium of the left atrium along the line of a regurgitant jet (Fig. 4.9). It may be impossible to tell if infection has spread from the aortic to the mitral valve or vice versa if both valves are involved. Kissing lesions on contiguous surfaces of cusps are another example of local spread.

The vegetations in bacterial endocarditis usually are polyploid masses adherent to the surface of the cusp. In some circumstances, however, infection also extends inward into the paravalvar tissues (Arnett and Roberts 1976). Organisms which have a considerable capacity for tissue destruction such as *Staphylococcus aureus*

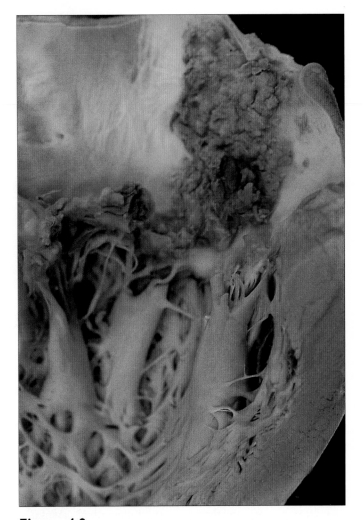

Figure 4.9
Mitral valve – bacterial endocarditis. The mitral valve posterior cusp is covered by vegetations which have spread up the posterior wall of the left atrium following the line of a regurgitant jet.

may extend outward from the aortic sinuses (Byrd *et al.* 1990). In the left coronary sinus an abscess forms in the tissues of the adjacent atrial septum and causes atrioventricular block by destroying the AV node. A

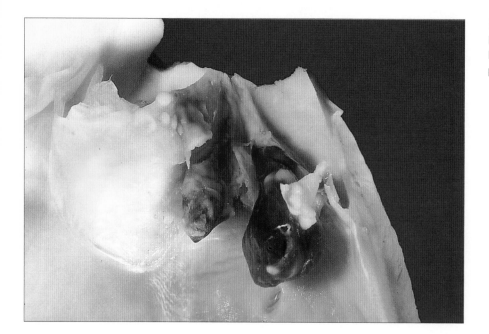

Figure 4.10
Pulmonary valve – bacterial endocarditis. A large mass of vegetations hangs from the pulmonary valve cusps.

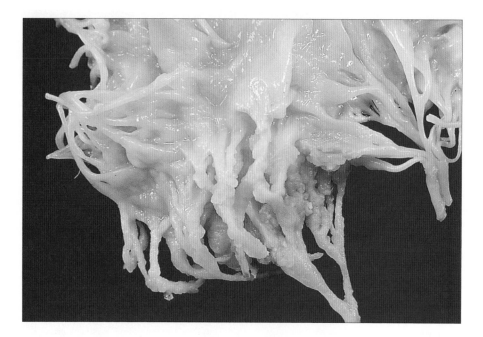

Figure 4.11
Anterior cusp of mitral valve – post-bacterial endocarditis. There are multiple ruptures of the chordae which are covered by many small calcified nodules representing the sites of previous vegetations.

fistula may develop between the aortic root and the right atrium. More rarely an aneurysm may develop in the right coronary sinus with an associated acute pericarditis and risk of haemopericardium following rupture. Native mitral valve endocarditis rarely causes perivalvar abscesses; the exception is when infection enters the ring of annular calcification seen in older subjects. Annular abscesses are however a very common feature of prosthetic valve endocarditis (Watana-kunakorn 1979). Infection spreads in the tissue plane surrounding the sewing ring of the valve and rapidly forms an abscess which extends around the whole annulus. The sutures often dehisce and the prosthetic valve tears away from the annulus over part or all of its circumference leading to paraprosthetic leaks.

Bacterial endocarditis on prosthetic valves usually begins on the valve ring and in addition to spreading

into the adjacent tissues also causes vegetations which protrude out into the valve orifice. Such vegetations may become large enough to cause obstruction or to hinder the mechanical movement of the valve causing regurgitation. Obstruction to flow by vegetations is far more common in prosthetic valves compared to native valves where the predominant haemodynamic abnormality is regurgitation.

Tricuspid valve endocarditis usually has large pedunculated vegetations attached to the anterior cusp (Figs 4.4, 4.5) which can be seen clearly to impinge on the outflow tract of the right ventricle by echocardiography in life. Tricuspid endocarditis is a complication of either intravenous drug abuse (Dressler and Roberts 1989) or an indwelling intravascular catheter or pacing wire left *in situ* across the valve for some time. Pulmonary valve endocarditis is very rare (Fig. 4.10) and also is related

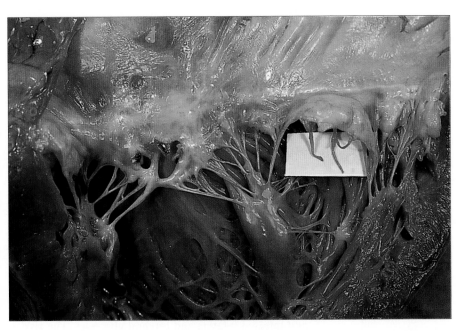

Figure 4.12
Mitral valve – post-bacterial endocarditis. The anterior cusp of the mitral valve shows central perforations typical of healed bacterial endocarditis. The posterior cusp is dome-shaped and has ruptured chordae not associated with any evidence of previous vegetations indicating this was a floppy valve with regurgitations which became infected.

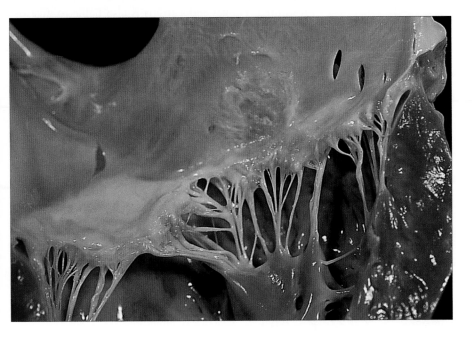

Figure 4.13
Mitral regurgitation – post-bacterial endocarditis. The chordae to the anterior cusp of the mitral valve at its medial end appears relatively normal. The chordae to the medial end of the cusp are thickened and there is some irregular thickening of the cusp. On the posterior wall of the left atrium there is an area of endocardial thickening where a regurgitant jet hit the wall. It is not possible to be dogmatic on whether this valve had prior mild rheumatic disease before developing S. *viridans* endocarditis.

to the passage of catheters across the valve and drug abuse.

Healing processes in infective endocarditis

The result of the healing process after successful treatment of bacterial endocarditis depends on the amount of cusp damage that occurred in the acute phase. Vegetations are reduced in size and organise from the base leading to fibrous nodules which often calcify (Fig. 4.11). Considerable cusp fibrosis occurs leading to thickening and retraction of the cusps. Infections which destroyed cusp tissue in the acute phase leave irregular indentations along the free edge of the cusp, chordal ruptures or smooth edged perforations through the body of the cusp (Figs 4.12). It is often impossible in the late stage of healed bacterial endocarditis to recognise if the valve was normal or abnormal before infection occurred (Fig. 4.13). Some conditions such as bicuspid aortic valves or floppy mitral valves can be still identified (Fig. 4.12) but fibrosis and vascularisation of the valve cusps are processes common to both healed infective endocarditis and chronic rheumatic disease. In the absence of a previous known clinical history of a valve murmur it is therefore often impossible to be certain whether mild chronic rheumatic disease was a predisposing factor.

Complications of endocarditis

The mortality of treated bacterial endocarditis remains high largely because of a number of serious complications (Table 4.3).

Cardiac failure

Cardiac failure is due to both the rapid increase in volume overloading of the left ventricle as mitral or

Table 4.3

Potentially fatal complications of infective endocarditis

Complication	Mechanism
Cardiac failure	Acute left ventricular volume overload due to aortic/mitral regurgitation Embolic/immune myocardial damage
Cerebral infarction Myocardial infarction Gastrointestinal infarction	Non-infected emboli
Abscesses (including brain)	Infected emboli (septic emboli)
Cerebral haemorrhage	Infectious arteritis (mycotic aneurysms)
Renal failure	Renal emboli Immune mediated glomerulonephritis
Pulmonary infarction	Emboli from tricuspid valve endocarditis

aortic regurgitation increases, coupled with a degree of myocardial damage due to intramyocardial microemboli and/or an immune mediated coronary vasculitis. The left ventricle tolerates sudden increases in volume overload very poorly as perforations develop in the aortic or mitral cusps and mitral chordae rupture. In aortic valve endocarditis, small platelet microemboli into the myocardium are common and cause microscopic foci of ischaemic necrosis. With virulent organisms the microemboli can lead to local microabscess formation. In many cases of bacterial endocarditis there is a low grade vasculitis in small intramyocardial vessels with an infiltrate of chronic inflammatory cells around veins.

Emboli and aneurysms

A major cause of mortality in infective endocarditis is cerebral or myocardial infarction due to emboli from the vegetations (Fig. 4.14). Virulent organisms such as *Staphylococcus aureus* lead to septic emboli (Fig. 4.14) and infected infarcts and cerebral abscesses. The risk of cerebral emboli persists for some weeks after therapy is instituted. Fungal endocarditis is also liable to give rise to emboli which contain numerous hyphae and occlude

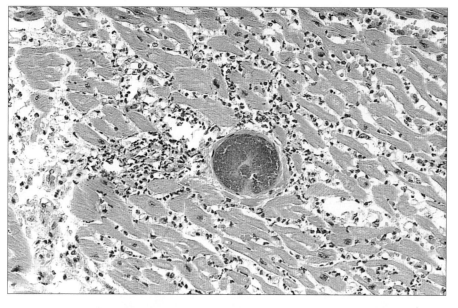

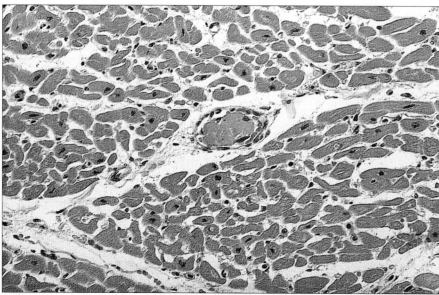

Figure 4.14 a,b

Coronary emboli – bacterial endocarditis. (a) A small intramyocardial artery is occluded by a mass of thrombus which appears deeply basophilic, due to huge numbers of *Staphylococcus aureus* organisms. The adjacent myocardium shows infarction with a pronounced polymorph infiltrate (H&E ×35). (b) In contrast to 18a, this case of infective endocarditis shows emboli in a small intramyocardial artery which do not contain organisms.

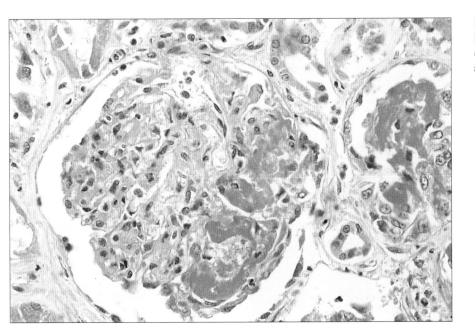

Figure 4.15
Focal glomerulonephritis – bacterial endocarditis. The glomerulus shows a focal area of brightly eosinophilic necrosis (H&E ×140).

medium-sized arteries such as the coronaries and cerebral vessels.

The term mycotic aneurysm is often applied to the intracerebral aneurysms which develop in infective endocarditis and closely resemble ordinary berry aneurysms. Subarachnoid and intracerebral haemorrhage follows their rupture. More rarely large saccular aneurysms occur in the aorta or its major branches in bacterial endocarditis. The term mycotic aneurysm covers aneurysms with a number of different pathogenetic mechanisms. In all, the media is locally destroyed. It may be as the direct effect of an inflammatory response to viable organisms in the embolus itself or due to an immune mediated antigen/antibody complex deposition without viable organisms being present. Emboli lodging in a vasa vasorum causing medial infarction in the aortic wall leading to a saccular aneurysm is another postulated mechanism.

Renal complications of bacterial endocarditis

The incidence of renal infarction at autopsy varies from 38–91%. Tiny emboli can produce local infarcts in glomeruli, but most focal glomerular lesions (Fig. 4.15) are thought to be the result of immune complex deposition. Focal segmental glomerulonephritis is the most common and is seen particularly in streptococcal viridans group infections where there is antibody excess giving rise to large complexes. Usually, less than half the glomeruli seen on sections are affected, but renal failure may develop if the majority are affected. Lesions may be of varying age. At the beginning an area of necrosis is seen accompanied by a polymorphonuclear leucocyte exudate, fibrin thrombi in adjacent capillaries and swelling and proliferation of both endothelial and mesangial cells. There may be adhesions between the glomerulus and Bowman's capsule. Occasionally, crescents may develop. At electron microscopy, electron-dense deposits may or may not be demonstrable in the mesangium.

An acute diffuse endocapilliary glomerulonephritis is caused by an antigen excess with small complexes. Electron-dense deposits are usually seen between the endothelial cells and the glomerular basement membrane and within the mesangium. This form of glomerular disease can usually be encountered in virulent infections such as *Staphylococcus aureus* and lead to renal failure. On immunofluorescence, the most consistent finding is a diffuse, granular staining of C3 along capillary walls. In addition, immunoglobulin deposits, primarily IgG, are often present in the capillary walls, mesangium or both. Fibrinogen is also seen in crescents and areas of necrosis. Specific antigens related to infecting organism may also be located in the glomeruli.

Immunological complications of infective endocarditis

The prolonged bacteraemia that occurs in infective endocarditis is accompanied by circulating immune complexes (Bayer and Theofilopolos 1990). Using a binding assay to Clq almost 100% of patients with infective endocarditis will have such circulating complexes (Garnier *et al.* 1984) which are thought to cause arthritis, purpuric skin rashes and subungual splinter haemorrhages. Skin biopsies show vasculitis with deposition of immunoglobulins in the vessel wall (Kauffman *et al.* 1981) and bacterial antigens are present in the tissues and in the complexes (Inhan *et al.* 1982). Ostler's nodes are subcutaneous tender lumps up to 4 cm across and are thought to be due to small emboli with a superadded vasculitic component.

NON-BACTERIAL THROMBOTIC ENDOCARDITIS (NBTE)

In non-bacterial thrombotic endocarditis (NBTE) thrombotic vegetations that do not contain microorganisms

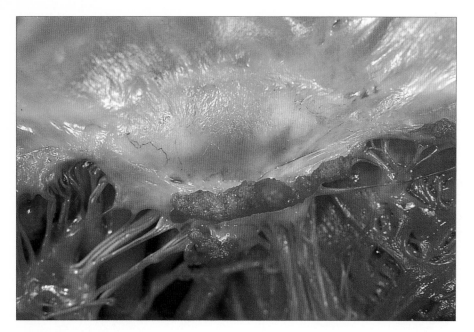

Figure 4.16
Non-bacterial thrombotic endocarditis – mitral valve. Red vegetations are distributed along the apposition lines of both the anterior and posterior cusps. The vegetations are however large and the clue to this being NBTE rather than infection is the even nature of the vegetations. Infected vegetations by this stage would have spread. Another clue is that the patient had terminal cancer.

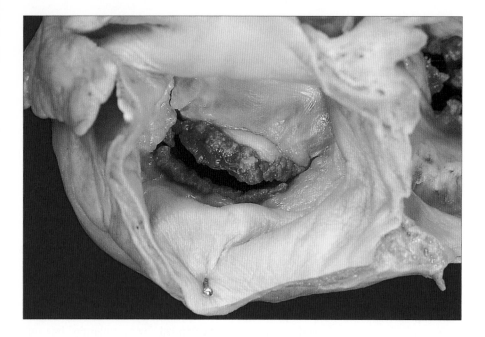

Figure 4.17
Non-bacterial thrombotic endocarditis – mitral valve. The vegetations are evenly distributed along the apposition line of the cusps. Terminal cancer patient.

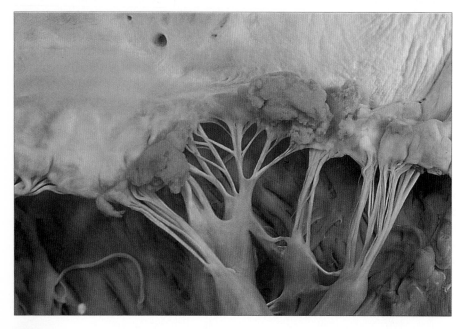

Figure 4.18
Non-bacterial thrombotic endocarditis – mitral valve. This is the form of NBTE in which the vegetations are large and polyploid rather than being arranged in an even manner on the apposition lines. Such thrombi are impossible to distinguish from infective endocarditis without histology and culture.

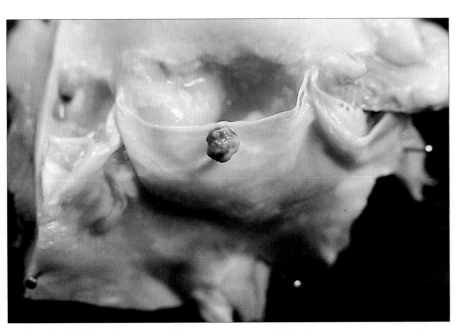

Figure 4.19
Non-bacterial thrombotic endocarditis – aortic valve. NBTE is less usual on the aortic valve than the mitral valve and the vegetations are smaller and attached to the nodulii Aranti of the cusp.

develop on heart valves. They are found in 1–2% of autopsies, are usually larger than the 1–2 mm diameter vegetations found, for example, in acute rheumatic fever and are most frequently attached at the line of closure. They are thought to have developed during the terminal phase of a patient's life (marantic vegetations) and are usually incidental findings. However, vegetations are present for some time prior to death and act as a source of bland thrombo-emboli that may cause clinical symptoms and signs. The incidence of visceral emboli in non-bacterial thrombotic endocarditis has been reported to be as high as 40% (Olney et al. 1979). Because non-bacterial thrombotic endocarditis is usually a condition found in terminally ill patients with widespread malignant disease, the clinical features suggesting emboli are often missed or ignored.

The macroscopic appearances are varied and there may be real difficulty in distinguishing these vegetations from infective endocarditis without histology (Figs 4.16–4.19). The vegetations may be smooth-surfaced and firmly attached, or become quite bulky, nodular and friable and spread over the adjacent surface of a cusp. 'Kissing' lesions affect adjacent sites on cusps. The aortic valve is most often affected singly, and is followed in frequency by the mitral and tricuspid valves. Multiple valve involvement may occur. Non-bacterial thrombotic endocarditis may occur at any age, but most commonly affects patients from the 40–80 years. There is an equal sex predilection. Histologically the vegetations consist of platelets admixed with fibrin and red blood cells. The adjacent valve may show little damage or contain some fibrin and a few leucocytes. Subsequent healing may occur with calcification. The vegetations of non-bacterial thrombotic endocarditis may become infected and the case transformed into infective endocarditis.

The exact pathogenesis of non-bacterial thrombotic endocarditis is not known, but is probably related to endothelial injury. Up to 50% occur in patients with hypercoagulable states such as disseminated intra-vascular coagulation (DIC) (Kim et al. 1977). The lesions follow stress-related oedema and swelling of the valve cusps. The thrombotic lesions can be seen frequently in patients with terminal malignant disease, especially with mucin producing adenocarcinomas of the lung, pancreas or colon. Occasionally the vegetations in malignant disease may contain tumour cells when examined histologically.

References

Arnett E, Roberts W. Valve ring abscess in acute infective endocarditis. Frequency, location and clues to clinical diagnosis from a study of 95 necropsy patients. *Circulation* 1976;54:140–5.

Baddour L, Christensen G, Lowrance J, Simpson W. Pathogenesis of experimental endocarditis. *Rev Infect Dis* 1989;11:452–63.

Banks T, Fletcher R, Ali N. Infective endocarditis in heroin addicts. *Am J Med* 1973;55:444–51.

Bayliss R, Clark C, Oakley C. Incidence, mortality and prevention of infective endocarditis. *J Roy Coll Phys* 1983;20:15.

Bayliss R, Clarke C, Oakley C, Sommerville W, Whitefield A, Young S. The microbiology and pathogenesis of infective endocarditis. *Br Heart J* 1983;50: 513–19.

Bayer AS, Theofilopoulos AN. Immunopathogenetic aspects of infective endocarditis. *Chest* 1990;97: 204–12.

Bouvet AM, Acar J. New bacteriological aspects of infective endocarditis. *Eur Heart J* 1984;5:45–8.

Byrd B, Shelton M, Wilson B, Schillig S. Infective perivalvular abscess of the aortic ring: Echocardiographic features and clinical course. *Am J Cardiol* 1990;66:102–5.

Caputo GM, Archer GL, Calderwood SB, DiNubile MJ, Karchmer AW. Native valve endocarditis due to coagulase-negative staphylococci. Clinical and microbiologic features. *Am J Med* 1987;**83**:619–25.

Cohen P, Maguire J, Weinstein L. Infective endocarditis caused by gram-negative bacteria: a review of the literature 1945–1977. *Prog Cardiovasc Dis* 1980;**22**: 205–42.

Dismukes W, Karcher A, Buckley M. Prosthetic valve endocarditis: analysis of 38 cases. *Circulation* 1973;**48**:365–77.

Dressler F, Roberts W. Infective endocarditis in opiate addicts: analysis of 80 cases studied at necropsy. *Am J Cardiol* 1989;**63**:1240–57.

Durack DT, Lukes AS, Bright DK. New criteria for diagnosis of infective endocarditis utilization of specific echocardiographic findings. *Am J Med* 1994; **96**:200–9.

Etienne J, Eykyn SJ. Increase in native valve endocarditis caused by coagulase-negative staphylococci: an Anglo–French clinical and microbiological study. *Br Heart J* 1990;**64**:381–4.

Etienne J, Ory D, Thouvenot D, Ed F *et al*. Chlamydial endocarditis: a report of ten cases. *Eur Heart J* 1992; **13**:1422–6.

Freeman R, Hall RJC. Infective endocarditis in *Diseases of the Heart*, 2nd edn. Julian DG, Camm AJ, Fox KM, Hall RJC, Poole-Wilson PA (eds). London: WB Saunders, 1996.

Garnier J, Touraine J, Colon S. Immunology of infective endocarditis. *Eur Heart J* 1984;**5**:3–10.

Guntheroth WG. How important are dental procedures as a cause of infective endocarditis? *Am J Cardiol* 1984;**54**:797–801.

Inhan R, Redecha P, Knechtle S, Schnede S, van de Rijn I, Christian C. Identification of bacterial antigens in circulating immune complexes of infective endocarditis. *J Clin Invest* 1982;**70**:271–80.

Karchmer A. Prosthetic valve endocarditis: a continuing challenge for infection control. *J Hosp Infect* 1991;**18**:355–66.

Kauffman R, Thompson J, Valentin R, Daha M, van Es L. The clinical implications and pathogenetic significance of circulating immune complexes in infective endocarditis. *Am J Med* 1981;**71**:17–25.

Kim H, Suzuki M, Lie J, Titus J. Non-bacterial thrombotic endocarditis (NBTE) and disseminated intravascular coagulation (DIC). *Arch Pathol Lab Med* 1977;**101**:65–8.

Malquarti V, Saradarian W, Etienne J, Milon H, Delahaye J. Prognosis of native valve infective endocarditis: a review of 253 cases. *Eur Heart J* 1984;**5**:11–20.

Olney B, Schattenberg T, Campbell J, Okazaki H, Lie J. The consequences of the inconsequential: marantic (non-bacterial thrombotic) endocarditis. *Am Heart J* 1979;**98**:513–22.

Perry T, Belter L. Brucellosis and heart disease. 11 fatal brucellosis: A review of the literature and a report of new cases. *Am J Pathol* 1969;**36**:673.

Tunkel A, Kaye D. Endocarditis with negative blood cultures. *N Engl J Med* 1993;**326**:1215–6.

Sanabria T, Alpert J, Goldberg R, Pape L, Cheeseman S. Increasing frequency of staphylococcal infective endocarditis. *Arch Intern Med* 1990;**150**:1305–9.

Skehan J, Murray M, Mills P. Infective endocarditis: incidence and mortality in the North East Thames region. *Br Heart J* 1988;**59**:62–8.

Reisberg B. Infective endocarditis in the narcotic addict. *Prog Cardiovasc Dis* 1979;**22**:193–204.

Uwaydah M, Weinberg A. Bacterial endocarditis: a changing pattern. *N Engl J Med* 1965;**273**:1231–5.

Vandenesch F, Etienne J, Reverdy ME, Eykyn SJ. Endocarditis due to *Staphylococcus lugdunensis*: report of 11 cases and review. *Clin Inf Dis* 1993; **17**:871–6.

Wahl MJ. Myths of dental-induced endocarditis. *Arch Int Med* 1994;**154**:137–44.

Wall T, Peyton R, Corey G. Gonococcal endocarditis: A new look at an old disease. *Medicine (Baltimore)* 1989;**68**:375–80.

Walsh T, Hutchins G, Bulkley B, Mendelsohn G. Fungal infections of the heart: analysis of 51 autopsy cases. *Am J Cardiol* 1980;**45**:357–66.

Watanakunakorn C. Prosthetic valve endocarditis. *Prog Cardiovasc Dis* 1979;**22**:181–92.

Wolff M, Regnier B, Witchitz S, Gibert C, Amoudry C, Vachon F. Pneumococcal endocarditis. *Eur Heart J* 1984;**5**:77–80.

FIVE

CARDIAC HYPERTROPHY, MYOCARDITIS AND CARDIOMYOPATHY

CARDIAC HYPERTROPHY

MACROSCOPIC CHANGES

The myocardium responds to an increased workload by hypertrophy. Initially this is a physiological response aimed at maintaining normal cardiac function – it may ultimately not be able to achieve this aim and cardiac failure supervenes.

Physiological, and what is known as pathological, hypertrophy are a continuum. For practical purposes hypertrophy is clinically regarded as pathological when it is fixed, i.e. does not regress when the stimulus is removed. This is best seen in athletes; in many when they cease to train to high levels of fitness the heart size declines. In some, however, the heart remains large and hypertrophy has become pathological. In life echocardiography is now an established means of estimating left ventricular mass (LV) and well-established formulae relate the values to body size. Clinicians are well aware that a major determinant of LV mass is body size.

Myocardial hypertrophy has a number of components. The first component is an increase in right or left ventricular muscle mass. This is achieved by an increase in mean myocyte volume, i.e. individual myocytes are larger. A second component of hypertrophy is a shape change (remodelling) in the ventricle (Grossman *et al.* 1975). In pressure-determined hypertrophy, the ventricular wall becomes thicker but the cavity is not affected (Fig. 5.1) or even becomes smaller. This response is seen in hypertension and aortic valve stenosis. In this form of hypertrophy the mean myocyte diameter rises, i.e. the myocytes add sarcomeric material laterally and the myocardial cells are thicker not longer. In volume determined hypertrophy (aortic regurgitation, left to right shunts) the myocytes increase in volume by increasing their length by adding additional sarcomeres (Gerdes *et al.* 1992). The cavity of the left ventricle increases in size and the wall thickness remains the same (Fig. 5.2)

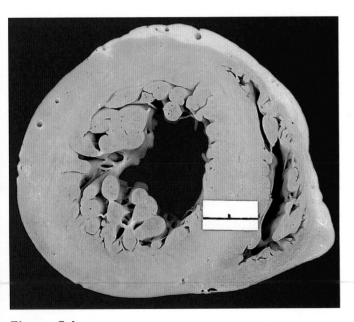

Figure 5.1
Pressure load hypertrophy – aortic valve stenosis. Short axis slices of the left and right ventricles at the mid septal level allow the left ventricular cavity size to be compared to the wall thickness. Here in aortic valve stenosis the LV wall is thickened symmetrically measuring over 2 cm. The cavity diameter is normal.

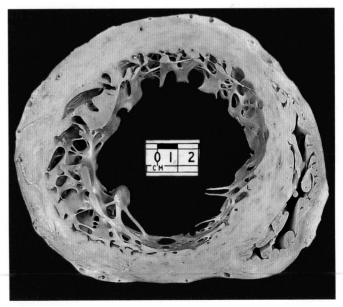

Figure 5.2
Volume load hypertrophy – aortic regurgitation. The total heart weight was increased to the same degree as in Fig. 5.1. The LV cavity diameter is greatly increased, but the LV wall thickness is unchanged.

or is even reduced. The increase in chamber volume and decrease in wall thickness is also associated with slippage of myocytes relative to each other (Anversa *et al.* 1991) and alterations in the supporting collagenous matrix of the ventricular myocardium. This change is probably irreversible. Pathologists can, by examining the macroscopic morphology in short axis transverse cuts of the ventricles, determine something about function in life. The right ventricular changes in response to volume and pressure overload are similar to those in the left ventricle.

Microscopic changes in myocardial hypertrophy

The most striking change observed in myocytes is nuclear enlargement. Numerous studies have shown that with increasing age even in normal hearts there is a rise in the DNA content of individual nuclei with a proportion of the cells becoming 4n or 8n (Vliegen *et al.* 1991; Van der Laarse *et al.* 1989). With hypertrophy this shift is accentuated and the myocytes become 4, 8, 16 or even 32n. The increase in individual myocyte volume is less easy to appreciate by routine histology. In pressure–load hypertrophy, myocyte width rises by up to twice normal, and this can be measured. It is however difficult to measure myocyte length, because the intercalated discs are not easy to see in routine stains and the state of contraction of the myocytes after death varies widely. The reduction in myocyte width that occurs with volume overload is sometimes known as attenuation.

It is still debatable as to whether myocyte division can occur in adult mammalian hearts (Anversa *et al.* 1991; Olivetti *et al.* 1994). DNA synthesis occurs with the development of polyploidy and immunohistochemistry staining is often positive for proliferating cell nuclear antigen (PCNA) in myocyte nuclei when hypertrophy is developing (Mann *et al.* 1992). The cell cycle is however arrested between S and G2 or G2 and M. One group (Anversa *et al.* 1991) has however always argued that total myocyte cell numbers are increased in hypertrophy. The number of binucleated myocytes increases in hypertrophy (Shozawa *et al.* 1990). A major objection to this view is that mitotic figures in myocytes are not seen in human hearts after the immediate neonatal period. Mitotic figures can, however, occur in young rodent hearts. The quantification of total myocyte numbers in the whole human heart is fraught with technical difficulty and the consensus is still that myocytes do not divide. Studies of apoptosis in myocytes in ageing mammalian hearts suggest, however, that some myocyte loss is occurring. To balance this and remain neutral in myocyte numbers, Anversa calculates that in a 2 cm^2 section of human myocardium there would be five mitotic figures in myocytes. This does not appear to be so, with the implication that with increasing age myocyte numbers, like that of neurones, fall. In myocardial hypertrophy there is no doubt that interstitial connective tissue cells undergo hyperplasia and contribute to a rise in total DNA content of the myocardium. The amount of interstitial collagen also rises as hypertrophy develops.

Methods of assessing cardiac hypertrophy

Many pathologists make a subjective assessment of cardiac hypertrophy and use the words mild, moderate and severe. These opinions should be reinforced by objective measurements, particularly if the opinion has to be defended in clinical meetings or in a legal opinion.

The objective of any measurement of hypertrophy is to determine either left or right ventricular muscle mass and to predict to what extent the weights are abnormal. Left ventricular mass in normal individuals is determined by at least three variables, the total body size, the degree of physical exercise that the individual takes, and the level of blood pressure. There is also increasing evidence of genetic influences on LV mass.

It is easy at autopsy to measure total fresh heart weight after washing blood clot out of the chambers. This measurement is a valid predictor of LV hypertrophy providing allowance is made for body size. It is valid for the simple reason that there is a linear relation between isolated LV mass and total heart weight. In contrast, the right ventricular mass makes up a minor component of total heart weight and therefore does not bear a direct relation to it; total heart weight therefore cannot give any useful information on the presence or absence of right ventricular hypertrophy.

Published pathology data on the normal range of total heart weight in relation to body size are not entirely consistent. One thing is however certain – it is of little use to record in an autopsy report total heart weight unless it can be related to body weight.

In a very simple formula Hudson (1965) stated that total heart weight in males was 0.45% of total body weight and 0.4% in females. Thus an 80 kg male has a heart weight of 360 g, but there is no allowance for physical activity and no indication of the confidence limits of such a weight. In a large series of in-hospital deaths (Kitzman *et al.* 1988) gave rather higher figures (Table 5.1). In this method, an 80 kg male has a mean heart weight of 349 g with the 95% upper limit of the population being 461 g.

Another approach (Hangartner *et al.* 1985) has been to use a regression equation determined by the relation of total heart weight to body weight in deaths outside hospital (Tables 5.2, 5.3). In this method an 80 kg male has a predicted normal weight of 3.44 × 80 + 144 = 419 g. To be reasonably certain that hypertrophy was present, at autopsy in a normally active person the heart weight would need to be more than 20% above the predicted value. If the subject undertook regular running, the heart weight could only be regarded as abnormal if it was 30% above the predicted value.

Table 5.1

Predicted total fixed heart weight for body weight in males and females (95% confidence upper limit in brackets).

	Body weights (kg)	Fixed total heart weight (g)
Female	30	196 (287)
	40	221 (324)
	50	243 (356)
	60	262 (385)
	70	280 (411)
	80	297 (435)
	90	312 (457)
	100	326 (478)
	110	339 (497)
Male	40	247 (325)
	50	276 (364)
	60	302 (399)
	70	327 (431)
	80	349 (461)
	90	371 (489)
	100	391 (516)
	110	410 (541)

Kitzman *et al.* 1988

Table 5.2

Prediction equations for fixed heart weight (FHW), isolated LV weight (LVW) and isolated right ventricular weight (RVW) for normal males and females in grams (x = body weight in kg). Fixed total heart weight exceeds that of the fresh heart by approximately 5%. Isolated ventricular weights are always based on fixed material.

	Males	Females
FHW	3.44x + 144	4.45x + 85.4
LVW	1.80x + 43.5	1.18x + 64.3
RVW	0.64x + 12.8	0.39x + 19.9

Hangartner *et al.* 1985

Table 5.3

Predicted total fixed heart weight, isolated left ventricular (LVW) and isolated right ventricular weight (RVW) for body weight in males and females.

	Body weight (kg)	FHW (g)	LVW (g)	RVW (g)
Females	30	219	99	32
	40	264	110	36
	50	308	122	39
	60	352	131	43
	70	396	145	47
Males	40	282	116	38
	50	336	134	45
	60	350	152	51
	70	385	170	58
	80	419	188	64
	90	454	206	70
	100	488	223	77

Hangartner *et al.* 1985

Table 5.4

Prediction of normal heart weight.

Body weight (kg)	Male 1.	2.	3.	Female 1.	2.	3.
30	135	247	213 (282)	120	219	196 (287)
40	180	282	247 (325)	160	264	216 (317)
50	225	316	276 (364)	200	308	243 (356)
60	270	350	302 (399)	240	352	262 (385)
70	315	385	327 (431)	280	396	282 (411)
80	360	419	349 (461)	320	441	297 (435)
90	405	454	371 (489)	360	485	312 (457)
100	450	488	391 (516)	400	525	326 (478)

1. Hudson 1965
2. Hangartner *et al.* 1985
3. Kitzman *et al.* 1988

The three approaches are compared in Table 5.4. That of Hudson should be considered obsolete, since it makes no allowance for individual variability. Many mortuaries do not have the facility to weigh bodies, but in hospital deaths the notes will contain this information. The correlation of heart weight to body height is far less precise, but should be recorded if weighing is impossible. The published series do not contain appreciable numbers of females in the upper weight ranges and in the event of a 100 kg female being encountered, the male data will have to be used. The published series in Table 5.4 are not entirely consistent with each other.

Normality of heart size in both males and females of body mass over 80 kg is not clear cut. What is certain however, is that the frequency of cardiac hypertrophy in such subjects is overestimated by many pathologists who adopt arbitrary upper limits of, for example, 400 g. The Kitzman figures are valuable in that they give 95% confidence limits showing that a heart of 500 g in a male of 100 kg body weight is still within the normal range of 95% of a population.

A more accurate measurement of ventricular mass can be made by weighing each ventricle separately after removing the atria and epicardial fat in the fixed heart. The interventricular septum is regarded as an integral part of the left ventricle. This technique described by Fulton *et al.* (1952) is the only reliable method of measuring right ventricular hypertrophy, particularly in the presence of left ventricular hypertrophy. The technique is really used to give a firm indication of the presence of right ventricular hypertrophy and thus uses a single rather high upper limit figure.

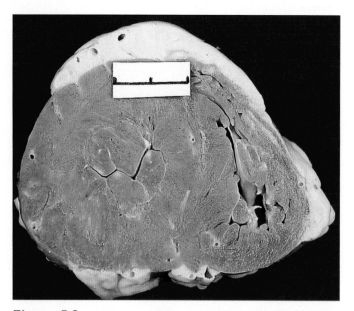

Figure 5.3
Myocardial rigor. This heart was totally within the normal limits of heart size for body size and there was no history of hypertension or valve disease. Myocardial histology was normal. The LV cavity is obliterated and the LV wall thickness therefore high. This phenomenon of rigor is referred to as a stone heart by surgeons who encounter it in subjects after cardiac bypass or in resuscitation attempts after cardiac arrest. Its pathophysiology is uncertain.

The normal values for the Fulton technique are:

1. An isolated right ventricular weight less than 65 g.
2. An isolated left ventricular weight of less than 190 g.
3. A left to right weight ratio of 2.3–3.3.

The Fulton technique requires the heart to be fixed; it takes at least 10 minutes and the specimen is destroyed. These facts mean the method is relatively little used.

The ease with which left or right ventricular wall thickness can be measured has beguiled pathologists into believing it can accurately measure hypertrophy. When isolated left ventricular mass is taken as the gold standard, left ventricular wall thickness has no predictive power for detecting hypertrophy. The same applies to the right ventricle. The reason for this is that chamber size is a second variable controlling wall thickness. The problem can be highlighted by comparing aortic stenosis with regurgitation (Figs 5.1, 5.2). Each valve abnormality can produce very heavy left ventricles; in aortic stenosis the wall thickness may be 1.8–2.0 cm, in aortic regurgitation 1.0–1.2 cm. Complex methods of measuring LV muscle volume as a surrogate for mass from the surface area of a series of transverse ventricular slices have been tried but are too complex for routine use. Some hearts, normal as judged by the absence of any history of cardiac disease and a normal LV weight for body size, develop myocardial rigor as an agonal phenomenon. At autopsy the chamber size is very small and the wall up to 2 cm thick (Fig. 5.3), but this does not indicate hypertrophy. The phenomenon appears to be particularly common in elderly subjects.

Another method of assessing hypertrophy is myocyte diameter. This can be measured by taking the diameter of the myocyte at the nuclear level. At least 100 randomly selected myocytes have to be measured to obtain reliable figures. Normal right ventricular myocytes have a diameter up to 14 μm and left ventricular myocytes 18 μm. In pressure–load hypertrophy, large diameters are obtained and give some indication of the degree of abnormality. In aortic regurgitation the diameters are low and uninformative. Myocyte length can only be measured by good quality electron microscopy in hearts fixed at known cavity pressure. This precludes accurate routine studies in human material.

HEART FAILURE

The term heart failure can be used in many different ways. There have however been major advances in the clinical understanding of 'heart failure' and pathologists will need to become more exact in their word usage. A modern working definition of heart failure is that of a clinical syndrome caused by an abnormality of the myocardium in which there are characteristic haemodynamic, renal, neural and hormonal responses (Poole-Wilson 1996). The clinical syndromes are:

1. acute heart failure in which there is the sudden onset of pulmonary oedema;
2. circulatory collapse in which there is a sudden onset of poor peripheral perfusion including hypotension and oliguria;
3. chronic heart failure (Table 5.5).

Circulatory collapse, when due to a failure of myocardial contractile function, is also known as cardiogenic shock. This is to distinguish it from peripheral circulatory failure due to profound vasodilation, caused by, for example, endotoxaemia. Pathologists should try to use the three terms in a credible clinical context. The term acute heart failure, for example, is inappropriate for a subject who is in good health, dies very suddenly,

Table 5.5
Syndromes of heart failure.

Syndrome	Clinical and pathological features
Acute heart failure	Sudden dyspnoea and pulmonary oedema. Left-sided cardiac disease
Circulatory collapse	Hypotension, oliguria, poor peripheral circulation, cold blue extremities.
(a) Cardiogenic	(a) Acute left ventricular disease, usually infarction

(b) Peripheral
   – Blood loss
   – Gram-negative septicaemia
	(b) No cardiac muscle disease

Chronic heart failure	Dyspnoea, poor exercise tolerance Peripheral oedema Cardiac disease or chronic lung disease

and does not have pulmonary oedema at autopsy. The latter usually indicates acute left ventricular heart failure but will also occur in some cases of extra-cardiac peripheral circulatory collapse, for example, in endotoxaemia where the pulmonary vascular bed is affected in the same way as the peripheral resistance vessels. In effect this is the first step toward an adult respiratory distress lung. Chronic heart failure is, in essence, a failure of the left ventricle to provide enough blood flow to satisfy the needs of the body relative to demands such as exercise. On exercise in subjects with chronic heart failure, the blood pressure falls and the reflex renal and humoral responses are exactly the same as those which follow haemorrhage. In this situation they are beneficial, but in chronic heart failure they lead to neurohumoral phenomena, which are in large part responsible for the clinical symptoms and signs.

Secondary responses to chronic heart failure

The principal changes occur in the myocardium itself, in the peripheral circulation and in the skeletal muscles.

The myocardium in heart failure

In chronic heart failure the myocardium undergoes hypertrophy. This hypertrophy reflects the increased demand on the ventricular myocardium. The great majority of cases have biventricular hypertrophy, but in certain circumstances one ventricle alone is involved. The best example of univentricular involvement is the right ventricle in pure mitral stenosis where the left ventricle remains small being protected by low filling pressures.

The hypertrophic response in the myocardium is an attempt to normalise cardiac function and may initially be successful. It is however followed by a further decline in function and the onset of heart failure. There are no morphological correlates that will tell the pathologist using light microscopy that the borderline between hypertrophy and failure has been crossed. Changes in phenotypic expression by myocytes, structural changes and functional changes do occur, but are probably secondary to failure rather than its cause (Table 5.6). A

Table 5.6
Myocardial changes in hypertrophy/failure.

Structural
Changes in myocyte shape/arrangement
Myofibrillary reduction in myocyte
Interstitial fibrosis
Permanent change in LV shape

Phenotypic expression
Change in isoforms of troponin T, myosin light chain
Reduction β Adrenergic receptors on myocyte

Functional
Reduced contractile protein response to calcium
Reduced uptake of calcium ions by sarcoplasmic reticulum

spiral of failure inducing changes which further depress function is likely.

A major change in the myocardium in hypertrophy/failure is the increase in interstitial fibrosis (Huysman et al. 1989). Interstitial fibrous tissue is usually defined as a material stained red by the Van Gieson or Sirius red methods. By surface area in histological sections, it makes up about 5% of the myocardium. The majority of the collagen is type III with about 15% being type I and a very minor component type IV collagen on the surface of the myocytes. In hypertrophy an increase in the number of interstitial fibroblastic cells occurs and the concentration of collagen rises. The surface area proportion of the myocardium staining as collagen may reach 25% in severe hypertrophy, and is distributed both as coarse strands and a more diffuse fine interstitial fibrosis. As hypertrophy increases, a point is reached when hyperplasia of the interstitial cells and collagen production becomes disproportionate to the increase in myocyte mass. At its extreme, in hearts weighing over 750 g, all the subsequent increase in mass may be collagen. The degree of interstitial fibrosis is significantly greater in pressure-overload hypertrophy such as aortic valve stenosis or hypertension than in volume-overload such as aortic regurgitation. Studies which compare the amounts of interstitial fibrosis in the myocardium with the degree of functional disability in the subject show that there is a direct correlation of increasing fibrosis with declining myocardial function. The degree of inter-subject and inter-cause variation, however, is so great that a pathologist cannot look at a myocardial section and categorically say that chronic heart failure was present.

The most widely used methods of measuring myocardial fibrosis is by surface area in sections stained to differentiate myocytes from collagen. The simplest method is to use a visual observer point-counting system, or a quantifying microscope which measures collagen as a percentage of the total field. These methods are easily introduced into any laboratory which should establish their own normal range for the method and stain they adopt. Sirius red stains rather more collagen than the Van Gieson method. The interstitial spaces contain components other than collagen, and an alternative method is to measure the surface area of the section occupied by myocytes and consider the rest as the percentage occupied by interstitial tissue. This will give higher values than for collagen alone. All methods based on histological sections will be subject to some subjective bias and are dependent on rigid discipline in selecting fields by a random method. Biochemical analysis in which hydroxyproline concentrations are measured after digesting the tissues with cyanogen bromide are less subject to bias, but are time-consuming. The data are expressed as the amount of hydroxyproline per gram wet weight of the myocardium.

The mechanisms by which fibrosis develops in myocardial hypertrophy are just beginning to be understood. There is evidence that altered mechanical forces on the myocardium will induce an increase in mRNA for

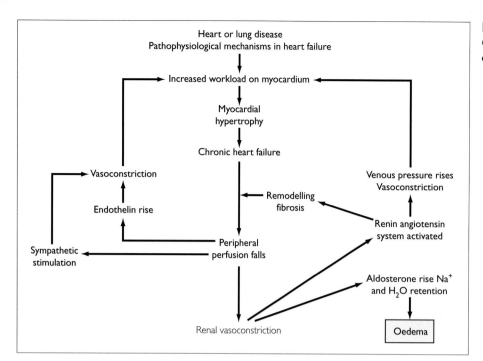

Figure 5.4
Consequences of a decline in cardiac output.

collagen (Komuro *et al.* 1990). Any myocyte death would invoke interstitial fibrosis. It is becoming clear that in very thick-walled left ventricles the subendocardial myocytes are subject to hypoxia and cell death occurs which would trigger fibrous repair. Finally, a number of neurohormonal factors which are activated in heart failure have direct stimulatory effects on myocardial interstitial cells – these include angiotensin II and growth hormone (Weber and Brilla 1991).

Another morphological change associated with cardiac failure is a reduction in the density of myofibrils within the myocyte. As with fibrosis, there is a good statistical link to poor LV function (Zimmer *et al.* 1992), but individual variation is considerable and the change is probably a late result of heart failure rather than its cause.

Neurohormonal responses in heart failure

A decline in cardiac output triggers a series of neuro-humoral responses (Fig. 5.4) which, while they to some extent increase blood pressure and cardiac output, do so at the cost of other effects which often lead to symptoms. In patients with heart failure who are at rest, plasma noradrenalin and adrenalin are raised, the renin angiotensin system is enhanced and endothelin levels increased. All these factors tend to increase peripheral vasoconstriction. Increased secretion of atrial natriuretic factor (Saito *et al.* 1989) induces natriuresis. The clinical signs of chronic heart failure, including raised central venous pressure and peripheral oedema are due to the kidneys retaining salt and water.

Skeletal muscle changes in heart failure

Skeletal muscle weakness and fatigue are a second component in addition to dyspnoea in limiting exercise capacity in subjects with chronic heart failure. Considerable loss of muscle bulk may occur and in addition there are atrophic changes with muscle fibre loss and changes in the distribution of fibre types.

Progression in heart failure

Most patients with chronic heart failure will progress albeit at widely differing rates. Exercise capacity and ventricular dysfunction pass through mild, moderate to severe heart failure. The final event in subjects with chronic heart failure is now most commonly death due to a ventricular arrhythmia. The mechanisms of progression are varied. In some causes of heart failure such as ischaemic heart disease, further myocardial damage occurs often in an episodic manner. Three separate mechanisms may enter into spirals in which adaptive changes beget further ventricular dysfunction. These are neurohormonal responses which cause increased peripheral resistance leading to further elevation of wall stress on the myocardium, neurohormonal activation which leads to fluid retention and the changes in the myocardium including fibrosis which is in part mediated by angiotensin (Fig. 5.4).

A further view is now emerging that there is progressive loss of myocytes. In ischaemic heart disease this is well recognised, but loss of individual myocytes by apoptosis is now thought to be a feature of any cause of heart failure. Heart failure leads to the induction of nitric oxide synthetase both by myocytes and interstitial macrophages. TNFα production within the myocardium is also induced. The internal production of such factors both depresses myocardial function and may trigger apoptosis of myocytes (Narula *et al.* 1996).

THE CARDIOMYOPATHIES

Terminology

The term cardiomyopathy has undergone radical changes in the last 25 years. In 1982 the World Health Organization (WHO) recommended that the term

Table 5.7
Cardiomyopathy – heart muscle dysfunction due to a wide variety of causes.

Specific	Primary myocardial
Ischaemic	Dilated
Valvar	Hypertrophic
Hypertensive	Restrictive
Inflammatory (myocarditis)	Obliterative
Systemic disorders	ARV cardiomyopathy

Table 5.8
Acute non-specific myocarditis.

Morphological features
Myocyte necrosis (individual cells)
T-lymphocyte infiltrate

Clinical features
Sudden death
Acute onset CCF/arrhythmias
Fever
Acute pericarditis ±

Table 5.9
The Dallas Convention reporting system for biopsies in myocarditis.

First biopsy
1. Acute myocarditis
2. Pathologist uncertain – re-biopsy
3. No myocarditis – record fibrosis if present

Second biopsy
1. Continuing myocarditis
2. Resolving myocarditis
3. Healed myocarditis*

*Used only if an earlier biopsy showed acute myocarditis

should be used for myocardial dysfunction which was not the result of coronary artery disease, valve disease, hypertension or congenital shunts. The term cardiomyopathy implied that the functional abnormality lay within the myocardium itself.

A recent major revision of this definition has broadened the use of the word cardiomyopathy. The WHO (Richardson 1996) has now adopted the term specific cardiomyopathy to encompass the entities in Table 5.7. The primary cardiomyopathies (those unrelated to hypertension, ischaemic, valvular or inflammatory disease) fall into those in which there is a thick-walled left ventricle (hypertrophic); a dilated poorly-contracting ventricle in systole (dilated); and restrictive in which the left ventricle fails to relax, impeding filling from the left atrium. The classification thus remains predominantly functional. This system of classification remains imperfect, and as more knowledge is gained is likely to be replaced within 10 years by a system based on genetic and pathogenetic mechanisms.

The use of the word cardiomyopathy for the dilated left ventricle with poor contraction due, for example, to long-standing aortic regurgitation, is a radical departure from the 1982 WHO nomenclature. This change was partly enforced by the continued usage of words such as ischaemic cardiomyopathy by clinicians. However, the change is also a recognition that after a period of hypertrophy, functional changes occur in the myocardium which impair contraction and lead to heart failure. These become self-perpetuating, irrespective of the nature of the initial disease. An example is the recognition that in heart failure myocytes are induced to produce inducible nitric oxide synthetase (iNOS) and TNFα which in turn have a negative inotropic effect on the heart.

Inflammatory cardiomyopathy – acute myocarditis

The wide variation in the proportion of cardiac biopsies reported to show acute myocarditis in patients who had a sudden onset of cardiac arrhythmias and/or cardiac failure associated with fever has led to a reassessment of the morphological criteria for the diagnosis. A group of cardiovascular pathologists met in Dallas (McManus

and Kandolf 1991; Aretz 1987; Aretz *et al.* 1987) and defined acute myocarditis (Tables 5.8, 5.9) as a condition which must have myocyte death and an interstitial inflammatory cell infiltrate in which T-lymphocytes are predominant (Chow *et al.* 1989) (Figs 5.5–5.8). The implication is that the myocyte damage is due to the action of cytotoxic lymphocytes. Myocyte death inevitably means that there is also an interstitial macrophage infiltrate. This constellation of features goes under the name of acute non-specific myocarditis.

In patients who die after some days of cardiac failure, the left ventricle may be dilated and the cut surface of the myocardium show marked variation in colour, but in cases which present as sudden death the heart may be macroscopically close to normal. Pericarditis may or may not be present. Acute myocarditis is *not* a diagnosis which can be accurately made, or excluded, without histology. In fatal cases the histology is striking and diffuse, being found in the myocardium of all four chambers.

Pathogenesis of acute myocarditis

The human pathology described above is mirrored by myocarditis in animals in which viral infection is known to be the cause (McManus *et al.* 1993). The best examples are the Coxsackie group of viruses in mice and papovavirus infection in the dog. The implication is that viruses are the likely cause of human acute myocarditis. Potentially, cardiotoxic viruses fall into two groups. In one, myocarditis is an inconstant feature

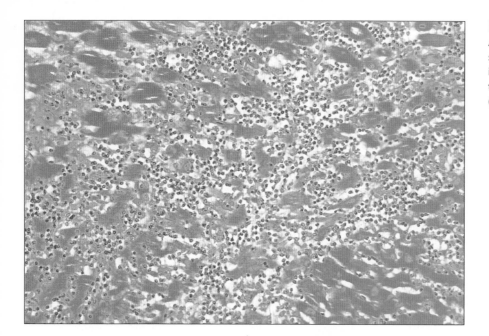

Figure 5.5
Acute non-specific myocarditis. The section shows the intense interstitial lymphocytic inflammatory cell infiltrate between the myocytes. Sudden death in an adult (H&E ×35).

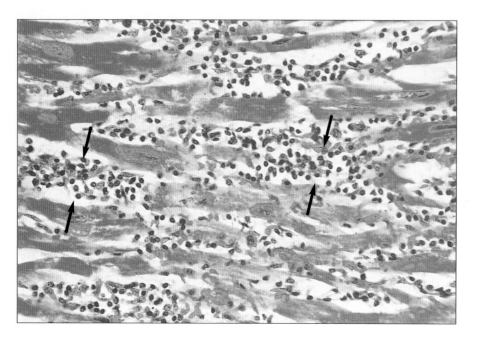

Figure 5.6
Acute non-specific myocarditis. There is an intense interstitial chronic inflammatory cell infiltrate between individual myocytes. Some myocytes have been lost, their position being recognised as areas in which there is a gap filled with lymphocytes and histiocytes (arrows). Sudden death in an adult (H&E ×56).

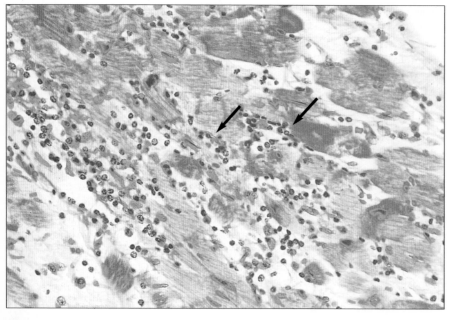

Figure 5.7
Acute non-specific myocarditis. This cardiac biopsy taken from a male of 32 with a short history of cardiac failure without obvious cause shows an easily recognisable interstitial infiltrate of lymphocytes which are adherent in places to the edge of myocytes. Focal loss of myocytes has occurred (arrows) (H&E ×87.5).

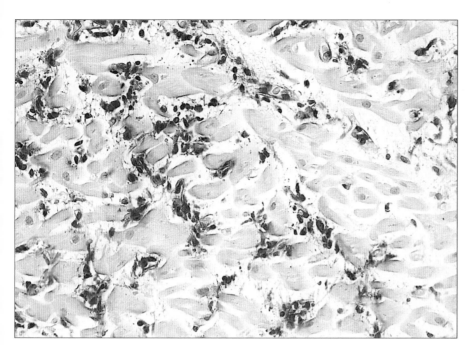

Figure 5.8
Acute non-specific myocarditis. The myocardium has been stained to show T-cells by immunohistochemistry (CD3) using alkaline phosphatase (red) as the marker (×56).

of a known systemic viral infection (Table 5.10). Acute myocarditis in this group is rarely the cause of death, but cardiac involvement can be detected by minor ECG changes. Practical problems exist for the pathologist in the rare fatal case in deciding the relative contribution made to death by pulmonary as distinct from myocardial involvement. This is particularly true in influenza and chicken pox where viral pneumonitis is common. Myocarditis should only be considered as an important contributor to the death if there are diffuse histological changes. Myocyte necrosis in the subendocardial areas associated with a neutrophil polymorph and not a T-cell infiltrate is cell death due to terminal hypoxia and must not be misinterpreted as a direct viral effect.

The second group of viruses are cardioselective and cause myocarditis either in isolation or in association with skeletal muscle involvement. In epidemics of fever and myalgia due to Coxsackie infection, about 5% of individuals develop acute pericarditis and in 1% pericarditis with myocarditis (Grist and Read 1992). In those who do develop myocarditis however, up to 50% die in the acute phase. In infants adenoviruses are now also recognised as an important cause of acute myocarditis. The conventional histological picture of acute myocarditis may occur in infants with a heavy T-cell infiltrate; there is however an equally common histological picture in which myocyte necrosis predominates and the infiltrate is macrophage in type. Evidence is emerging that such cases are due to adenovirus infection. Infants who survive a few days with either histological type of myocarditis may develop focal myocyte calcification and often have superimposed ischaemic myocardial necrosis due to terminal hypoperfusion. The different histological patterns in Coxsackie compared with adenovirus infection may indicate that, in the former, myocyte death is mediated by cytoxic T-cells targeted to virally infected cells, while in the latter it is direct viral lysis of myocytes.

Table 5.10
Viruses causing human myocarditis.

In isolation	As part of systemic disease	
Coxsackie B1–6	Polio	Rubella
Coxsackie A4, 9, 16	Influenza	Respiratory syncytial virus
ECHO 4, 9, 16, 22	Mumps	Vaccinia
Adenovirus	Measles	Varicella
	Herpes simplex	CMV
	Hepatitis A	EB virus

In cases of acute myocarditis, it is very rare to isolate viruses using tissue culture from the myocardium at autopsy. Rising IgM titres to the virus in the last few days of life are a more usual way of making the diagnosis. *In situ* hybridisation or polymerase chain reaction (PCR) for Coxsackie and adenovirus genomic material within the myocardium is far more sensitive and reported to be positive in a significant proportion of cases of human myocarditis at autopsy. Positive rates are highest in young infants and fall to about 30% in adults.

The histological diagnosis of fatal acute myocarditis at autopsy is not usually difficult. Biopsy interpretation is more difficult due to the less severe and focal nature of the disease in subjects who are still alive. The changes may not be present in every biopsy fragment. For this reason at least six separate biopsy fragments are needed to exclude acute myocarditis. It is also mandatory to use immunohistochemistry to demonstrate that T-lymphocytes are present. The density (absolute number per square millimetre of section) of T-lymphocytes needed to make the diagnosis of acute myocarditis is contentious (Tazelaar and Billingham 1986). It has now been set by some workers as low as a mean of three

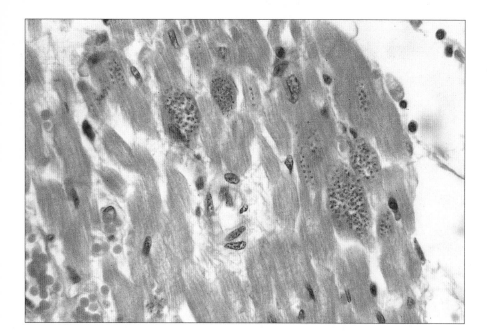

Figure 5.9
Toxoplasmosis of myocardium. Several myocytes in the myocardium contain toxoplasma organisms. Each myocyte is a so-called pseudocyst. From a child with a congenital immune system deficiency (H&E ×56).

per × 40 high-power field (Kuhl *et al.* 1996). It should be emphasised that this is a mean figure for randomly selected fields throughout the whole biopsy. The number of fields which need to be counted to achieve a reliable mean will vary depending on how evenly the cellular infiltrate is distributed. It is likely that there will continue to be considerable centre-to-centre variation over the diagnosis of acute myocarditis on biopsies. The increasing availability of reliable T-cell markers which will allow formalin fixed material to be studied by routine laboratories may alter the definitions based at the moment on frozen sections. The Dallas group strongly emphasised two negative points. Fibrosis indicates a long-standing process and excludes a diagnosis of acute myocarditis on biopsy. Second, the term 'resolving' or 'resolved acute myocarditis' must not be used unless there has been a previous biopsy showing acute myocarditis.

Prognosis of acute non-specific myocarditis

A large recent trial of the treatment of acute non-specific myocarditis diagnosed by biopsy (Mason *et al.* 1996) shows that the outcome may be recovery with good LV function, death from circulatory failure in the acute phase, or initial partial recovery followed by a progressive decline of LV function over some months or years to end in the clinical picture of chronic cardiac failure and dilated cardiomyopathy (see below). Immunosuppression or anti-viral therapy in the acute phase is not, so far, of proven benefit.

Non-viral causes of human acute myocarditis

The protozoan parasites *Trypanosoma cruzei* and *Toxoplasmosa gondii* (Fig. 5.9) both cause acute myocarditis. *T. cruzei* (Higuchi *et al.* 1987; Koberle 1968) which causes Chagas disease is confined to areas of South and Central America, since it needs the reduviid bug as a vector. In these geographic areas however, *T. cruzei* infection is the commonest cause of cardiac disease. Up to 3 months after infection a

proportion of cases (about 4%) develop acute myocarditis and/or meningoencephalitis and a proportion (up to 15%) die. In such cases the organism can be easily identified by histology, and this finding separates the condition from other causes of acute non-specific myocarditis. The more common cardiac complication, however, is long-term chronic heart failure developing after some years, often without a history of an acute infection. Such chronic cases macroscopically resemble dilated cardiomyopathy (see below). Histologically there are focal areas of myocarditis alongside areas of fibrous replacement. A very specific and striking feature is apical LV aneurysms. In chronic cases it is often very difficult to find the organism, although the percentage of cases which are positive can be increased by use of immunofluorescence. The paucity of the organism, despite the clear presence of progressive myocyte loss and replacement fibrosis, raises the possibility that the myocardial damage has an autoimmune component. In theory the organism needs a vector for transmission to man, and carrying out an autopsy on a chronic case of Chagas disease is no risk to the dissector, but similar precautions as those adopted for hepatitis autopsies are advisable.

Toxoplasmosis causes an acute non-specific myocarditis predominantly in infants. The organism can be seen within myocytes both in areas of inflammation and in apparently normal areas. Acute toxoplasma myocarditis in immune-competent subjects is very rare outside infants, but very many asymptomatic infections occur. In immune-compromised individuals, myocarditis occurs as infection is reactivated (Luft *et al.* 1986).

The spirochete *Borrelia burgdorferi* which is spread from deer or sheep to man by tick bites can cause myalgia, myocarditis, arthritis and acute lymphadenopathy (Lyme disease) (van der Linde *et al.* 1990). Clinically severe acute myocarditis is rare, but it does have a high incidence of atrioventricular heart block.

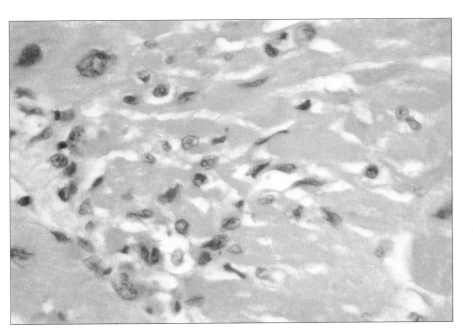

Figure 5.10
Myocardial lesions due to phaeochromocytoma. There is a focal area of myocyte death in which the stromal tissue has survived. In this area there is a range of inflammatory cells. Such focal necrosis is a ubiquitous response to a wide range of drugs and in particular those which have positive inotropic effects (H&E ×87.5).

The organisms can be demonstrated if special silver staining methods are used, but they can easily be missed. Serological studies however suggest that currently in the UK this organism is a very rare cause of acute myocarditis.

Toxic myocarditis

A number of drugs are directly toxic to myocytes in a cumulative dose related response (Billingham 1985; Buja *et al.* 1974). Focal myocyte death occurs and initiates a predominantly macrophage response. Drugs in this group include arsenic, emetine, fluorouracil and lithium. Many antidepressant drugs are also cardiotoxic, but at levels far in excess of the usual therapeutic range. Many drugs associated with inotropic effects including dopamine and noradrenalin in high dosage can cause small foci of necrosis of individual myocytes in which the stroma survives. A florid inflammatory response occurs with macrophages as the predominant cell. Identical myocardial changes occur with phaeochromocytomas (Fig. 5.10). The appearance of focal myocyte necrosis associated with a florid inflammatory response in both catecholamine and cocaine-mediated myocardial damage has led to the term 'myocarditis' being used. The predominant macrophage response and the presence of numerous contraction bands following cocaine abuse (Isner and Chokshi 1991), however, differ from viral myocarditis. Once focal myocardial necrosis has developed, sudden death can occur. In cocaine abuse the myocardial changes are also, in part, due to intense vasospasm both of epicardial and intramyocardial vessels. The small foci of necrosis heal by fibrosis, and if the damage continues a scarred myocardium is produced. If ventricular dilatation develops, a morphological picture arises which is indistinguishable from other causes of dilated cardiomyopathy.

Acute diphtheria is associated with an often fatal acute myocarditis. The histological picture is somewhat different from those described so far. Myocyte necrosis predominates and the cell response is largely macrophage/histiocytic. Necrosis is due to the direct action of the diphtheria toxin on the myocyte.

Hypersensitivity myocarditis

All of the forms of acute myocarditis described so far have acute myocyte death as an essential component, and it is this which produces the acute symptoms and often causes death. There are however cases, usually following drug therapy, in which there is an interstitial inflammatory infiltrate without any evidence of myocyte damage. The inflammatory cell infiltrate is often heaviest in the fibrous trabeculae of the myocardium and around blood vessels rather than related to myocytes. The infiltrate is often very pleomorphic with histiocytes, eosinophils and basophils. Small histiocytic giant cells also can occur.

Myocarditis and sudden death

When there is no other cause of sudden death and the inflammatory infiltrate is heavy and diffuse throughout the ventricular myocardium and is associated with myocyte damage, it is entirely reasonable to ascribe death to myocarditis. The diffuse infiltrate seen in drug hypersensitivity does seem occasionally to cause death. More problems in interpretation arise if the inflammatory infiltrate is focal and not associated with myocyte damage (Chapter 8). If blocks of myocardium are taken from hearts with other well-established causes of death, the frequency of finding one focus of interstitial inflammatory cells rises directly with the number of blocks examined. It does not seem logical to give a single focus of interstitial inflammatory cells, particularly if in the atria alone, as a sole cause of death.

Giant cell myocarditis

Several forms of myocarditis (Table 5.11) occur in which there is myocyte death and a diffuse inflammatory infiltrate with giant cells being present.

Table 5.11
Myocarditis with giant cells.

Idiopathic acute giant cell myocarditis
– in isolation
– in association with thymoma
–immune disorders
Sarcoidosis
Wegener's granulomatosis
Drug hypersensitivity
Acute rheumatic fever
Tuberculosis

In idiopathic giant cell myocarditis (Cooper *et al.* 1995) there is a short history of a very sudden onset of arrhythmias, often with left ventricular failure. The clinical history differs from that of acute non-specific myocarditis only in the very rapid onset and progression to death. The striking feature macroscopically at autopsy is of diffuse irregular linear or serpigenous yellow areas of necrosis in the myocardium. Histologically the areas of necrosis show widespread myocyte death with a dense pleomorphic inflammatory cell infiltrate, often containing numerous eosinophils. At the margins of the necrotic zones of myocardium there are striking giant cells (Figs 5.11, 5.12). These giant cells are within the sarcolemmal sheath of the original myocyte and in longitudinal sections the giant cells appear strap-like often with up to 30 nuclei. In other planes the giant cells appear round. The relation of the cells to the original sheath of the myocyte led to speculation that the giant cells were of myogenic origin but immunohistochemistry shows them to be of macrophage lineage (Davies *et al.* 1975; Theaker *et al.* 1985; Kodama *et al.* 1991). It is unknown why there is this unusual macrophage giant cell response, and a viral

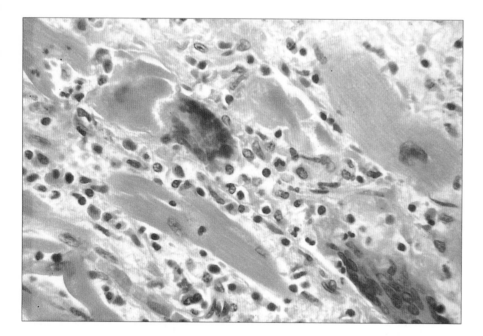

Figure 5.11
Idiopathic giant cell myocarditis. The section taken at the edge of an area of necrosis shows elongated strap-shaped giant cells. Numerous eosinophils are present. Autopsy specimen (H&E ×87.5).

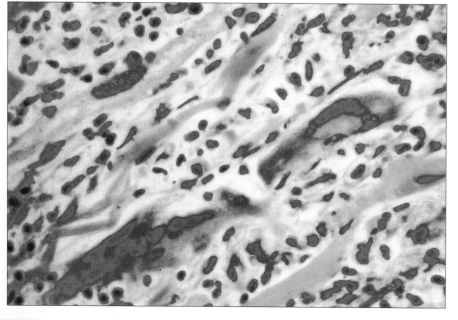

Figure 5.12
Idiopathic giant cell myocarditis. The section shows a giant cell associated with myocyte loss and a dense inflammatory interstitial infiltrate which contains lymphocytes, plasma cells and eosinophils. Biopsy specimen. Eight days sudden cardiac failure – died while awaiting urgent transplantation (H&E ×42).

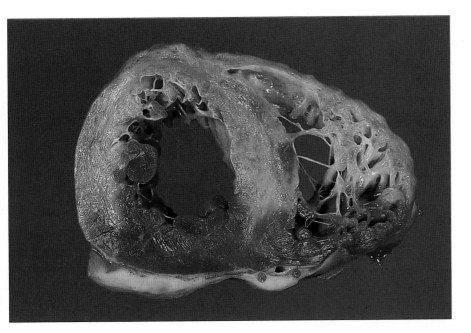

Figure 5.13
Sarcoid heart disease. The whole of the anterior wall of the left ventricle, much of the septum and the lateral wall in the mid-septal transverse plane shows the myocardium to be replaced by white fibrous tissue. This tissue on histology is made up of confluent giant cell granulomas (Explanted heart for cardiac sarcoid).

aetiology has not been shown. The rapid progression of this form of myocarditis is typical, but occasional less acute cases are now coming to transplantation. The diffuse involvement of the myocardium means that cardiac biopsy is a useful diagnostic procedure. The only facts known about the pathogenesis of idiopathic giant cell myocarditis are rare associations with organ-specific autoimmune disease, myasthenia gravis and thymomas (Burke *et al.* 1969).

Sarcoid heart disease

Sarcoid disease involving the heart produces a spectrum of morphological features (Valentine *et al.* 1987; Silverman *et al.* 1978; Fleming and Bailey 1981) (Table 5.12). The frequency with which systemic sarcoid involves the heart is reported as very variable and depends on how thorough a search is made for small cardiac granulomas. Symptomatic cardiac sarcoid is very frequently isolated with other organ involvement being trivial. The expanding regional masses of granulomas (Fig. 5.13) which are typical of acute cardiac sarcoid, are common in the septum and cause AV block and sudden death. Their rapid expansion leads to ECHO misdiagnosis as tumours. Expanding masses ultimately heal by fibrosis and lead to aneurysms (Fig. 5.14).

The histological features are those of sarcoid elsewhere, with discrete giant cell granulomas without central

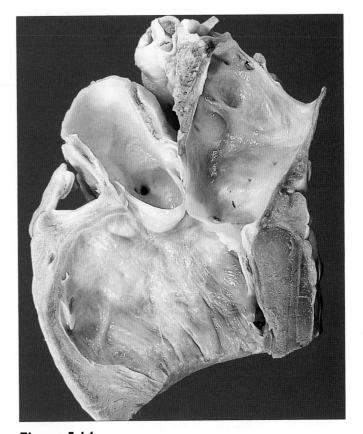

Figure 5.14
Myocardial sarcoid. The upper interventricular septum is the most common site for a mass of granulomas in cardiac sarcoid. With healing, the area thins to give an aneurysm of the upper interventricular septum.

caseation (Fig. 5.15). Eosinophils are not present in large numbers. Cardiac biopsy is only occasionally positive in myocardial sarcoid due to the regional nature of the ventricular involvement. When biopsy is positive (Fig. 5.16) the discrete round follicular granulomas distinguish sarcoid from giant cell myocarditis of the idiopathic type. While most cases of giant cell

Table 5.12
Morphological forms of cardiac sarcoid.

| Coincidental microscopic granulomas |
| Diffuse granulomas/fibrosis – restrictive cardiomyopathy |
| Regional expanding mass of granulomas |
| Regional scars |
| Regional LV aneurysm |

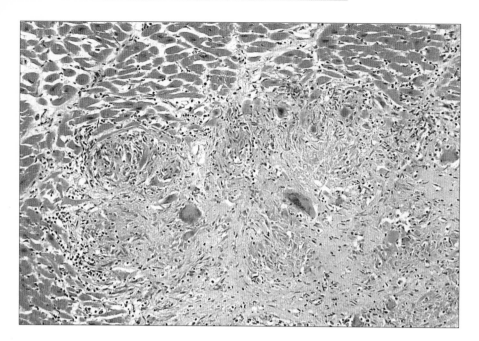

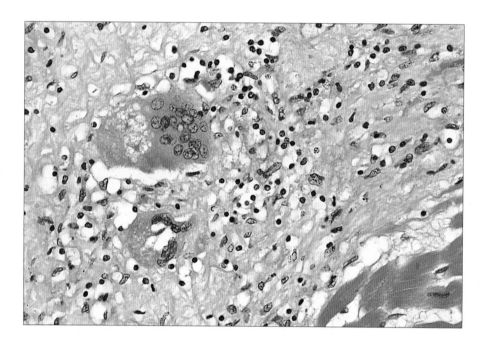

Figure 5.15 a,b
Myocardial sarcoid. This histology is taken from the edge of the white solid area of myocardium in Fig. 5.13. At this low power it is possible to see that the mass is built up of contiguous but still distinct round shaped giant cell granulomas (H&E ×56). In (b) at high power (×140) the granulomas are seen to have no necrosis and typical sarcoid giant cells.

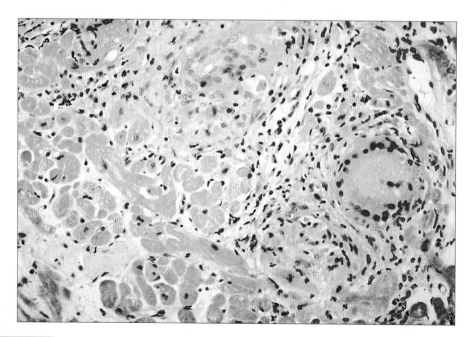

Figure 5.16
Myocardial sarcoid. An individual sarcoid granuloma from a cardiac biopsy. The biopsy granuloma is round and non-caseating (H&E ×140).

Table 5.13

Features of sarcoid contrasted to giant cell myocarditis.

Sarcoid	Giant cell myocarditis
Macroscopic	
Regional mass	Diffuse serpigenous
Regional scar	Yellow myocardial necrosis
Diffuse fibrosis	
Microscopic	
Follicular granulomas	Giant cells adjacent to necrosis
Necrosis absent	Eosinophilis abundant
Eosinophils scanty	No extra-cardiac granulomas
Extra-cardiac granulomas	

Table 5.14

Criteria for diagnosis of acute rheumatic fever.

Major
Carditis
– Pericarditis (audible rub)
– Myocarditis (long PR interval)
– Endocarditis (murmurs)
Polyarthritis
Sydenham's chorea
Erythema marginatum
Subcutaneous nodules
Minor
Fever, raised ESR, Raised C-reactive protein
Positive culture throat swab
Rising antistreptococcal antibodies (ASO titre)

myocarditis can be ascribed to either sarcoid or idiopathic giant cell myocarditis using the features listed in Table 5.13, there is some cross-over. Cases of acute non-specific giant cell myocarditis occasionally show typical sarcoid granulomas in other organs. Whether this means that both conditions have a similar pathogenesis is unknown.

Other forms of giant cell myocarditis

Acute rheumatic fever produces highly characteristic and specific interstitial granulomas (see below). In infants, calcification of myocytes may occur both in hypercalcaemia and following myocyte necrosis due to any cause. Such calcified myocytes may invoke a giant cell response. Perivascular intramyocardial granulomas are also a feature of Wegener's disease, but the arteritis is the histological feature providing the diagnosis.

Acute rheumatic fever

The disease is now virtually extinct in developed countries, but remains endemic in many parts of the third world, in particular those which are semi-tropical.

The geographic distribution of the disease today reflects socioeconomic factors rather than climatic effects and the disease thrives in crowded deprived communities with a high proportion of infants in the population, examples being South America and the Middle East (Garcia-Palmiere 1962).

The disease occurs most frequently in children between 6 and 15 years of age and is initiated by a sore throat due to infection with group B haemolytic streptococci. After a latent period of 2–6 weeks the patient develops fever, a flitting arthropathy and skin rashes or nodules. Concomitant with this there is a pericarditis. Guidelines have been drawn up to unify the diagnosis of acute rheumatic fever (Table 5.14) and there should be serological or culture evidence of prior streptococcal infection plus one major and two minor criteria or two major criteria. The criteria originally laid down by Duckett and Jones have been regularly revised and are the gold standard for diagnosis (Kaplan 1993).

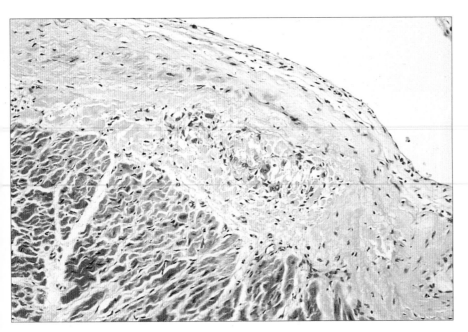

Figure 5.17

Acute rheumatic fever – left atrium. In this low power picture the endocardium is seen to be thickened with a diffuse but mild infiltrate of non-specific chronic inflammatory cells. A single giant cell granuloma (Aschoff body) is present at the junction between the myocardium and the endocardium (H&E ×14).

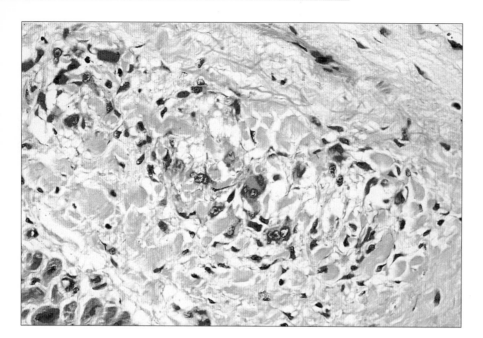

Figure 5.18
Acute rheumatic fever – Aschoff body. The Aschoff body is a loose conglomeration of giant cells and histiocytes around a central focus of blurred but not brightly eosinophilic connective tissue (H&E ×56).

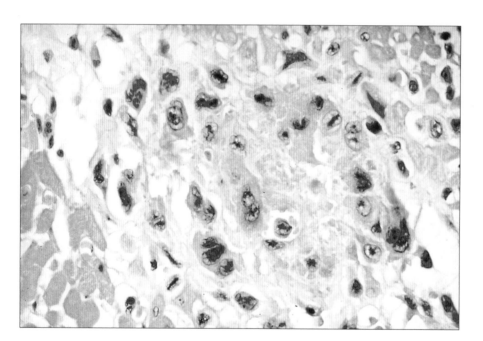

Figure 5.19 a,b
Acute rheumatic fever – Aschoff body. In this higher power picture (a) the detailed morphology of the cell types can be seen. Aschoff cells have large open nuclei and are often multi-nucleated. Anitschkow cells (b) have single nuclei with a central band of chromatin (H&E ×140).

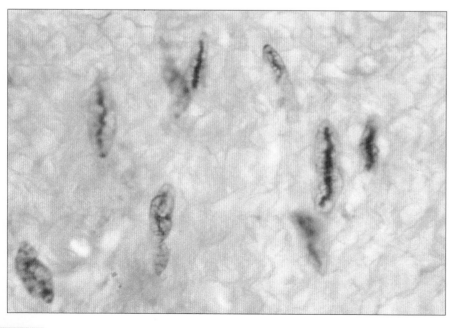

Acute rheumatic fever – pericarditis

Pericarditis is acute and has non-specific histology. While it is a very common component of the disease recognised by the appearance of a pericardial rub, in life it is not clinically important and causes no long-term sequelae.

Acute rheumatic fever – myocarditis

Myocarditis is important in that it is responsible for the acute phase mortality which may be as high as 3%, but it causes no long-term effects. The specific histological feature, which does not occur in any other disease and cannot be exactly reproduced in an experimental model, is the Aschoff body (Figs 5.17–5.19). This is a microscopic structure occurring in the fibrous trabeculae of the myocardium, in perivascular tissues and in the subendocardium. Each Aschoff body has a central focus of rather blurred, smudged connective tissue which is not as brightly eosinophilic as in fibrinoid necrosis. Immune deposits with IgG are not found in the Aschoff bodies. Around the central focus are arranged small giant cells (Aschoff giant cells) and histiocytic cells with a long central bar of nuclear chromatin (Anitschkow cells). There is also a diffuse non-specific interstitial myocarditis in the acute phase. Anitschkow cells in isolation have no specificity for acute rheumatic fever. This form of connective tissue cell arises in the myocardium, and particularly the atria, in children with a wide range of cardiac diseases.

Aschoff bodies may persist for 20 or more years before becoming small fibrous scars. The presence of Aschoff bodies in atrial appendages removed at mitral valve surgery does not indicate current active rheumatic carditis – merely that the patient has had rheumatic fever sometime in the past.

Acute rheumatic fever – endocarditis

Endocarditis is the least of the acute clinical problems but is the ultimate cause of the chronic long-term morbidity and mortality associated with chronic rheumatic valve disease. Mitral regurgitation during the acute phase disease is due to dilatation of the left ventricle, not due to cusp disease per se.

The valve cusps in the acute phase are swollen and oedematous with small flat brown vegetations arranged along the closure line of the mitral (Fig. 5.20) and aortic valve cusps. Histologically the vegetations are predominantly platelets and the underlying cusp is infiltrated by histiocytic cells and lymphocytes. Aschoff bodies in the cusp itself do occur but are very rare. As acute valvulitis develops, vessels extend into the cusps from the base. This is followed by the development of fibrosis which begins to efface the cusp architecture.

Pathogenesis of acute rheumatic fever

The disease is clearly an aberrant immune response to the streptococcus, but it must be emphasised that no bacteria or even bacterial antigens reach the heart. Acute rheumatic fever is totally different from acute streptococcal glomerulonephritis, which is due to local immune complex deposition. Antigenic similarities between certain streptococcal wall components and cardiac connective tissue led to the concept of 'molecular mimicry' for rheumatic fever (Williams 1985). This hypothesis is based on a fortuitous sharing of antigens by the streptococcus and the heart (Cunningham et al. 1989) which allow a humoral antibody to cause the tissue damage. It is certainly true that streptococcal antigens invoke a brisk antibody response. High titres of ASO haemolysin are used to diagnose acute rheumatic fever. However, the theory has major inconsistencies – for example humoral antibody is not bound within Aschoff bodies. The concept of antigens being shared by the streptococcus and the heart is likely to be important, and there is now evidence for a T-cell mediated immune response against cardiac components.

Natural history of acute rheumatic fever

The great majority of cases occur in children between 6 and 15 years of age between 10 days and 6 weeks

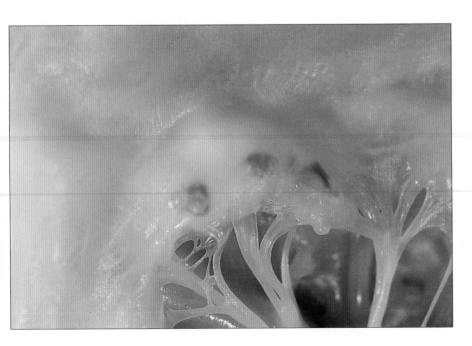

Figure 5.20
Acute rheumatic fever – endocarditis. On the apposition line of the anterior cusp of the mitral valve is a number of sessile brown vegetations.

after a streptococcal sore throat. It is estimated that only 3% of streptococcal sore throats, even in children in communities where acute rheumatic fever is endemic, develop a carditis (Siegel *et al.* 1961). This implies that there is either an element of individual susceptibility, or that certain strains of streptococci have a greater capacity to cause carditis than others. Both are likely to occur – individual susceptibility is indicated by a predilection of acute rheumatic fever to run in families and be related to certain MHC subtypes. The proportion of patients who have had acute rheumatic fever who will ultimately develop chronic rheumatic valve disease is difficult to ascertain. Wood in 1954 suggested that the mean latent period was 19 years. Today in developed countries the latent period appears longer. Recurrent attacks of acute rheumatic fever in childhood both increase the risk of chronic valve disease in later life, and radically reduce the latent period.

The decline in acute rheumatic fever in developed countries over the period since 1940 has been linked both to major improvements in living conditions and the introduction of penicillin as a routine treatment for sore throats. There is some evidence that acute rheumatic fever may be once again increasing in developed countries (Kaplan 1993) based on the emergence of new strains of rheumatogenic group A streptococci (Bisno 1991).

CARDIOMYOPATHY – NON-INFLAMMATORY

The classification of the primary cardiomyopathies – that is those not associated with other systemic diseases, hypertension, valve disease or ischaemic disease – is currently made by the functional effect on the ventri-

cles. While this is clinically satisfactory, different functional effects may be produced by the same aetiological and pathogenetic factors in different subjects. Increasingly the genetic causes of cardiomyopathies are being defined; a single abnormal gene can produce very diverse phenotypes. We are probably within 10 years of a full genetic and pathogenetic classification of the cardiomyopathies, but for the moment a functional system is still in use.

Functional forms of cardiomyopathy

The commonest clinical pattern is dilated cardiomyopathy (DCM) (Fig. 5.21). This is predominantly a failure of systolic contraction leading to an increase in left ventricular end-systolic volume, and a decline in ejection fraction. Left ventricular end-diastolic volume also rises, and the left ventricular cavity increases in size with a decrease in wall thickness to produce a globular heart (Figs 5.22). In hypertrophic cardiomyopathy (HCM) systolic contraction is forceful, but early and not coordinated. In conjunction with this there is abnormal diastolic relaxation making the ventricle difficult to fill. The result is a thick-walled left ventricle with a small cavity (Figs 5.23, 5.24). In restrictive cardiomyopathy (RCM) the abnormality is entirely in diastole. The ventricle fails to relax, necessitating very high left atrial pressures to achieve filling. The effect on the heart is rather like that of mitral valve stenosis; the left ventricle is externally normal with a normal cavity proportion, but the left atrium is dilated. Pulmonary hypertension develops giving severe right ventricular hypertrophy (Fig. 5.25). In obliterative cardiomyopathies (OCM) thrombosis and fibrosis obliterate the cavities of one or both ventricles (Fig. 5.26). In right ventricular dysplasia (RVD) the right ventricle is dilated and thin-walled, with arrhythmias being the striking clinical feature (Fig. 5.27).

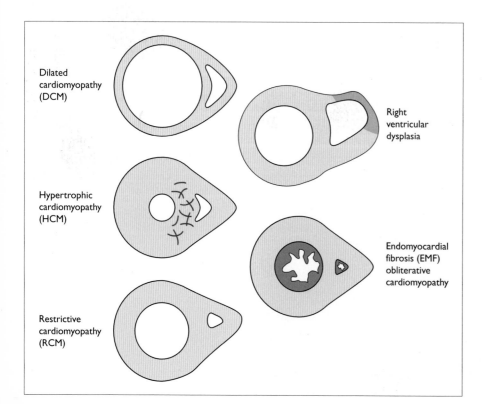

Figure 5.21
Morphological expression of different functional forms of cardiomyopathy. Ventricular shape is best appreciated in transverse cuts through both ventricles at mid-septal level. This allows assessment of the wall thickness of the ventricular myocardium in relation to cavity dimensions.

Dilated cardiomyopathy (DCM)

Right ventricular dysplasia

Hypertrophic cardiomyopathy (HCM)

Endomyocardial fibrosis (EMF) obliterative cardiomyopathy

Restrictive cardiomyopathy (RCM)

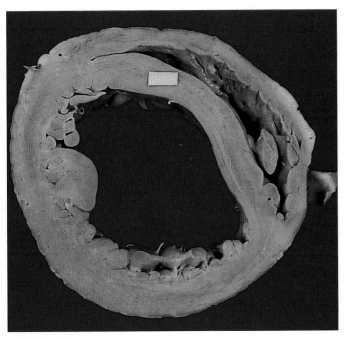

Figure 5.22
Dilated cardiomyopathy. The transverse slice of the ventricles shows marked LV cavity dilatation with a wall thickness throughout the whole circumference of the left ventricle of 1 cm. No mural thrombus is present. No macroscopic myocardial scarring is present.

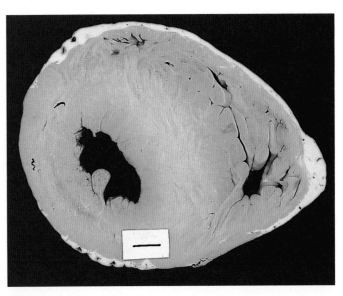

Figure 5.23
Hypertrophic cardiomyopathy – asymmetric form. The transverse slice of the ventricles shows a very thick interventricular septum (4.3 cm) compared with the posterior wall of the left ventricle (1.9 cm) giving a septal posterior wall ratio of 2:3:1. The cut surface of the septum shows a whorled pattern similar to that of a uterine fibroid. The case is from a family originally described by Donald Teare and subsequently found to have a β heavy chain myosin mutation.

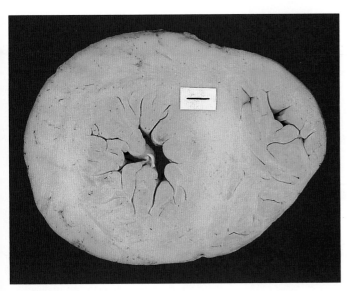

Figure 5.24
Hypertrophic cardiomyopathy – symmetric form. The heart weighed over 750 g. The left ventricle has a tiny cavity and symmetric wall thickening (4.6 cm). The right ventricle is also uniformly thickened with a small cavity.

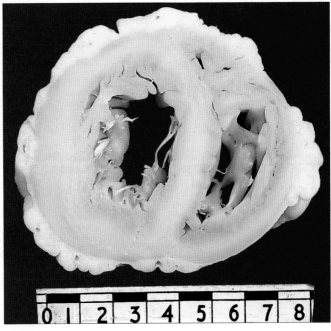

Figure 5.25
Restrictive cardiomyopathy. The left ventricular wall thickness is not more than mildly thick-walled with a ventricular cavity which is in proportion. There is a striking degree of right ventricular wall thickening.

A number of entities do not fit this system of classification. Hearts are encountered in which there is no history of cardiac failure and arrhythmias are the dominant clinical manifestation. This clinical picture is associated with widespread myocardial fibrosis, but no alterations in ventricular shape. We prefer the term idiopathic fibrosis heart (IF) for this entity which usually presents to pathologists as sudden death (*see* Chapter 8).

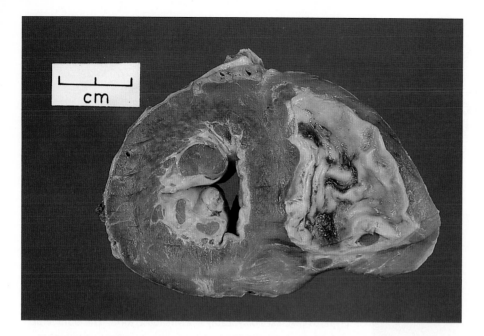

Figure 5.26
Obliterative cardiomyopathy –
endomyocardial fibrosis. The cavity of each
ventricle is being obliterated by a shaggy
coat of thrombus superimposed on white
endocardial thickening.

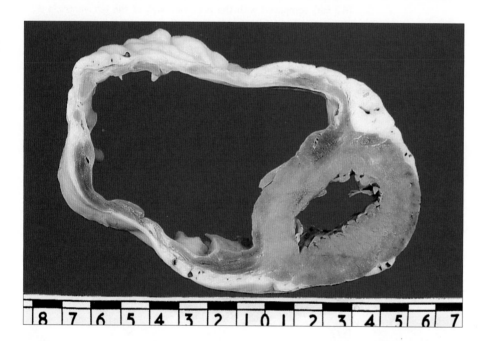

Figure 5.27
Right ventricular dysplasia. The right
ventricle is extremely dilated and thin
walled with a macroscopically normal left
ventricle.

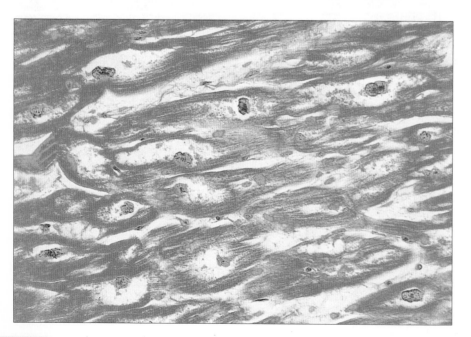

Figure 5.28
Dilated cardiomyopathy – histology. In this
case the striking feature is the loss of
myofibrils giving the myocytes an unduly
vacuolated appearance (H&E ×25).

Table 5.15
Dilated cardiomyopathy.

LV mass	↑	LV cavity	↑	LV wall thickness	↓
		Interstitial fibrosis			
		Myocyte nuclear hypertrophy			
		Myocyte width decreased			
		Myofibrillary loss			
		T-lymphocyte count increased			

Dilated cardiomyopathy

This term should be strictly used to indicate a genuine abnormality of ventricular structure combined with a clear history of left ventricular dysfunction and chronic

cardiac failure in life. The macroscopic and microscopic features are shown in Table 5.15.

Dilated cardiomyopathies may have any combination of these histological features (Figs 5.28–5.33) or even only one of them alone and look histologically close to normal. There is some correlation between the degree of myofibrillary loss and fibrosis with the degree of left ventricular dysfunction (Zimmer *et al.* 1992). Cases of dilated cardiomyopathy with an increase in the number of T-lymphocytes are sometimes called chronic myocarditis. To use the term dilated cardiomyopathy accurately, a pathologist thus needs knowledge of the clinical picture and the macroscopic and microscopic features. The case-to-case variability is less with end-stage cases at autopsy, but those coming to transplant are less advanced and rarely show all the pathology features. While dilated cardiomyopathy is a rather general term it should not be used as a 'rag bag' to

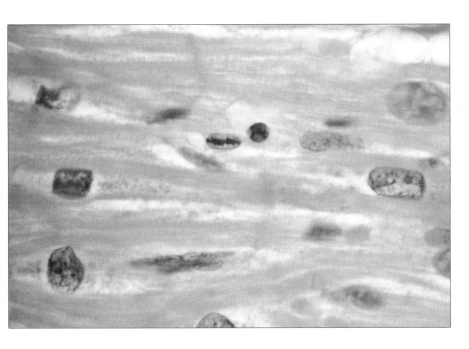

Figure 5.29
Dilated cardiomyopathy – histology. In this case from a child the striking feature is the nuclear enlargement within myocytes. An Anitschkow cell with a long bar of nuclear chromatin is present in the interstitial tissue. Such cells are a non-specific response in children (H&E ×140).

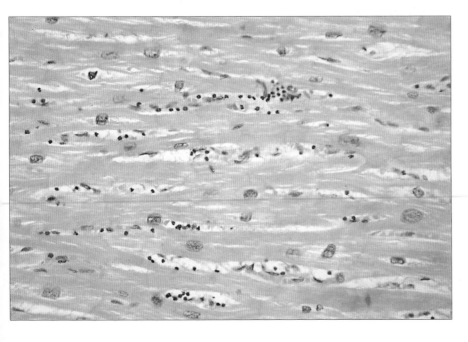

Figure 5.30
Dilated cardiomyopathy – histology. The features here are of an increase in nuclear size within myocytes and an increase in the number of interstitial lymphocytes (H&E ×56).

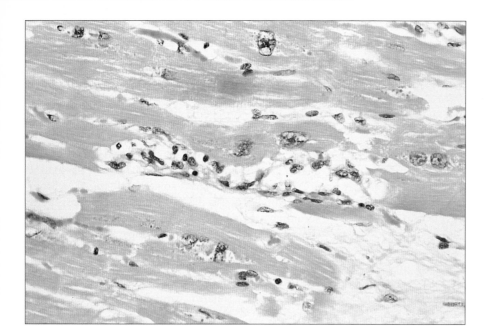

Figure 5.31
Dilated cardiomyopathy – histology. A single myocyte has undergone cell death and the sarcolemmal sheath contains macrophages (H&E ×87.5).

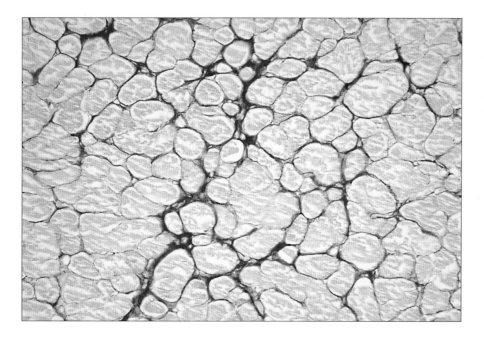

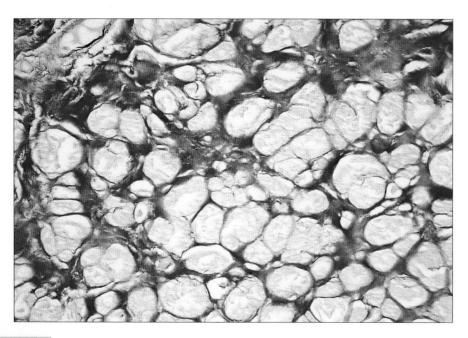

Figure 5.32 a,b
Dilated cardiomyopathy – histology. The characteristic pattern of fibrosis in dilated cardiomyopathy starts in a fine perimyocyte distribution and (a) passes into a more dense honeycomb of fibrosis within which myocytes are embedded (b) (EVG ×140).

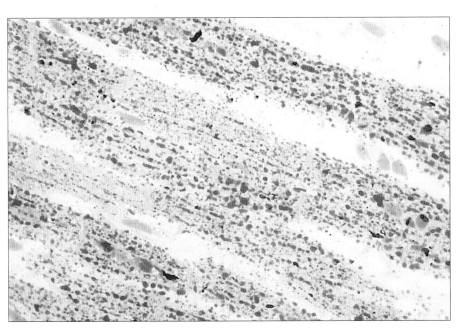

Figure 5.33
Fatty change in myocytes. There is widespread accumulation of fatty droplets within all the myocytes. The change can occur in a very wide range of diseases and has no specificity for alcoholic ingestion (Sudan red ×56).

explain unexplained sudden death. For example, it is no help to anyone to call a slightly enlarged heart which is otherwise normal, but where the pathologist is seeking a cause of sudden death in a subject without cardiac failure, a dilated cardiomyopathy.

Pathogenesis of dilated cardiomyopathy

The pathogenesis of dilated cardiomyopathy is very heterogeneous (Table 5.16). None of the morphological features described above allow the pathogenesis to be determined with the exception of haemachromatosis and amyloid which are sometimes called infiltrative cardiomyopathies. The great majority of dilated cardiomyopathy is idiopathic in origin; in a recently reported series of 673 cases of dilated cardiomyopathy (Kaspar *et al.* 1994) 47% of cases were regarded as idiopathic. Provided alcohol can be excluded, two main views, namely, viral and autoimmune, are held concerning pathogenesis. Whatever the relative importance of these two mechanisms, up to a third of cases have a familial factor, as shown by detailed study of the relatives of index cases of dilated cardiomyopathy (Michels *et al.* 1992; Mestroni *et al.* 1990). Dilated cardiomyopathy may be the long-term result of viral myocarditis. The evidence is suggestive, but by no means conclusive. Comparison of cases with controls shows a higher proportion of subjects with dilated cardiomyopathy to have serological evidence of Coxsackie infection in the form of increased titres of IgM antibodies. Viral genomic material in the myocardium from DCM cases can be shown by PCR and/or *in situ* hybridisation in about 10–20% of cases. The difficulty is that a proportion of totally normal individuals have similar evidence of persistent Coxsackie carriage, and very few human cases of dilated cardiomyopathy follow documented acute myocarditis. Many cases of dilated cardiomyopathy have raised titres to a variety of cardiac-specific antigens including heavy chain myosin, the β adrenergic receptor, heat-shock protein and mitochondrial

Table 5.16
Dilated cardiomyopathy – pathogenesis.

Genetic
Mitochondrial
Chromosomal – Protein kinase gene
– Dystrophin gene
Post viral
Autoimmune
Toxic
Alcohol
Others
Peripartum
Idiopathic

components (Latif *et al.* 1993). This has led to a hypothesis which suggests autoimmune mechanisms act against myocytes, possibly initially triggered by a virus (Schultheiss 1992). There is an association of dilated cardiomyopathy with certain HLA Class II phenotypes. There now seems no doubt that part of the progression of dilated cardiomyopathy is determined by persistent individual myocyte death, possibly mediated by the T-lymphocytes which are present.

Alcohol-related heart muscle disease

There is a wide spectrum of pathological change in the heart related to high alcohol intake. It is difficult to define at which point in this spectrum the term cardiomyopathy becomes applicable. Alcohol-related cardiac damage is more idiosyncratic and less clearly related to total alcohol intake than liver damage. Alcoholic heart muscle disease is usually seen in subjects without cirrhosis, and for unknown reasons there appears to be a negative relation between alcohol-related liver and heart disease. It is very difficult to determine exactly the incidence of alcoholic heart muscle disease in the population. It is common to find living patients with 'idiopathic' dilated cardiomyopathy whose alcohol intake is high from the perspective of a non-drinking doctor. The best test to confirm the role of alcohol is whether left ventricular function improves on total abstinence.

The spectrum of alcohol-related heart muscle disease begins at the bottom end of the scale with an excess of sudden deaths without cause in alcoholics with fatty livers, but morphologically normal hearts. The spectrum continues through increases in left ventricular mass, increases in interstitial fibrosis, fatty change in myocytes (Fig. 5.33), isolated marked myofibrillary loss and culminates at the extreme end of the spectrum in hearts with all the features of a dilated cardiomyopathy. It must be emphasised again that there are no specific histological features of alcohol-related heart muscle disease.

The toxicity of alcohol is related to its degradation to acetaldehyde which has widespread effects on the myocyte including interfering with myosin ATPase and calcium binding, inhibiting mitochondrial oxidation, reducing protein synthesis and allowing lipid droplets to accumulate in the cell (Guarnieri and Lakatta 1990). Ultrastructural changes include the appearance of many membrane-bound myelin figures within myocytes.

Toxic cardiomyopathy

Heavy metals may cause a dilated cardiomyopathy. This fact was first recognised in North America following the addition of cobalt to beer to maintain its frothy head in the drinking glass (Alexander 1969). The striking feature histologically is vacuolation of myocytes with many appearing empty due to myofibrillary loss. Fibrosis then follows myocyte death.

The anthracyline groups of drugs and doxorubicin are widely used cytotoxic agents, particularly used for malignant tumours in children. Regrettably they have considerable cardiotoxic potential which has to be monitored with care. The effect of the drugs is dose-related and if 550 mg/m^2 of body area is exceeded, 30% of patients develop cardiac failure. Even lower doses reduce ventricular contraction and late cardiac failure up to 10 years after a course of therapy can occur. The light microscopy changes appear late, and if the effects of the drug on the myocardium are being monitored by cardiac biopsy, electron microscopy is essential (Billingham and Bristow 1984; Rowan et al. 1988). At least 10 EM blocks from three separate biopsy fragments need to be examined. Sarcotubular dilatation is easily recognised on EM and ultimately leads to some myocytes appearing finely vacuolated under light microscopy. Another change is myofibrillary loss leaving a ghost myocyte containing a few mitochondria. Both changes are indicative of drug toxicity and can be very focal. Ultimately focal myocyte necrosis occurs, leading to replacement fibrosis. A grading system on

biopsies is used to aid in adjusting dosage; the use of cardiac biopsies to monitor therapy is a specialised field needing experience and it should not be attempted on an occasional basis. The increasing use of these drugs may mean many pathologists are faced with hearts from subjects whose therapy was given some or many years previously. The late changes are predominantly of diffuse interstitial fibrosis replacing myocytes, and without a clinical history are not distinguishable from other dilated cardiomyopathies.

Genetic causes of dilated cardiomyopathy

Known genetic defects causing dilated cardiomyopathy can be divided into those which are mitochondrial and those involving chromosomal DNA mutations. In both there is often, but not inevitably, concomitant skeletal muscle involvement. The majority of currently recognised cases present with the skeletal muscle problems and may or may not develop cardiac manifestations in later life. It is becoming increasingly clear that differential tissue expression of genes may occur, and some cases may present purely with cardiac disease or even conduction disease alone. These cases may be sporadic in families where in other members the more usual skeletal problems predominate, or families in all of whose members cardiac disease predominates. The genotype–phenotype relation in both nuclear DNA mutation and chromosomal DNA mutations is not yet well-defined. A complex mixture of phenotypes ranging from macroscopically normal to dilated to hypertrophic cardiomyopathy may occur.

Myotonic dystrophy is due to an increase in a repetitive sequence of base pairs in the protein kinase gene located on chromosome 19. The number of repeats in the gene tends to increase in successive generations, leading to what is known as anticipation, i.e. each generation experiences a successively worse clinical disease. This autosomal dominant condition is characterised by muscle weakness and atrophy with frontal baldness and cataracts. In up to 85% of cases the ECG is abnormal with prolonged atrioventricular conduction. 15–20% of cases have symptomatic cardiac disease and sudden death is a frequent phenomenon, being the final event in 30% of affected individuals. Anaesthetics in subjects with myotonic dystrophy are a high-risk procedure (Olofsson et al. 1988; Harper 1989). Sudden death may occur before any structural disease of the heart is apparent and create difficulties in diagnosis for the pathologist unless the family history is known.

Duchenne's and Becker's muscular dystrophy are due to deletions or mutations in the gene coding for dystrophin on the X chromosome. Reduced amounts or absence of the normal protein or an abnormal protein product may be produced. Dystrophin is a component of the sarcolemma of the muscle cells and is complexed with glycoproteins; it is concerned with both membrane flexibility and calcium ion transport. The gene encodes for both cardiac and skeletal muscle dystrophin and in the majority of families both tissues are equally

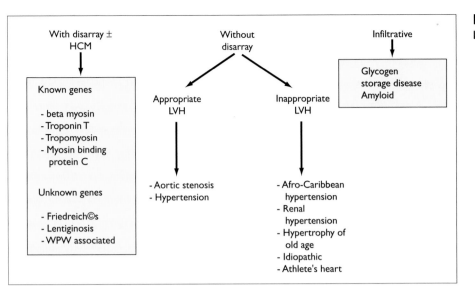

Figure 5.34
Increased LV mass and wall-thickness.

affected. Cardiac disease ultimately develops in 80% of cases of Duchenne's dystrophy, although only 10% of cases actually die of cardiac disease (Sanyal and Johnson 1982). This is due to the high mortality from respiratory muscle weakness and pneumonia in relatively young individuals.

The Becker form of the disease is due to mutations in the dystrophin gene which allow the production of a somewhat less abnormal protein. The clinical manifestations are milder with regard to skeletal muscle disease, but cardiac disease still occurs. Mutations in the promotor gene for cardiac expression of dystrophin are now recognised (Muntoni *et al.* 1993). Some mutations are selective for expression of dystrophin in conduction tissue (Beggs 1997).

Skeletal muscular dystrophies which have cardiac involvement are characterised by replacement of both conduction and contractile myocytes by a mixture of adipose tissue and fibrous tissue. In the conduction system the AV and SA nodes may virtually vanish, being replaced by fat. Fibrous scarring has a predilection for the posterior basal segment of the left ventricle and is subepicardial. In many cases the heart is not dilated and death is due to arrhythmias rather than chronic cardiac failure (Frankel and Rosser 1976). This suggests that selective promoter genes exist for the conduction system and provide the genetic basis for a phenotype in which selective conduction tissue loss occurs.

There is now growing recognition of genetic defects in the cytoskeleton of myocytes which lead to progressive myocyte loss and end as a dilated cardiomyopathy. Dystrophin is the best characterised (Beggs 1997); metavinculin is another (Maeda *et al.* 1997).

Other dilated cardiomyopathies are associated with defects in the mitochondrial respiratory and oxidative systems due to mutations in mitochondrial DNA, and are therefore maternally transmitted. Most mitochon-

drial genetic defects predominantly affect skeletal muscle, but the conduction system of the heart is also very susceptible. In the Kearns–Sayre syndrome (Butler and Gadoth 1976) for example, ocular paralysis is associated with progressive loss of conduction tissue leading to heart block without any myocardial contraction loss. The phenotypic expression of mitochondrial cardiac disease is very wide-ranging, from purely conduction tissue loss to a conventional dilated cardiomyopathy (Suomalainen *et al.* 1992) to a hypertrophic cardiomyopathy (Sengers *et al.* 1985). While in the mitochondrial myopathies the mitochondria under electron microscopy may appear large and abnormal, the ease with which fixation artefacts can distort the structure means that cardiac biopsy to confirm or exclude the diagnosis of a mitochondrial abnormality is not reliable. The pattern of inheritance down the female line provides the clue to proceed to formal genetic analysis of mitochondrial DNA.

Peripartum cardiomyopathy

This is defined as a dilated cardiomyopathy in which cardiac failure appears either within the 3 months prior to delivery, or within the 6 months following delivery (O'Connel *et al.* 1986). The condition is extremely heterogeneous and is unlikely to be a specific entity (Homans 1985). Care should be used by pathologists in applying the term; peri-partum cardiomyopathy should not be used as an explanation of death when the heart is morphologically normal and the mode of death was a sudden arrhythmia or circulatory collapse. Any peri-partum death needs coordination of the clinical data and the histology of many organs including the heart. Pathologists should record accurate data on the heart (i.e. total heart weight, LV wall thickness etc) to assist enquiry into the death. Morphologically the heart may be indistinguishable from any other dilated cardiomyopathy with an increase in total heart weight, a dilated left ventricle with wall thinning, and marked interstitial fibrosis. Such cases may represent the haemodynamic stresses of pregnancy, unmasking a pre-existing

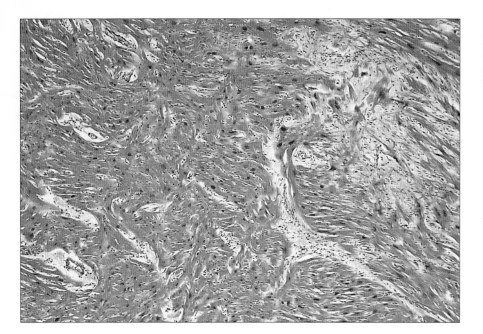

Figure 5.35
Myocyte disarray in hypertrophic cardiomyopathy. In low power histology the overall impression is of myocytes arranged in a whorled criss-cross pattern (H&E ×35).

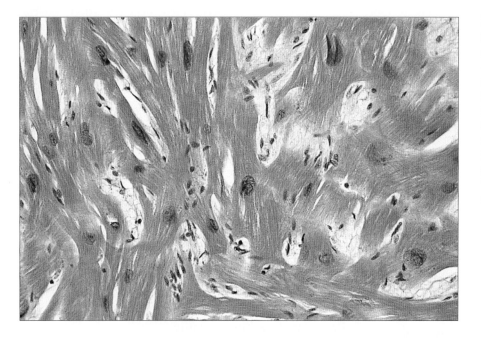

Figure 5.36
Myocyte disarray in hypertrophic cardiomyopathy. In addition to a disorganised myocyte arrangement the concordance of wide myocytes with very large nuclei and width is a feature. Note the variation in myocyte nuclease size in this one field. This irregular hypertrophy contrasts with that found in reactive hypertrophy due to, for example, aortic stenosis where the response is more even. There are small foci of rather cellular loose connective tissue (H&E ×87.5).

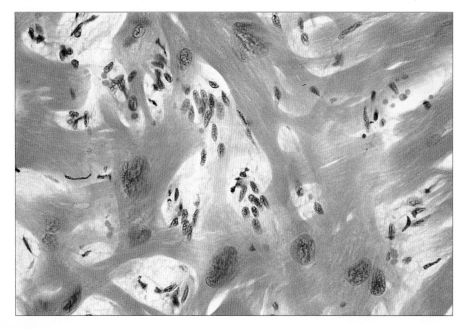

Figure 5.37
Myocyte disarray in hypertrophic cardiomyopathy. Myocytes are arranged in circular fashion around foci of connective tissue. Myocyte nuclei are very large. Even in a conventional H&E section, the myofibril disarray within myocytes is noted (H&E ×140).

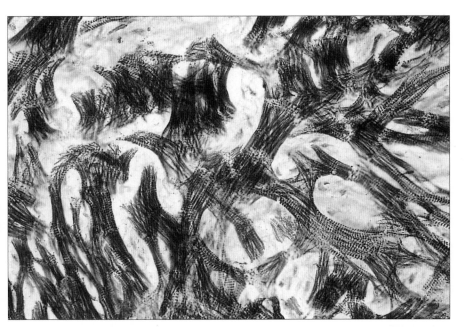

Figure 5.38
Myocyte disarray in hypertrophic cardiomyopathy. Staining of the myofibrils accentuates the disarray since it shows both the disorganisation and criss-crossing of myofibrils within the cell and the abnormal cell-to-cell arrangement (PTAH ×87.5).

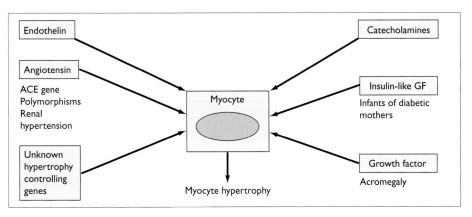

Figure 5.39
Inappropriate hypertrophy.

subclinical dilated cardiomyopathy (Cunningham *et al.* 1986). Other cases show less hypertrophy and dilatation and histology which is characterised by either inflammatory cell infiltrate of sufficient degrees to use the term myocarditis, or marked myofibrillary loss with vacuolisation of myocytes. Virus infection, autoimmune damage and vitamin deficiencies have all been postulated, but there is likely to be a marked variation in pathogenesis between different socioeconomic or geographic populations.

Hypertrophic cardiomyopathy (HCM)

Hearts in which there is an increase in left ventricular mass with a thick wall and a normal or reduced left ventricular cavity fall into several categories (Fig. 5.34). Those in which the increase in size is due to infiltrative conditions such as amyloid or glycogen storage disease must be identified. The remaining cases can then be subdivided. In a large group there is a clear and appropriate cause for hypertrophy such as aortic stenosis (Fig. 5.1). The remaining cases are then divided into those in which myocyte disarray (Figs 5.35–5.38) is present and those in which it is absent. Histology is essential to go through this sequence.

Hypertrophy without disarray

The hypertrophy of the myocytes in this group is 'normal'. This means the myocyte increases in size and in particular the diameter increases; myocyte nuclei increase in size and ploidy. Myofibrillary organisation within the myocyte is normal and there is no disarray. Hypertrophy of this type may be appropriate; namely, there may be a clear cause such as athletic training, hypertension or aortic stenosis. However, the hypertrophy may be inappropriate, in that the left ventricular mass is increased without a clear cause, or is disproportionate to a cause such as mild hypertension.

There is increasing recognition that hypertrophy is dependent on a number of growth factors including angiotensin, endothelin and insulin-like growth factors (Fig. 5.39). An excess of these factors will cause inappropriate left ventricular hypertrophy. In renal hypertension, the degree of left ventricular hypertrophy is often far greater than expected, due to excess circulating angiotensin. Of the three forms, II, ID, DD, of the angiotensin converting enzyme gene (ACE), the deletion/deletion polymorphism has higher circulating

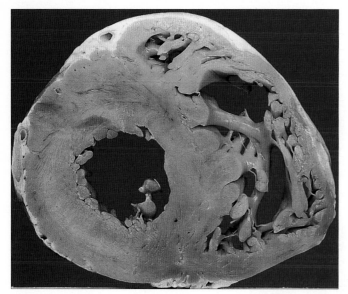

Figure 5.40
Excessive LV hypertrophy. The patient of Afro-Caribbean origin had mild hypertension well-controlled by drugs. Death was sudden. The heart weighed 590 g and had a symmetric left ventricle with a thick wall. No disarray was present.

Table 5.17
Myocyte disarray.

Myocardial bundle disorganisation
Myocyte-to-myocyte disorganisation – whorls around connective tissue
Myofibrillary disorganisation within myocyte

angiotensin levels and thus individuals who possess this form develop more hypertrophy in response to hypertension than individuals who are insertion/insertion (II). In subjects of Afro-Caribbean origin, the degree of left ventricular hypertrophy often exceeds that which would be expected for any given level of hypertension in Caucasians (Frohlich *et al.* 1992) (Fig. 5.40). Sufficient left ventricular hypertrophy may be present to lead to sudden death (*see* Chapter 8). While this hypertrophy was originally thought to reflect less rigorous control of blood pressure, a genetic cause operating through control of hypertrophy is more likely. In some elderly subjects the left ventricle also becomes thick-walled with a moderate increase in mass. The ventricular septum when viewed in its long axis is sigmoid in shape, and in these elderly hearts the curvature is accentuated so that the septum bulges out below the aortic valve, simulating clinically a true obstructive hypertrophic cardiomyopathy. Disarray and a familial tendency are not described as present, and the response is another example of inappropriate hypertrophy possibly initiated by rising blood pressure.

In infants born to diabetic mothers the heart may show marked hypertrophy with a thick-walled left ventricle due to insulin-like growth factors crossing the placenta to act on the foetal heart. The change may take up to 2 years to regress.

For both clinicians and pathologists the hearts of athletes present a major challenge in interpretation (Pelliccia *et al.* 1991). Trained athletes develop considerable physiological cardiac hypertrophy which will regress if they stop physical training (Maron *et al.* 1993). Isometric exercise such as that which occurs in short bursts in weight lifters or shot putters leads to a thick-walled left ventricle; short-term rises in blood pressure

up to 300 mm Hg are recorded in such athletes. Long distance runners and cyclists develop an equivalent degree of left ventricular hypertrophy, but the cavity is larger and the wall only moderately thickened. If the hypertrophy does not regress on rest or becomes excessive in life there are inevitably questions, at the moment unanswered, about prognosis and advice with regard to further athletic activity. A small number of athletes with large hearts die suddenly without clear cause and become a problem for pathologists. The possibilities are first that the individual is in fact carrying one of the known hypertrophic cardiomyopathy genes. If so, disarray will be present histologically. If disarray is absent, the question of steroid abuse arises and can only be resolved by a detailed retrospective history. If the heart is above 600 g and both these possibilities are excluded, the individual must be regarded as having had a genetic propensity to excessive hypertrophy.

Hypertrophic cardiomyopathy with disarray

Central to the constellation of conditions going under the name of hypertrophic cardiomyopathy are cases with the histological features listed in Table 5.17 and shown in Figs 5.35–5.38.

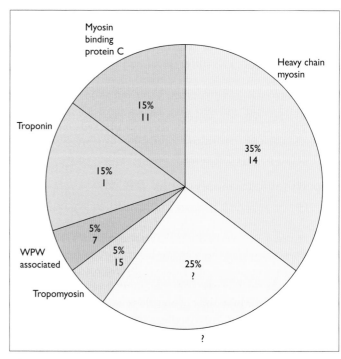

Figure 5.41
Genetic basis of HCM.

Five genes are now recognised to cause three quarters of this condition (Fig. 5.41). The most frequent are point mutations or deletions in the heavy chain myosin gene on chromosome 14. The family originally described by Donald Teare in 1958 which initiated recognition of the disease have such a mutation. The other genes responsible for an identical phenotype are those controlling troponin T, tropomyosin and a myosin-binding protein. A fifth gene on chromosome 7 causes hypertrophic cardiomyopathy conjointly with pre-excitation. All the genes identical so far produce their phenotypic expression by interfering with myofibrillary organisation within the myocyte leading to a misshapen cell with both abnormal contraction and relaxation (Thierfelder *et al.* 1994; Watkins *et al.* 1992). Diagnosis can be made in life from DNA extracted from peripheral blood lymphocytes or from wax-embedded tissue by PCR.

Phenotypic and clinical features of hypertrophic cardiomyopathy with disarray

The striking and still largely unexplained feature is a very marked variation in the clinical picture, echocardiographic appearances and macroscopic autopsy appearances (Davies and McKenna 1995; Maron *et al.* 1984) between cases. This is even true of members of one family who all carry the same gene mutation. Family-to-family variation is even more pronounced.

The first facet of the phenotypic range of hypertrophic cardiomyopathy to be described was asymmetric hypertrophy of the interventricular septum (Fig. 5.23). Ratios of septal width to posterior wall thickness in the left ventricle exceed a ratio of 2:1. The septal asymmetry can be best appreciated in short axis transverse sections of the ventricles. Such tissue slices also show macroscopically a characteristic whorled cut surface reflecting a combination of the myocyte malarrangement and fibrosis. One striking feature of this type of asymmetric case is the apparent normality of the left ventricular free wall. In hypertrophic cardiomyopathy, echocardiography in life shows that, as ventricular contraction begins, the anterior cusp of the mitral valve moves forward to hit the expanded ventricular septum with considerable force, thus narrowing the left ventricular outflow. This phenomenon leads to a patch of endocardial thickening on the ventricular septum just below the aortic valve (Fig. 5.42). The endocardial lesion (subaortic mitral impact lesion) is a very specific feature and occurs in no other disease. The thickening forms an exact mirror image of the mitral cusp and has a very sharply defined lower border. More diffuse endocardial thickening is not a specific feature of hypertrophic cardiomyopathy, being found in dilated ventricles from many causes. While the sub-mitral impact lesion is specific for hypertrophic cardiomyopathy it occurs only in one third of cases at autopsy, i.e. it has a low sensitivity for the diagnosis. The physical force with which the mitral cusp hits the septum also causes thickening of the valve and chordal rupture can occur. There is also a risk of bacterial endocarditis developing on the thickened mitral valve.

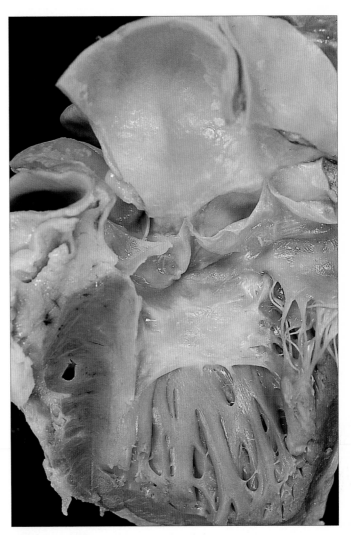

Figure 5.42
Sub-mitral impact lesion in hypertrophic cardiomyopathy. On the interventricular septum just beneath the aortic valve there is a sharply demarcated patch of endocardial thickening which is an exact mirror image of the anterior cusp of the mitral valve. To be pathognomonic of hypertrophic cardiomyopathy there must be a sharp lower edge which is exactly opposite the lower border of the mitral cusp.

Hypertrophic cardiomyopathy is often symmetric involving the whole of the left ventricle to produce an even, thick-walled chamber with a small cavity (Fig. 5.24).

It is now recognised that the segment of most abnormal muscle can involve any region of the left ventricle, can be in discontinuous segments, and will often involve the right ventricle. Disarray of myocytes is most pronounced in macroscopically thick segments of muscle, but also occurs focally elsewhere in the ventricle. It is also usual to be able to find segments of ventricular muscle which do not show hypertrophy or disarray. This regional distribution within the heart of the phenotypic expression when the gene is presumably expressed by every myocyte, is unexplained.

Management of large numbers of patients carrying the hypertrophic cardiomyopathy genes has allowed the

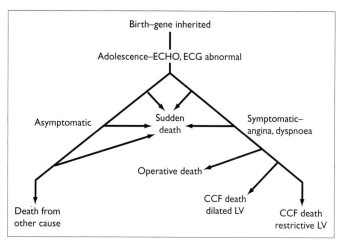

Figure 5.43
Hypertrophic cardiomyopathy.

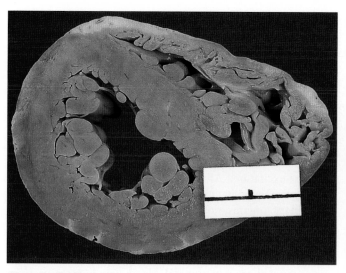

Figure 5.44
Hypertrophic cardiomyopathy in children. The transverse slice is from the ventricles of a girl of 9 who dropped dead while playing. The transverse section is macroscopically normal although widespread disarray was present histologically. Scale is 2 cm long.

natural history of the disease to be defined (Fig. 5.43). The heart becomes structurally abnormal only during the adolescent growth phase (Maron *et al.* 1986). Before this, sudden death is rare but does occur and the heart will be macroscopically normal at autopsy (Fig. 5.44). After adolescence, patients develop LV wall thickening either with symptoms such as angina or remain symptom-free for many years. However, sudden death is always a risk, both in symptomatic and asymptomatic individuals. The average risk for a group of patients with HCM is that sudden deaths occur from between 0.6% to 1.5% per year. However, some families with the abnormal troponin T gene and some of the mutations of the myosin gene involving a change in charge have a far higher risk (Maron *et al.* 1978) leading to the curious term 'Malignant' hypertrophic cardiomyopathy.

Troponin T mutations produce far less striking macroscopic changes than heavy chain myosin gene defects (Fig. 5.45). There is widespread disarray, however, and a high risk of sudden death. In view of the absence of striking macroscopic abnormalities in patients dying before adolescence, and in the troponin T mutation group, it is wise never to be too dogmatic that hypertrophic cardiomyopathy is absent until histology is available.

A small proportion of patients with hypertrophic cardiomyopathy go on to develop congestive cardiac failure and may require transplantation. This subgroup develop a ventricle which dilates and the thick-walled segment thins (Spirito *et al.* 1987). Part of the thinning reflects replacement of the abnormal muscle by fibrosis and large fibrous scars may develop. Many cases of hypertrophic cardiomyopathy develop very abnormal intramyocardial small arteries (Tanaka *et al.* 1987). These have an external diameter which is greater than normal and develop very thick walls with extreme disorganisation of the medial smooth muscle and intimal thickening (Fig. 5.46). These vascular changes in intramyocardial arteries are thought to contribute

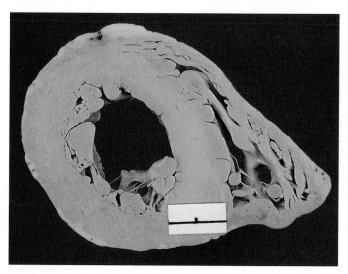

Figure 5.45
Hypertrophic cardiomyopathy due to troponin T mutation. The transverse slice of the ventricles shows symmetric mild LV wall thickening (1.5 cm) but until histology showed widespread disarray was not diagnosable as hypertrophic cardiomyopathy.

both to the fibrous scars and to the symptoms of angina in life.

Diagnostic problems with hypertrophic cardiomyopathy and disarray

Cases with the extreme of the phenotypic expression of hypertrophic cardiomyopathy are easy to recognise at autopsy. Others are less easy, particularly those in which the increase in heart weight is modest and the left ventricular involvement symmetric. It is often impossible at autopsy to exclude by naked eye examination hypertrophic cardiomyopathy in children, because before hypertrophy develops the heart may macroscopically be normal; there are also families in

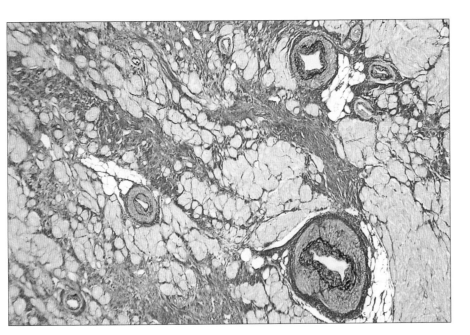

Figure 5.46
Intramyocardial arteries in hypertrophic cardiomyopathy. Many of the intramyocardial arteries show altered lumen to external diameter ratios due to wall thickening by medial hypertrophy and disorganisation. There is a severe degree of myocardial fibrosis (EVG ×22.4).

whom the heart remains macroscopically normal despite widespread disarray and sudden death (McKenna *et al.* 1990). Disarray by microscopy is quantitatively not qualitatively diagnostic (Maron *et al.* 1981). All normal hearts will show small foci of disarray, particularly where the right ventricular myocardium interdigitates with the septum anteriorly and posteriorly. Thus judgement has to be exercised. Most cases of hypertrophic cardiomyopathy will have more than 20% of the myocardium showing disarray in at least two tissue blocks of 4 cm². The characteristic changes are nearly always regional, and the whole circumference of a left ventricular slice at mid-septal level has to be examined to be sure that disarray is present or absent.

The myocyte disorganisation that occurs in small focal areas in normal hearts is different in a number of ways from true disarray. In the latter, there are foci of cellular connective tissue in the centre of whorls of myocytes. Marked nuclear enlargement within myocytes related to the disarray is also seen; this absent in normal hearts.

Subaortic septal resection in hypertrophic cardiomyopathy

To relieve outflow obstruction in the left ventricle, a shallow saucer-shaped segment of the left side of the ventricular septum just below the aortic valve is often surgically removed. A submitral impact lesion on the septum is often included in the specimen. The resection is shallow, and its benefit may be as much in producing left bundle branch-block, thus slowing ventricular activation, as in debulking the septum. The resection is often not deep enough to show the myocyte disarray; fibrosis and hypertrophy alone will be present. Two conditions, desmin myopathy and Fabry's disease, both lead to subaortic septal hypertrophy which may be resected and can be diagnosed on surgical material (see below).

For pathologists, problems are created in that a proportion of cases of 'normal' hypertrophy developing in response to aortic stenosis also develop an accentuation of the subaortic bulge of the ventricular septum, and the surgeon resects this at the time of valve replacement. The question is then asked if this is concomitant hypertrophic cardiomyopathy. If disarray is present in large amounts, the answer is 'yes', but finding such disarray is rare even when the diagnosis is known to be HCM by genetic studies. Exclusion of concomitant hypertrophic cardiomyopathy is best made by echocardiography, but may need genetic study of the patient and family to be certain. Pathologists should not hesitate to say that the question cannot be answered on what was resected.

Other genetic forms of hypertrophic cardiomyopathy with disarray

A number of other genes (known and unknown) can cause thick walled, small cavity left ventricles with myocardial disarray which simulate almost exactly the appearances of those due to the five hypertrophic cardiomyopathy genes described above.

In desmin myopathy, the disease is mainly expressed in skeletal muscle, but cardiac involvement does occur and in rare families cardiac involvement is predominant (Stoeckel *et al.* 1981). The features are exactly as described above with the addition that myocytes contain eosinophilic conglomerates of fibrillary material staining by immunohistochemistry for desmin. The similarity of the disease to the five known hypertrophic cardiomyopathy genes is not surprising since again myofibril formation is abnormal.

In Friedreich's ataxia cardiac involvement (Harding and Langton 1983) can produce the full range of phenotypic expression described above with the exception that the diversity is even more pronounced, and cases with widespread disarray but a relatively macroscopically normal heart are common. The condition initially presents with its central nervous symptoms of dysarthria and incordination before puberty. Progressive spinocerebellar degeneration follows. Many cases have kyphoscoliosis. About 50% of cases die of cardiac disease in the 3rd and 4th decades. Some have cor pulmonale, some hypertrophic cardiomyopathy phenotype, and others are described as more akin to a dilated cardiomyopathy with fibro-fatty replacement of the myocardium (Boehm *et al.* 1970; Berg *et al.* 1980). The gene responsible is on chromosome 9 and codes for a 210 amino acid protein frataxin. This protein is expressed by cardiac myocytes, but its function is unknown. The genetic abnormality is an unstable expansion of the gene involving a repeat sequence. The length of the repeat sequence is directly related to the degree of left ventricular hypertrophy (Isnard *et al.* 1997).

Lentiginosis and Noonan's syndrome are also associated with cardiac involvement, with all the features of hypertrophic cardiomyopathy. The fully expressed phenotype of Noonan's syndrome is characterised by short stature, a webbed neck, low set ears, some retardation of intellect and pulmonary valve stenosis in 70% of cases. Features of hypertrophic cardiomyopathy are present in 20% of patients. Many cases have Factor XI deficiency. The gene is on chromosome 12, but the chromosomal segment involved is very long, containing many genes, none of which is an obvious candidate for this very wide-ranging phenotype. How the gene produces the phenotypic change which affects both mesenchymal tissues in valve cusps and the myocyte is at present unknown (Burch *et al.* 1992; 1993).

Restrictive cardiomyopathy

In the archetypal form of restrictive cardiomyopathy, the left ventricle retains its normal dimensions while the left atrium becomes thick-walled and may dilate as the disease progresses. Right ventricular hypertrophy develops. Restriction is the rarest cause of a cardiomyopathy and will be encountered by pathologists most frequently in biopsies taken to elucidate the cause of abnormal left ventricular diastolic function or in explanted hearts from transplantation.

Biopsy studies of restrictive cardiomyopathy show that several main groups exist. Restrictive cardiomyopathy is an area where cardiac biopsy provides clear clinical benefit in arriving at a diagnosis. Amyloid in myocardial biopsies is usually easily identified by cutting somewhat thicker sections than usual (12 μ) and staining with Congo red, viewing under polarised light. Some cases develop considerable associated fibrosis and electron microscopy may be needed to identify the characteristic fibrils. For this reason, in cases of restrictive cardiomyopathy, it is good practice to place one biopsy into gluteraldehyde. Perimyocyte diffuse fibrosis produces a characteristic lattice of collagen surrounding every myocyte. The pathogenesis is unknown. A

proportion of cases have myocyte hypertrophy and mild disorganisation of the arrangement of muscle bundles. Such cases are often familial, but the gene responsible is unknown. In restrictive cardiomyopathy, if the biopsy is reported to be normal, the clinician will need to reconsider if the diagnosis is not one of constrictive pericarditis rather than a myocardial disease.

Amyloid heart disease

Two morphological forms of cardiac amyloid occur. The first is 'senile' cardiac amyloid confined to the atrium (amyloid IAA – isolated atrial amyloid). With increasing age, small nodules of material staining as amyloid appear in the left atrial myocardium and beneath the endocardium (Steiner 1987). In formalin-fixed specimens, the subendocardial deposits can be seen with the naked eye as small brown nodules 1–3 mm across. These deposits of amyloid are a natural ageing process (Cornwall *et al.* 1983), and can be found in all subjects over 80 years of age if enough sections of atria are taken. There is, however, very considerable variation in degree – a small number of individuals replace virtually all their atrial muscle by amyloid. The amyloid is thought to derive from atrial natriuretic factor produced by atrial myocytes, and does not occur in the ventricle. Unless present in large amounts when it contributes to the development of atrial fibrillation, this form of amyloid is not clinically important. Extra-cardiac deposition does not occur.

The second morphological form of cardiac involvement by amyloid has deposition in both the atria and the ventricles (Hesse *et al.* 1993). The amyloid may be immunoglobulin in origin (amyloid AL); secondary to chronic infection where the amyloid is a part of the acute phase serum amyloid A (amyloid AA); or familial forms in which transthyretin proteins (Hesse *et al.* 1993) (amyloid AF) are deposited. In all these forms extra-cardiac deposits are usually widespread by the time cardiac involvement is apparent. In the ventricular myocardium, amyloid is deposited on the external surface of the myocyte leading to a lattice of amyloid rather like a honeycomb (Fig. 5.47). In each cell there is a myocyte. Ultimately myocyte death occurs, and the mass of amyloid coalesces into nodules (Roberts and Waller 1983). Small vessel involvement is also striking. Ultimately considerable fibrosis develops in association with the amyloid. In the ventricle, the dominant clinical picture is of a restrictive abnormality due to splinting of the myocyte by amyloid deposited on its surface. Atrial involvement by AL, AF or AA amyloid has a pattern identical to that of isolated atrial amyloid, but is often more extensive. Nodules of amyloid may develop in the cusps of any of the valves.

Macroscopically, ventricular involvement with amyloid gives anything from close to normal shape to symmetric wall thickening with a hard rubbery feel. The firm nature of the atrial walls is often striking and subendocardial brown nodules may be visible (Fig. 5.48). A small proportion of cases develop very thick-walled asymmetric ventricles (Fig. 5.49). The similarity

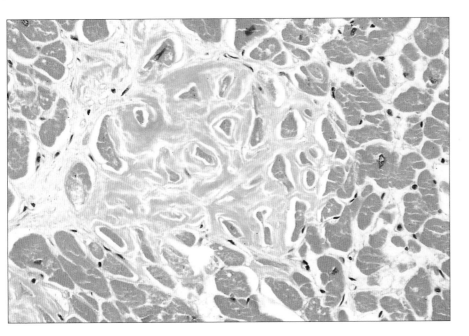

Figure 5.47a
Cardiac amyloid. In sections stained with haematoxylin and eosin the amyloid is pale pink, but its distribution in a focal area with a lattice containing some surviving myocytes makes the appearance distinguishable from collagen (H&E ×87.5).

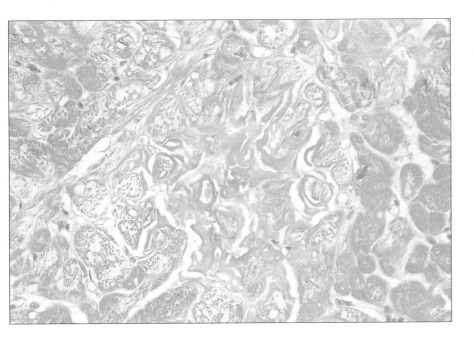

Figure 5.47b
In sections stained with trichrome methods the lattice appearance is more easily appreciated. Amyloid stains a grey/pale blue colour in trichrome stains (Trichrome ×87.5).

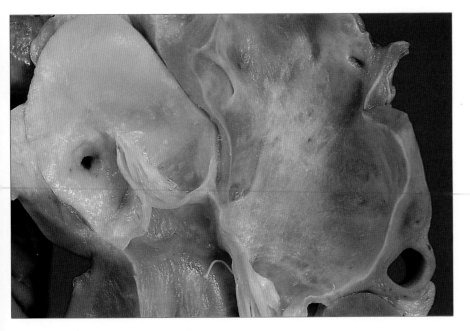

Figure 5.48
Amyloid heart disease. The left atrial endocardium in formalin-fixed specimens shows nodules of brown material arranged in a dot-like pattern or as more irregular shaped deposits. These deposits are translucent in the fresh specimen and very difficult to see until fixation has occurred.

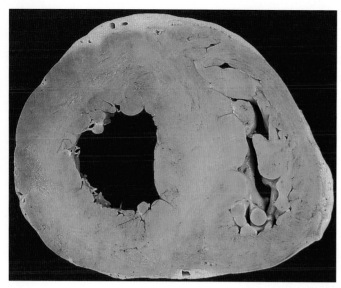

Figure 5.49

Amyloid heart disease. The transverse slice of the ventricles shows very marked LV wall thickening with disproportionate thickening of the septum mimicking hypertrophic cardiomyopathy.

between some cases of amyloid and hypertrophic cardiomyopathy on echocardiography in life is often striking. The histological and ultrastructural characteristics of amyloid are shown in Figs 5.50–5.52. The familial forms of amyloid can be treated by liver transplantation and it may be necessary to type the amyloid by immunohistochemistry to detect this type of case.

Obliterative cardiomyopathy

Two forms exist; one occurs in temperate climates and is closely associated with systemic eosinophilia; this is often a relatively acute disease. In tropical climates a more chronic form exists (endomyocardial fibrosis – EMF) which may, or may not be, related to eosinophilia. The end-stages of both diseases are identical, leading to a view that they are both the same disease seen at different stages. This view is however firmly denied by others (Kartha and Gupta 1993; Valiathon *et al.* 1993; Shaper 1993). Whatever the pathogenesis the two groups form a continuum for purposes of morphological description.

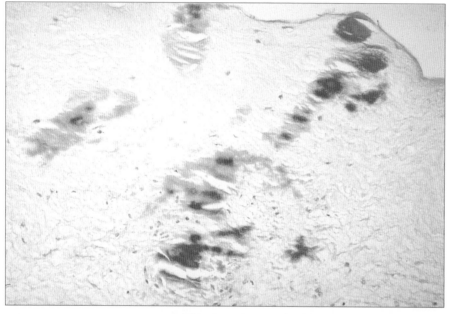

Figure 5.50 a,b

Cardiac amyloid. Stained with Congo red. Amyloid appears pale red (a) but when viewed under polarised light gives this apple green colour. (b) Not all the amyloid within the section gives a green colour. Collagen gives a different grey refractile colour.

These amyloid deposits are just beneath the left atrial endocardium (Congo red ×18.9).

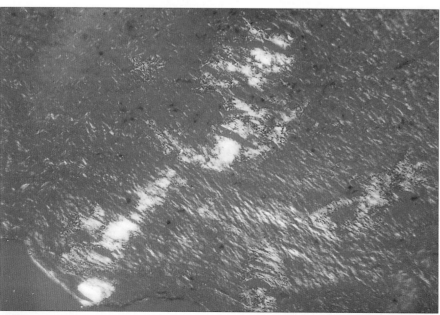

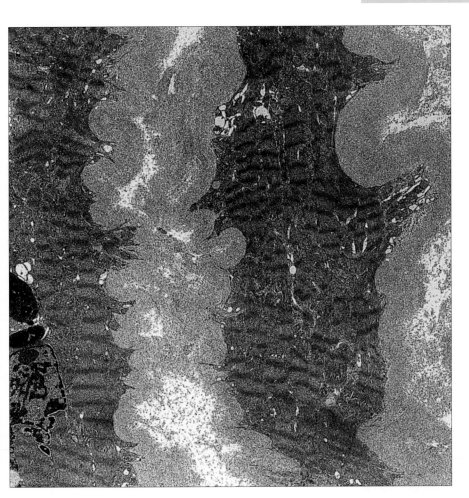

Figure 5.51
Cardiac amyloid. The characteristic ultrastructural appearance is of a layer of fibrillary material exactly coating the external surface of the myocytes. This distribution is unique and separates the appearance from interstitial fibrosis.

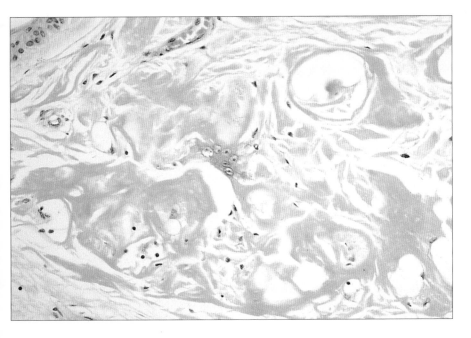

Figure 5.52
Amyloid heart disease. This intramyocardial focus is more advanced than that in Fig. 5.47. All the myocytes have been lost but the lattice appearance is still retained. A giant cell response has occurred (H&E ×87.5).

In temperate climates, a relatively acute onset is associated with any cause of eosinophilia in which the proportion of circulating degranulated cells is high. The cause of the eosinophilia is immaterial, and ranges through eosinophilic leukaemia, pulmonary eosinophilia, Churg–Strauss syndrome, idiopathic causes and ulcerative colitis. The disease represents damage to the endocardium by cationic proteins released by the eosinophils in the circulation (Sasano 1989).

In the acute phase, a shaggy coat of thrombus covers the endocardium of one or both ventricles (Figs 5.53). The usual sites are the inflow tracts and apical portions of the ventricle. Thrombus smoothes out the trabecular pattern and obliterates the apices of the ventricles on

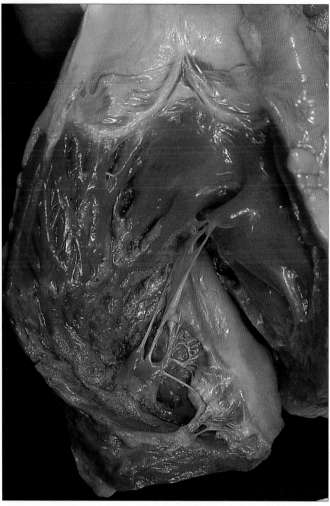

Figure 5.53
Endomyocardial fibrosis (non-tropical). This patient had idiopathic hypereosinophilia. The apex of the right ventricle is covered by a shaggy coat of thrombus.

organises from the base (Figs 5.54), ultimately covering the endocardium with a thick white sheet of fibrous tissue. In the acute phase the thrombus may contain numerous eosinophils, but these often vanish as the disease progresses. The thrombus extends down into the cracks and crevices of the endocardium, but there may also be some inflammatory infiltration and replacement fibrosis of the subendocardial myocardium. In a few cases the myocardial extension is more pronounced and eosinophils are very numerous. Such cases are known as Löeffler's eosinophilic endomyocarditis.

When the disease is burnt out, the endocardium is a dense white fibrous sheet which can be decorticated to improve ventricular function.

Tropical endomyocardial fibrosis

This condition has a striking geographic distribution within a 12° latitude band on either side of the equator in Africa, India and South America. Numerous unproven theories exist to explain the pathogenesis. These include a relation to hypereosinophilia, an aberrant response to streptococcal infection, autoimmunity induced by chronic malaria, deficiencies or excesses of trace elements and dietary toxins.

The macroscopic features are of dense white fibrosis effacing the trabeculae and obliterating the apex of one or both ventricles. Dense sheets of fibrous tissue may extend up toward the outflow tracts and involve both atrio-ventricular valves. Histologically there is dense fibrosis with some chronic inflammatory cells, but eosinophils and acute thrombus are very rare.

Arrhythmogenic cardiomyopathies

In these conditions, ventricular contraction is preserved and cardiac failure is absent leading to a normal exercise tolerance. However, the patients are troubled by episodic ventricular tachycardia and syncope, and have a high risk of sudden death.

angiography in life (Fig. 5.26). Thrombus surrounds the papillary muscles and may incorporate the chordae leading to mitral regurgitation. The layer of thrombus

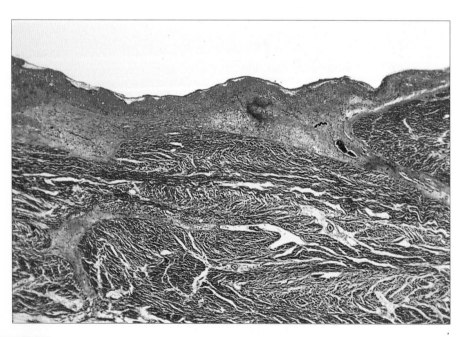

Figure 5.54
Endomyocardial fibrosis. The histology of the case in Fig. 5.50 shows that the layer of thrombus (red) is being organised from the underlying endocardium with new blood vessels and the deposition of collagen (blue) which begins to efface the trabecular pattern of the ventricle (Trichrome ×87.5).

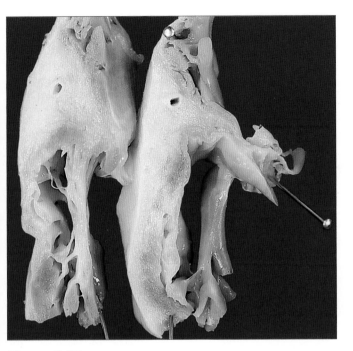

Figure 5.55
Arrhythmogenic right ventricular dysplasia. Two longitudinal sections of the right ventricle through the tricuspid valve show focal very localised replacement of the wall by fat and fibrous tissue. There is marked thinning of the wall. Sudden death, female aged 37. Previously well, other than fainted when became emotional.

The best-defined subgroup (Thiene *et al*. 1988; Gerlis *et al*. 1993) is right ventricular dysplasia (RVD) also known as arrhythmogenic right ventricular dysplasia (ARVD). Segments of the right ventricle show dilatation and thinning of the wall which is translucent (Figs 5.27, 5.29, 5.55). In these segments myocytes have vanished and been replaced by both adipose and fibrous tissue (Fig. 5.56). The thinned areas are often translucent. Rarely, the whole right ventricle is dilated and thin-walled, but mural thrombus does not usually occur. In

about half the cases associated with the myocyte loss there is a chronic inflammatory infiltrate.

The condition is strongly familial. Surveys of large families show that the degree of right ventricular abnormality is very variable and there are appreciable numbers of asymptomatic carriers. Sudden death can, however, occur in all. The lesser degrees of right ventricular dysplasia can easily be missed at autopsy in cases of sudden death. A European registry of fatal cases with autopsy data shows that in approximately one-third of cases there is some left ventricular involvement which takes the form of subepicardial posterior wall fibrosis and fatty infiltration and linear depressed scars in the septum. The pattern of fibrosis is totally different from that seen in coronary disease.

Care must be taken not to overinterpret fatty infiltration of the right ventricle. As an age-related change, particularly in women, adipose infiltration between atrial and right ventricular myocytes is common. Adipose tissue extends in as a finger-like protrusion from the epicardium. It is not associated with fibrosis, and myocytes are pushed apart rather than replaced. The ventricular wall becomes thick rather than thin.

A study which analysed right ventricular cardiac biopsies in a wide range of conditions including right ventricular dysplasia, highlights the difficulty facing the pathologist is assessing the significance of adipose tissue in the myocardium (Dembinksi *et al*. 1994). The presence of some adipose tissue in one fragment is almost universal when at least six fragments are taken at each biopsy session. In right ventricular dysplasia both the tissue area occupied by fat and the number of fragments containing fat are significantly greater than in any other condition. However, this study compared the biopsy findings in subjects with a clinical diagnosis of right ventricular dysplasia with conditions such as allografts (transplanted hearts) and dilated cardiomyopathy. It is a very

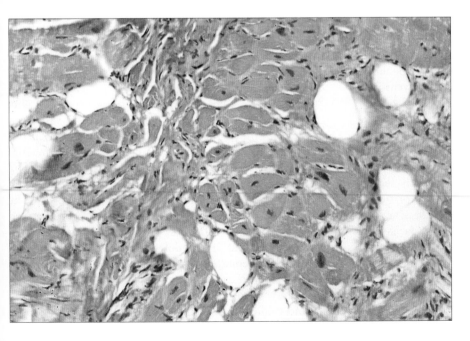

Figure 5.56
Arrhythmogenic right ventricular dysplasia. The histology shows replacement of the right ventricular myocytes with fat and fibrous tissue (Picro Mallory ×87.5).

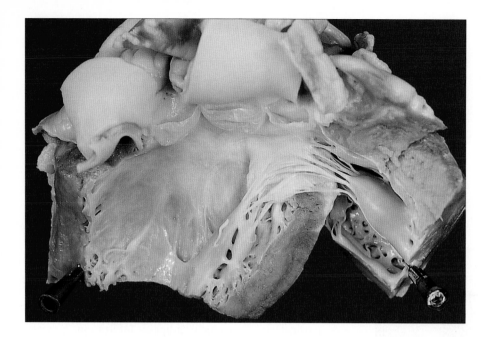

Figure 5.57
Endocardial fibroelastosis. The left ventricle is somewhat dilated and the endocardium, particularly over the septum, shows uniform white endocardial thickening. The right coronary artery was anomalous, rising from the pulmonary artery.

different matter to interpret fat in a biopsy taken for the investigation of an arrhythmia in a subject with normal right ventricular structure and function. The pathologist should record how many fragments contain fat and the approximate tissue area occupied by fat. These data can be used as one element in arriving at a diagnosis alongside other criteria such as a family history, in labelling the case right ventricular dysplasia.

Although very active studies searching for gene linkage in families with ARVD are underway in several centres, the gene or genes responsible are not yet known. In the UK the condition is far less common than hypertrophic cardiomyopathy, but in northern Italy the gene appears more common.

In a small number of cases the left ventricular changes predominate, suggesting that there may be a left ventricular dysplasia which is part of the phenotypic spectrum that the ARVD gene produces.

Idiopathic myocardial fibrosis

Myocardial fibrosis occurring both as macroscopic or microscopic scarring in subjects who do not have chronic cardiac failure but who present with ventricular tachycardia and/or sudden death present a pathological challenge. Fibrosis is the end-stage of a wide variety of mechanisms of cardiac damage. Some of these will be revealed by the previous medical history, i.e. radiation or scleroderma, in others their pathogenesis remains unknown. Ischaemic scarring is usually recognised by the presence of severe coronary artery stenosis, due to atheroma and at least some of the scars are regional and transmural in distribution. Ischaemic scarring is usually maximal in the subendocardial zones. In all hypertrophied hearts and in particular those due to pressure overload such as hypertension or aortic stenosis, subendocardial fibrosis develops even in the absence of coronary atherosclerosis. In normal weight

hearts idiopathic fibrosis takes a number of forms. Macroscopically the distribution is often strikingly different from ischaemic disease. Scars may be subpericardial and are often circumferential and linear with depression of the tissue in cross-sections of the ventricle. The septum and posterior wall are often maximally involved. Such scarring is often ascribed by default to previous acute myocarditis, but this hypothesis cannot be proven unless there has been a clear clinical history of an acute episode in the past. The scarring pattern is often very like the left ventricular involvement in right ventricular dysplasia, and the skeletal muscle dystrophies such as myotonia dystrophica. Some idiopathic fibrosis may therefore be genetic with the phenotypic expression being confined to the heart.

Endocardial fibroelastosis

This condition in which the endocardium in the left ventricle and/or left atrium becomes uniformly white and thick (Fig. 5.57) is a secondary response by the endocardial tissue to abnormal flow and pressure *in utero* or in the first few years of life (Fishbein *et al.* 1977). Histologically the endocardium contains many new elastic lamina, but fibrosis does not extend into the myocardium and thrombosis is not present in marked contrast to EMF. Endocardial fibroelastosis is now regarded as an endocardial response to a variety of stimuli, rather than being a discrete homogeneous entity. In infancy a range of congenital abnormalities are associated with endocardial fibroelastosis, including anomalous coronary arteries, aortic valve stenosis, aortic hypoplasia and mitral valve hypoplasia. The hypoplastic left heart syndromes all have pronounced endocardial fibroelastosis. Cases are encountered both in infancy and up to adolescence in which there is no associated congenital anomaly but the left ventricle is dilated. Such cases differ only from a dilated cardiomyopathy in the degree of white endocardial thickening and in the youth of the subject. These cases are proba-

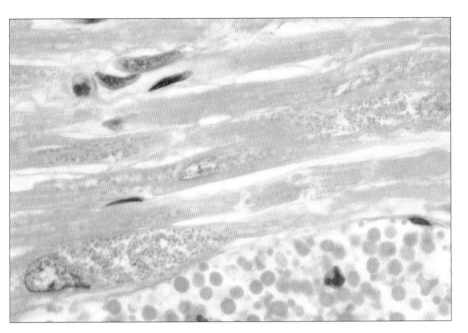

Figure 5.58
Haemochromatosis in the myocardium. There is a diffuse deposition of a brown pigment throughout many of the myocytes. Compare this to lipofuscin granules in Fig. 5.58 (H&E ×56).

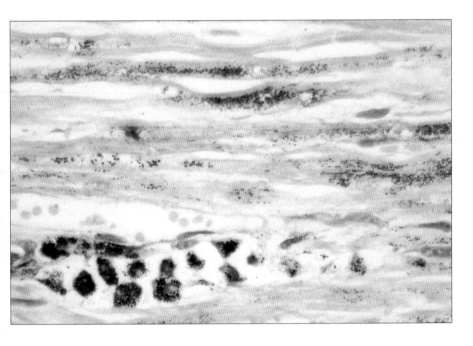

Figure 5.59
Haemochromatosis. In the Perls stain on the myocardium in Fig. 5.56 the brown intramyocardial pigment is shown to be iron. Iron pigment has also accumulated in macrophages following myocyte death (Perls stain ×56).

bly due to myocardial dysfunction during early life, and the morphological picture can occur in any metabolic genetic myocardial defect.

Other cases have been linked to mumps infection presumably with myocarditis *in utero* or in neonatal life (Ni *et al*. 1997). Studies have been made of the prognosis of cases diagnosed in life either by the echocardiogram demonstrating a thick endocardium, or by biopsy and in whom there was no congenital structural defect such as aortic hypoplasia. About a third of the patients died within 10 years and 50% had chronic cardiac failure (Ino *et al*. 1988). Sudden death may occur in adolescence.

Division of cases has been made into those with a dilated left ventricle akin to a dilated cardiomyopathy in pathophysiology, and those in whom the left ventricle remains small and the pathophysiology is restrictive

in type (Rowe *et al*. 1987). Dilated cardiomyopathy and endocardial fibroelastosis of the dilated type are a continuum in childhood cases; which label the pathologist applies is a personal choice. The possibility of a familial metabolic defect in the myocardium should always be considered.

Myocardial storage disease

Deposition of iron, glycogen, oxalates and a large number of other very rare metabolic substances may produce dilated, restrictive or hypertrophic functional abnormalities.

Iron storage disorders

In both primary haemochromatosis due to increased intestinal absorption of iron, and in chronic haemolytic anaemias treated by transfusion, excess iron may be

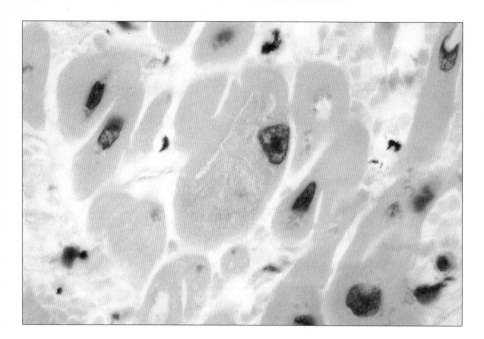

Figure 5.60
Mucoid (basophilic) degeneration of myocytes. An individual myocyte contains a blue grey amorphous inclusion within the cytoplasm. The adjacent myocytes contain lipofuscin as brown granules particularly in the perinuclear zone (H&E ×224).

deposited in the myocardium (Barosi *et al.* 1989). Iron is present within myocytes, particularly in the perinuclear zone (Figs 5.58, 5.59). Myocyte death develops leading to increasing interstitial fibrosis within which there is iron containing macrophages. The commonest functional changes are a dilated or restrictive physiology; conduction disturbances are common due to iron deposition in the atrioventricular node. At autopsy the heart in severe cases is mahogany brown in colour.

Basophilic degeneration of myocytes

Sections of myocardium stained with haematoxylin and eosin frequently show individual myocytes in which there is a slightly granular blue material (Fig. 5.60). This appearance has been called basophilic or mucoid degeneration (Tamua *et al.* 1995). The material is PAS positive and resistant to diastase, stains red with Best's carmine, is metachromatic with toluidine blue, and blue/green with alcian blue suggesting that it is a glycoprotein. The material is antigenically identical to the polyglucosan which accumulates in the type IV glycogen storage disease caused by branching enzyme deficiency.

Individual myocytes showing this change can be found in virtually all hearts, irrespective of the cause of death provided that enough sections are examined. There is however considerable variation in the number of myocytes showing this change from case to case. In some individuals every section will have some abnormal cells. The frequency rises with age, but to a less striking degree than lipofuscin or atrial amyloid. An increase in the number of abnormal myocytes is described in hypothyroidism, but is not specific for the condition.

Brown atrophy of the myocardium

Lipofuscin is present within the perinuclear areas of myocytes (Fig. 5.60) and steadily increases with age. The pigment results from lipid peroxidation of cell membranes and does not appear to be cytotoxic. Any disease process which causes myocyte death will release lipofuscin which will be ingested by macrophages in the interstitial tissues. In old age, the total heart weight often drops due to prolonged immobility and the accumulation of lipofuscin leads to a small brown heart macroscopically. It is very doubtful if this leads to any major functional abnormality and it should not be given as a primary cause of death.

Glycogen storage disorders

The classic Pompe 'cardiomegalia glycogenica' is due to the genetic lack of alpha-1,4 glucosidase, a lysosomal enzyme concerned with the conversion of glycogen into glucose. Glycogen accumulates within myocytes giving them a vacuolated appearance with a paucity of myofibrils (Fig. 5.61). The glycogen is brightly PAS positive. The heart often enlarges with a thick-walled asymmetric left ventricle simulating hypertrophic cardiomyopathy (di Sant'Agnese 1959).

Fabry's disease

Fabry's disease is a deficiency of the lysosomal enzyme galactosidase A that catabolises glycophosphophingolipids. These substances accumulate in the tissues leading to CNS disturbances, skeletal muscle weakness, renal tubular disease, skin nodules and cardiac abnormalities. The heart shows marked left ventricular hypertrophy which may be asymmetric due to septal thickening. The myocytes appear vacuolated and distorted. Unless the history is known or electron microscopy carried out to show the characteristic lysosomal accumulation of a granular and lamellar material, it is very easy to misdiagnose a case as hypertrophic cardiomyopathy.

ENDOCRINE DISORDERS AFFECTING THE MYOCARDIUM

A number of endocrine disorders will directly affect the myocardium contributing to a cardiac or sudden death.

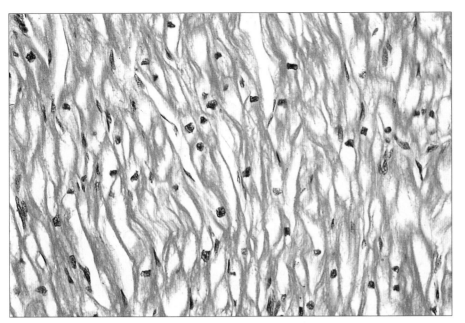

Figure 5.61
Glycogen storage disease. All the myocytes appear vacuolated due to the accumulation of glycogen (H&E ×35).

The thyroid hormones increase the activity of ATPase and enhance both myocardial contraction and oxygen consumption raising heart rate and stroke volume. The major clinical effect on the heart is tachycardia and atrial fibrillation. Clinical studies suggest that mild left ventricular hypertrophy may develop (Forfar *et al.* 1982). There are no specific cardiac morphological changes. Sudden deaths do occur occasionally in thyrotoxicosis, probably due to increased myocardial sensitivity to catecholamines. Hypothyroidism has been associated with more specific cardiac changes causing heart failure. The heart is often described as pale and flabby with mucoid oedema of the visceral pericardium and an effusion which may contain cholesterol crystals (Aber and Thompson 1963). The cholesterol levels in the plasma in long-standing myxoedema are often very high indeed and lead to accelerated coronary atherosclerosis which is a major cause of heart failure. In addition to disease in the major epicardial arteries, smaller epicardial arteries and intramyocardial arteries show intense foam cell infiltration of the intima narrowing the lumen. The myocardium in such cases will show focal acute and chronic ischaemic damage. Other changes in the myocardium include unduly vacuolated myocytes indicating some myofibrillary loss, interstitial oedema and basophilic mucoid degeneration of myocytes. This last change is not specific for myxoedema.

In acromegaly, the action of growth hormone leads to cardiac enlargement which is often disproportionate to other organomegaly. Cardiac complications occur in up to one-third of cases, and cause both cardiac failure and sudden death. In part, the cardiomegaly reflects coexistent hypertension which is found in up to 50% of cases. The heart in acromegaly is strikingly large with hearts over 1000 g in total weight being known (Lie 1980). Left ventricular wall thickness is usually markedly increased relative to the chamber size. Histologically, interstitial fibrosis is increased and myocyte diameters are increased. Although the term acromegalic cardiomyopathy is sometimes used, the heart failure which occurs is probably largely due to hypertension and the secondary changes such as fibrosis that inevitably occur with this degree of hypertrophy.

INTERPRETATION OF CARDIAC BIOPSIES

The potential indications for obtaining a cardiac biopsy are shown in Table 5.18. Cardiac biopsies are usually obtained by passing a bioptome into the right atrium and then across the tricuspid valve into the right ventricle. The tip of the catheter is impacted into the endocardium, the jaws closed and the catheter withdrawn to yield a sample of myocardium 1–4 mm in diameter. The process is usually repeated to give up to six specimens in each patient during the same

Table 5.18
Indications for cardiac biopsy.

Established as being of clinical use
Management of cardiac transplantation
Monitoring adriamycin therapy
Elucidation of cause of RCM – diagnosis of cardiac amyloid
Diagnosis of acute myocarditis
Confirmation iron storage disease – monitoring chelation therapy
Possible clinical use
Diagnosis of sarcoid heart disease
Investigation of DCM
Investigation of ventricular tachycardia
Obtain tissue diagnosis in tumours
Confirm endomyocardial fibrosis (EMF)

catheter session. The biopsy catheter is usually directed to the interventricular septum, but samples are often obtained from the free wall of the right ventricle indicating the difficulty in placing the catheter tip with accuracy. Some centres place a sheath across the tricuspid valve and pass the biopsy catheter through the sheath. The multiple biopsies obtained usually come from the same area where the tip of the sheath is wedged. It is possible to pass a sheath across the aortic valve to biopsy the left ventricular myocardium but this technique is not routinely used by most centres.

Complications of cardiac biopsy

The major complication is perforation of the right ventricular free wall. Perforation is relatively common and occurs in up to 1% of attempts to obtain cardiac biopsies. In the majority of cases, bleeding into the pericardium is self-limiting, but in an occasional case draining the pericardium to prevent tamponade is required. In a small number of these, open operation to close a hole in the right ventricle may be required. When a cardiac biopsy contains epicardial tissues, the clinicians should be informed at once in order that the patient is monitored closely to exclude progressive intrapericardial bleeding.

Morphological interpretation of cardiac biopsies

The very specialised interpretation needed to monitor cardiac rejection and adriamycin therapy (Billingham and Bristow 1984) means that experience in these areas is essential. These are not areas in which pathologists should try to interpret on an occasional basis and are not discussed here.

The pathological responses in myocardial tissue are somewhat limited, but the pathologist should have a check-list of different components to assess as normal or abnormal. Any report should indicate the number and size of the tissue fragments obtained at each catheter session. The larger the size and number of fragments the greater is the reliability of data.

The presence or absence of endocardium should be recorded and any increase in thickness noted. Many fragments do not have an endocardial surface, due to the bioptome tip penetrating into the myocardium before the jaws were closed.

Myocyte morphology should be assessed. The mean diameter of myocytes at the point where the cell contains a nucleus can be measured or a simple visual assessment made. A visual assessment should be made of whether the myocytes contain the usual amount of myofibrillary material, or whether they appear empty and vacuolated due to a reduction in myofibrillary content. The assessment of this feature is best carried out on H&E stained sections. The amount and distribution of collagen should be assessed visually, or

formally measured by point counting or in a quantification system. The stain used to demonstrate collagen depends on personal choice and can be variants of the trichrome method, Van Gieson staining or Sirius red. Fibrosis can be even and diffuse, surrounding individual myocytes, or be as focal course scars.

An important function of cardiac biopsy is to confirm or exclude acute myocarditis. In florid cases the increase in the number of nuclei and cells in the interstitial spaces is obvious in H&E staining of paraffin embedded material. Less florid cases are far more difficult to interpret in conventionally fixed and H&E sections. It is very easy to mistake endothelial nuclei for lymphocytes. For this reason it is now advisable, if acute myocarditis is the clinical diagnosis, to freeze at least two biopsies for immunohistochemical identification of interstitial cells. The rapidly improving antibodies to mark T-cells in paraffin embedded tissue will affect this need.

If any pigment is present, staining for iron should be used. Any suspicion of amyloid should prompt the use of Congo red staining on 7–8 μm thick sections, followed by examination of the biopsy under polarised light. Small amounts of amyloid mixed with collagen may be difficult to identify in biopsies, and if the original differential diagnosis includes amyloidosis, one biopsy should be fixed in a way suitable for electron microscopy.

Artefacts in cardiac biopsies

Myocardial biopsies are subject to some potentially misleading artefacts. As the biopsy is torn away from the beating heart, the myocytes undergo an intense injury-mediated hypercontraction. This appearance is identical to contraction band necrosis, and is maximal at the edges of the biopsy. When it extends throughout the biopsy and the myocytes are cut in the transverse plane, an appearance of empty vacuolated myocytes alongside dense brightly eosinophilic myocytes is produced. Blood vessels in the biopsies may show invagination giving the appearance of a vessel within a vessel.

Biopsy findings in cardiomyopathy

Myocarditis

Acute myocarditis is a diagnosis made by demonstrating an excess of lymphocytes in the interstitial tissues. This raises in turn the difficulty in recognising lymphocytes and the number needed to make a diagnosis of myocarditis. Recognition is best carried out in frozen sections using immunohistochemistry – the number of lymphocytes needed has been put as low as a mean of three per high power ($\times 40$) microscopy fields. Complementary immunohistochemistry to show inappropriate class II MHC expression ICAM and VCAM expression has been suggested to improve the sensitivity of the biopsy diagnosis of acute myocarditis (Kuhl *et al.* 1996). Nevertheless, it seems likely that there will be continuing discord between different laboratories over what is or is not acute myocarditis on biopsy.

Sarcoid heart disease can be recognised on biopsy by finding discrete non-caseating granulomas with giant cells (Ratner *et al.* 1986). Myocardial sarcoid is however a patchy rather than a uniform disease, and although a biopsy positive result is useful, there will be many false negative results. Personal experience suggests that the biopsy positive rate is less than 20%, even when the clinical diagnosis of myocardial sarcoid is a firm one.

Dilated cardiomyopathy

The morphological features of a dilated cardiomyopathy are neither consistent nor specific. Cardiac biopsies in dilated cardiomyopathy are usually done in the clinical context that ischaemic heart disease has been excluded by coronary angiography. All the pathologist can do is to record the presence of abnormal features and state whether these are consistent with a diagnosis of a dilated cardiomyopathy. It is not possible to make an absolute diagnosis of a dilated cardiomyopathy.

Hypertrophic cardiomyopathy

Hypertrophic cardiomyopathy is a myocardial disease which is seldom uniform throughout the myocardium. The sites at which maximum disarray occur are not easily reached by the bioptome and many biopsies would be false negatives. Biopsy is not the way to distinguish between ordinary hypertrophy and hypertrophic cardiomyopathy if there is clinical doubt. Nevertheless biopsies are often taken in hypertrophic cardiomyopathy and a small proportion will show disarray. Stains which delineate the myofibrillary structure within the myocyte such as PTAH are helpful in highlighting disarray.

Restrictive cardiomyopathy

Restrictive cardiomyopathy is a condition where cardiac biopsy has a defined clinical use. The causes of a restrictive cardiomyopathy include haemosiderosis, amyloid deposition, interstitial fibrosis and variants of hypertrophic cardiomyopathy. All of these can be recognised on biopsy. Fibrosis causing restriction is usually diffuse and each myocyte is surrounded by fine collagen. Familial restrictive cardiomyopathy is usually due to amyloid or to hypertrophy/disarray. Although disarray may not be present in a biopsy, marked myocyte hypertrophy suggests the diagnosis is the familial form related to hypertrophic cardiomyopathy. A totally normal biopsy in restrictive cardiomyopathy raises the possibility that the diagnosis is in fact pericardial constriction.

Biopsy in ventricular arrhythmias

Biopsies are sometimes taken in patients with ventricular tachycardia in order to exclude structural heart disease. The pathologist should record any abnormality, particularly concentrating on whether there is an excess of fibrosis. Fibrosis is a substrate for chronic re-entrant arrhythmias in the myocardium. The greater the amount of fibrosis the more likely is this to be causally related to the arrhythmia. The cause of the fibrosis, however, is not revealed by biopsy. In right ventricular dysplasia there is both fibrosis and replacement of myocytes by adipose tissue. Some infiltration of the right ventricular myocardium by adipose tissue is an age- and female-related phenomenon, not specifically related to any disease process. Fatty infiltration is, however, more pronounced in right ventricular dysplasia.

Rare indications for cardiac biopsy

Endomyocardial fibrosis is on occasion biopsied to try to confirm the diagnosis. In the late stage of the disease biopsies are difficult to obtain, due to the failure of the bioptome jaws to grip the thick fibrous tissue. If biopsies are obtained, these will show rather cellular fibrous tissue which contains some chronic inflammatory cells and often eosinophils and haemosiderin. Biopsy fragments of intracavity tumours are often attempted, particularly those in the right atrium or ventricle. The failure rate of achieving a fragment of tumour is very high, but an occasional case of haemangiosarcoma can be identified avoiding open exploration.

References

Aber C, Thompson G. Factors associated with cardiac enlargement in myxoedema. *Br Heart J* 1963;**25**:421.

Alexander C. Cobalt in the heart. *Ann Intern Med* 1969;**70**:411–3.

Anversa P, Olivetti G, Capasso J. Cellular basis of ventricular remodelling after myocardial infarction. *Am J Cardiol* 1991;**68**:7D-16D.

Aretz HT, Billingham ME, Edwards WD *et al.* Myocarditis: a histopathologic definition and classification. *Am J Cardiovasc Pathol* 1987;**1**:3–14.

Aretz H. Myocarditis: The Dallas Criteria. *Hum Pathol* 1987;**18**:619–24.

Barosi G, Arbustini E, Gavazzi A, Grasso M, Pucci A. Myocardial iron grading by endomyocardial biopsy. A clinicopathologic study on iron overloaded patients. *Eur J Haematol* 1989;**42**:383–8.

Beggs AH. Dystrophinopathy, the expanding phenotype. Dystrophin abnormalities in X-linked dilated cardiomyopathy. *Circulation* 1997;**95**:2344–7.

Berg R, Kaplan A, Jarrett P, Molthan M. Freidreich's ataxia with acute cardiomyopathy. *Am J Dis Child* 1980;**134**:390–3.

Billingham M, Bristow M. Evaluation of anthracycline cardiotoxicity: predictive ability and functional correlation of endomyocardial biopsy. *Cancer Treat Symp* 1984;**3**:71–6.

Billingham M. Pharmacotoxic myocardial disease: An endomyocardial study. In: Sekiguchi M, Olsen E, Goodwin J (eds). *Myocarditis and related disorders.* Heidelberg: Springer-Verlag, 1985; 282.

Bisno A. Group A streptococcal infections and acute rheumatic fever. *N Engl J Med* 1991;**325**:783.

Boehm T, Dickerson R, Glasser S. Hypertrophic subaortic stenosis in Friedreich's ataxia. *Am J Med Sci* 1970;**260**:279–84.

Buja L, Ferrans W, Roberts W. Drug-induced cardiomyopathies. *Adv Cardiol* 1974;**13**:330–48.

Burke J, Medline N, Katz A. Giant cell myocarditis and myositis associated with thymoma and myasthenia gravis. *Arch Pathol* 1969;**88**:359–66.

Burch M, Mann J, Sharland M, Shinebourne E, Davies M, McKenna W. Myocardial disarray in Noonan syndrome. *Br Heart J* 1992;**68**:586–9.

Burch M, Sharland M, Shinebourne E, Smith G, Patton M, McKenna W. Cardiological abnormalities in Noonan syndrome: Phenotypic diagnosis and echocardiographic assessment of 118 patients. *J Am Coll Cardiol* 1993;**22**:1189–92.

Butler I, Gadoth N. Kearns-Sayre's syndrome: A review of a multisystem disorder in children and young adults. *Arch Intern Med* 1976;**136**:1290–3.

Chow L, Ye Y, Linder J. Phenotypic analysis of infiltrating cells in human myocarditis. *Arch Pathol Lab Med* 1989;**13**:1357–62.

Cooper LT, Berry GJ, Rizeq M, Schroeder JS. Giant cell myocarditis. *J Heart Lung Transplant* 1995;**14**: 394–401.

Cornwall G, Murdoch W, Kyle R, Westermark P, Pitkanen P. Frequency and distribution of senile cardiovascular amyloid. *Am J Med* 1983;**75**:618–23.

Cunningham F, Pritchard J, Hankins G, Anderson P, Lucas M, Armstrong K. Peripartum heart failure: Idiopathic cardiomyopathy or compounding cardiovascular events. *Obstet Gynaecol* 1986;**67**:157–68.

Cunningham M, McCormack J, Fenderson P. Human and murine antibodies cross-reactive with streptococcal M protein and myosin recognise the sequence GLN-LYS-SER-LYS-GLN in M protein. *J Immunol* 1989;**143**:2677–83.

Davies MJ, McKenna WJ. Hypertrophic cardiomyopathy – pathology and pathogenesis. *Histopathology* 1995;**26**:493–500.

Davies M, Pomerance A, Teare R. Idiopathic giant cell myocarditis – a distinctive clinico-pathologic entity. *Br Heart J* 1975;**37**:192–5.

Dembinski A, Dobson J, Wilson J. Frequency, extent, and distribution of endomyocardial adipose tissue: morphometric analysis of endomyocardial biopsy specimens from 241 patients. *Cardiovasc Pathol* 1994;**3**:33.

di Sant'Agnese P. Diseases of glycogen storage with special reference to the cardiac type of generalized glycogenosis. *Ann NY Acad Sci* 1959;**72**:439.

Fishbein M, Ferrans V, Roberts W. Histologic and ultrastructural features of primary and secondary endocardial fibroelastosis. *Arch Pathol Lab Med* 1977;**101**:49–54.

Fleming H, Bailey S. Sarcoidosis of the heart. *J R Coll Physicians* 1981;**15**:245–53.

Forfar J, Muir A, Sawer S, Toft A. Abnormal left ventricular function in hypothyroidism. *N Engl J Med* 1982;**307**:1165–70.

Frankel K, Rosser R. The pathology of the heart in progressive muscular dystrophy: epimyocardial fibrosis. *Human Pathol* 1976;**7**:375–86.

Frohlich E, Apstein C, Chobanian A. The heart in hypertension. *Am Heart J* 1992;**327**:998–1008.

Fulton R, Hutchinson E, Morgan-Jones A. Ventricular weight in cardiac hypertrophy. *Br Heart J* 1952;**14**:413–20.

Garcia-Palmiere M. Rheumatic fever and rheumatic heart disease as seen in the tropics. *Am Heart J* 1962;**64**:577–83.

Gerdes A, Kellerman S, Moore J, *et al*. Structural remodelling of cardiac myocytes in patients with ischemic cardiomyopathy. *Circulation* 1992;**86**: 426–30.

Gerlis L, Schmidt-Ott S, Ho S, Anderson R. Dysplastic conditions of the right ventricular myocardium: Uhl's anomaly v arrhythmogenic right ventricular dysplasia. *Br Heart J* 1993;**69**:142–150.

Grist N, Reid D. Epidemiology of viral infections of the heart. In: Banatvala J (ed). *Viral infections of the heart*. London: Edward Arnold, 1992; 23–31.

Grossman W, Jones D, McLaurin L. Wall stress and patterns of hypertrophy in the human left ventricle. *J Clin Invest* 1975;**56**:56–64.

Guarnieri T, Lakatta EG. Mechanism of myocardial contractile depression by clinical concentration of ethanol. *J Clin Invest* 1990;**85**:1462–7.

Hangartner J, Marley N, Whitehead A, Thomas A, Davies M. The assessment of cardiac hypertrophy at autopsy. *Histopathology* 1985;**9**:1295–306.

Harding A, Langton A. The heart disease of Friedreich's ataxia: a clinical and electrocardiographic study of 115 patients with an analysis of serial electrocardiographic changes in 30 cases. *Q J Med* 1983;**52**: 489–502.

Harper P. Post operative complications in myotonic dystrophy. *Lancet* 1989;**ii**:1269.

Hesse A, Altland K, Linke R *et al*. Cardiac amyloidosis: a review and report of a new transthyretin (prealbumin) variant. *Br Heart J* 1993;**70**:111–5.

Higuchi M, De Morais C, Narreto A, Lopes E, Stolf N, Bellotti G. The role of active myocarditis in the development of heart failure in chronic Chagas' disease. A study based on endomyocardial biopsies. *Clin Cardiol* 1987;**10**:665–70.

Homans D. Peripartum cardiomyopathy. *N Engl J Med* 1985;**312**:1432–7.

Hudson R. Structure and function of the heart. In: *Cardiovascular pathology*, vol 1. London: Edward Arnold, 1965.

Huysman J, Vliegen H, VanderLaarse A, Eulderink F. Changes in nonmyocyte tissue composition associated with pressure overload of hypertrophic human hearts. *Pathol Res Pract* 1989;**184**:577–81.

Isnard R, Kalotka H, Dûrr A, Cossée M *et al*. Correlation between left ventricular hypertrophy and GAA trinucleotide repeat length in Friedreich's ataxia. *Circulation* 1997;**95**:2247–9.

Isner J, Chokshi S. Cardiovascular complications of cocaine. *Curr Probl Cardiol* 1991;**16**:89–123.

Ino T, Benson LN, Freedom RM, Rowe RD. Natural history and prognostic risk factors in endocardial fibroelastosis. *Am J Cardiol* 1988;**62**:431–4.

Kaplan ET. Duckett Jones Memorial Lecture: Global assessment of rheumatic fever and rheumatic heart disease at the close of the century: influences and dynamics of populations and pathogens: a failure to realize prevention. *Circulation* 1993;**88**:1964–72.

Kartha C, Gupta N. Pathological spectrum and possible pathogenesis of endomyocardial fibrosis. In: Valiathan M, Somers K, Chandrasekharan Kartha C (eds). *Endomyocardial fibrosis*. Delhi: Oxford University Press, 1993; 125–40.

Kasper E, Agema W, Hutchins G. The causes of dilated cardiomyopathy: a clinicopathologic review of 673 consecutive patients. *J Am Coll Cardiol* 1994;**23**: 589–90.

Kitzman D, Scholz D, Hagen P, Ilstrup D, Edwards W. Age-related changes in normal human hearts during the first 10 decades of life. Part II maturity: A quantitative anatomic study of 765 specimens from subjects 20 to 99 years old. *Mayo Clin Proc* 1988;**63**:137–46.

Koberle F. Chagas' disease and Chagas' syndrome: the pathology of the trypanosomiasis. *Adv Parasitol* 1968;**6**:63–116.

Kodama M, Matsumoto Y, Fujiwara M. Characteristics of giant cells and factors related to the formation of giant cells in myocarditis. *Circ Res* 1991;**69**: 1042–50.

Komuro I, Kaida T, Shibazaki Y et al. Stretching cardiac myocytes stimulates proto-oncogene expression. *J Biol Chem* 1990;**265**:3595–8.

Kuhl U, Noutsian M, Seeberg H, Schultheiss H-P. Immunohistochemical evidence for a chronic intramyocardial inflammatory process in dilated cardiomyopathy. *Heart* 1996;**75**:295–300.

Latif N, Baker C, Dunn M, Rose M, Brady B, Yacoub M. Frequency and specificity of antiheart antibodies in patients with dilated cardiomyopathy detected using SDS-PAGE and Western blotting. *J Am Coll Cardiol* 1993;**22**:1378–84.

Lie J, Grossman S. Pathology of the heart in acromegaly: anatomic findings in 27 autopsied patients. *Am Heart J* 1980;**100**:41–52.

Luft B, Billingham M, Remington J. Endomyocardial biopsy in the diagnosis of toxoplasmic myocarditis. *Transplant Proc* 1986;**18**:1871–3.

Maeda M, Holder E, Lowes B, Valent S, Bies RD. Dilated cardiomyopathy associated with deficiency of the cytoskeletal protein metavinculin. *Circulation* 1997;**95**:17–20.

Mann J, Jennison S, Moss E, Davies M. Assessment of rejection in orthotopic human heart transplantation using proliferating cell nuclear antigen (PCNA) as an index of cell proliferation. *J Pathol* 1992;**167**:385–9.

Maron B, Lipson L, Roberts W, Savage D, Epstein S. 'Malignant' hypertrophic cardiomyopathy: identification of a subgroup of families with unusually frequent premature death. *Am J Cardiol* 1978;**41**: 1133–40.

Maron B, Anan T, Roberts W. Quantitative analysis of the distribution of cardiac muscle cell disorganisation in the left ventricular wall of patients with hypertrophic cardiomyopathy. *Circulation* 1981;**63**: 882–8.

Maron B, Nicholas PI, Pickle L, Wesley Y, Mulvihill J. Patterns of inheritance in hypertrophic cardiomyopathy: assessment by M-mode and two dimensional echocardiography. *Am J Cardiol* 1984;**53**:1087–94.

Maron B, Spirito P, Wesley Y, Arce J. Development and progression of left ventricular hypertrophy in children with hypertrophic cardiomyopathy. *N Engl J Med* 1986;**315**:610–14.

Maron B, Pelliccia A, Spataro A, Granata M. Reduction in left ventricular wall thickness after deconditioning in highly trained Olympic athletes. *Br Heart J* 1993;**69**:125–8.

Mason JW, O'Connell JB, Herskowitz A et al. A clinical trial of immunosuppressive therapy for myocarditis. *N Engl J Med* 1995;**333**:269–75.

McKenna W, Stewart J, Niyannopoulos P, McGinty F, Davies M. Hypertrophic cardiomyopathy without hypertrophy: Two families with myocardial disarray in the absence of increased myocardial mass. *Br Heart J* 1990;**63**:287–90.

Michels W, Mills P, Miller F, Tajik A, Chu J, Driscoll D. The frequency of familial dilated cardiomyopathy in a series of patients with idiopathic dilated cardiomyopathy. *N Engl J Med* 1992;**326**:77–82.

McManus B, Kandolf R. Myocarditis: evolving concepts of cause, consequence and control. *Curr Opin Cardiol* 1991;**6**:418.

McManus B, Chow L, Wilson J et al. Direct myocardial injury by enterovirus: a central role in the evolution of murine myocarditis. *Clin Immuol Immunopathol* 1993;**68**:159–69.

Mestroni L, Miani D, Di L. Clinical and pathologic study of familial dilated cardiomyopathy. *Am J Cardiol* 1990;**65**:1449–53.

Muntoni F, Cau M, Ganau A, et al. Brief Report: Deletion of the dystrophin muscle-promoter region associated with X-linked dilated cardiomyopathy. *N Engl J Med* 1993;**329**:921–25.

Narula J, Haider N, Virmani R, DiSalvo TG, Kolodgie FD, Hajjar RJ et al. Apoptosis in myocytes in end-stage heart failure. *N Engl J Med* 1996;**335**:1182–9.

Ni J, Bowles NE, Kim Y-H, Demmler G et al. Viral infection of the myocardium in endocardial fibroelastosis. Molecular evidence for the role of mumps virus as an etiologic agent. *Circulation* 1997;**95**: 133–9.

O'Connell J, Costanzo-Nordin M, Subramanian R, et al. Peripartum cardiomyopathy: clinical, hemodynamic, histologic and prognostic characteristics. *J Am Coll Cardiol* 1986;**8**:52–6.

Olivetti G, Melissan M, Balbi T, Quaini F, Sonnenblick E, Anversa P. Myocyte nuclear and possible cellular hyperplasia contribute to ventricular remodelling in the hyertrophic senescent heart in human. *J Am Coll Cardiol* 1994;**24**:140–9.

Olofsson B, Forsberg H, Anderson S, Bjerle P, Hendriksson A, Wedin I. Electrocardiographic findings in myotonic dystrophy. *Br Heart J* 1988;**59**: 47–52.

Pelliccia A, Maron B, Spataro A, Proschan M, Spirito P. The upper limit of physiologic cardiac hypertrophy in highly trained elite athletes. *N Engl J Med* 1991;**324**:295–301.

Poole-Wilson P. Chronic heart failure: Definition, epidemiology, pathophysiology, clinical manifestations and investigations. In: Julian DG, Camm AJ, Fox KM, Hall RJ, Poole-Wilson PA (eds). *Diseases of the heart*. 2nd edn. London: W.B. Saunders, 1996; 467–81.

Ratner S, Fenoglio JJ, Ursell P. Utility of endomyocardial biopsy in the diagnosis of cardiac sarcoidosis. *Chest* 1986;**90**:528–33.

Richardson P. Report of the WHO/ISFC Task Force on the definition and classification of cardiomyopathy. *Circulation* 1996;**93**:341–2.

Roberts W, Waller B. Cardiac amyloidosis causing cardiac dysfunction: analysis of 54 necropsy patients. *Am J Cardiol* 1983;**52**:137–46.

Rowan R, Masek M, Billingham M. Ultrastructural morphometric analysis of endomyocardial biopsies: idiopathic dilated cardiomyopathy anthracycline cardiotoxicity and normal myocardium. *Am J Cardiovasc Pathol* 1988;**2**:137.

Rowe R, Benson L, Wilson G. Clinical diagnosis of left ventricular endocardial fibroelastosis of the dilated type: the Keith criteria and tissue confirmation. *Pediatr Cardiol* 1987;**8**:231.

Saito Y, Nakao K, Arai H, Nishimura K, Okumura K, Obata K. Augmented expression of atrial natriuretic polypeptide gene in ventricle of human failing heart. *J Clin Invest* 1989;**83**:298–305.

Sanyal S, Johnson W. Cardiac conduction abnormalities in children with Duchenne's progressive muscular dystrophy – electroncardiographic features and morphologic correlates. *Circulation* 1982;**66**:853– 63.

Sasano HRV. Eosinophilic products lead to myocardial damage. *Hum Pathol* 1989;**20**:850–7.

Schultheiss HP. Cardiomyopathy: a post-viral autoimmune disease? *Ann Med Int* 1992;**143**:387–90.

Sengers R, Stadhouders A, Lakwi-jk-Vondrovicoavan E, Kubat K, Ruitenbeek A. Hypertrophic cardiomyopathy associated with a mitochondrial myopathy of voluntary muscles and congenital cataract. *Br Heart J* 1985;**54**:543–7.

Shaper A. The aetiology of endomyocardial fibrosis. In: Valiathan M, Somers K, Chandrasekharan Kartha C (eds). *Endomyocardial fibrosis*. Delhi: Oxford University Press, 1993: 121–4.

Shozawa T, Kawamura K, Okada E, Sageshima M, Masuda H. Development of binucleated myocytes in normal and hypertrophied human hearts. *Am J Cardiovasc Pathol* 1990;**3**:27–36.

Siegel A, Johnson E, Stollerman G. Controlled studies of streptococcal pharyngitis in a pediatric population. I. Factors related to the attack rate of rheumatic fever. *N Engl J Med* 1961;**265**:559–64.

Silverman K, Hutchins G, Bulkley B. Cardiac sarcoid: a clinicopathological study of 84 unselected patients with system sarcoidosis. *Circulation* 1978;**58**: 1204–11.

Spirito P, Maron B, Bonow R, Epstein S. Occurrence and significance of progressive left ventricular wall thinning and relative cavity dilatation in hypertrophic cardiomyopathy. *Am J Cardiol* 1987;**59**: 123–9.

Steiner I. The prevalence of isolated atrial amyloid. *J Pathol* 1987;**153**:395–8.

Stoeckel M-E, Osborn M, Porte A, Sacrez A, Batzenschlager A, Weber K. An unusual familial cardiomyopathy characterized by aberrant accumulations of desmin-type intermediate filaments. *Virchows Arch* 1981;**393**:53–60.

Suomalainen A, Paetau A, Leinonen H, Majander A, Peltonen L, Somer H. Inherited idopathic dilated cardiomyopathy with multiple deletions of mitochondrial DNA. *Lancet* 1992;**340**:1319–20.

Tamua S, Tyakahashi M, Kawamura S, Ishihara T. Basophilic degeneration of the myocardium: histological, immunohistochemical and immuno-electro-microscopic studies. *Histopathology* 1995;**26**:501–8.

Tanaka M, Fujiwara H, Onodera T *et al*. Quantitative analysis of narrowings of intramyocardial small arteries in normal hearts, hypertensive hearts and hearts with hypertrophic cardiomyopathy. *Circulation* 1987;**75**:1130–9.

Tazelaar H, Billingham M. Leukocytic infiltrates in idiopathic dilated cardiomyopathy: a source of confusion with active myocarditis. *Am J Surg* 1986;**10**:405–12.

Teare D. Asymmetrical hypertrophy of the heart in young patients. *Br Heart J* 1958;**20**:1–8.

Thiene G, Nava A, Corrado D, Rossi L, Pennelli N. Right ventricular cardiomyopathy and sudden death in young people. *N Engl J Med* 1988;**318**:129–33.

Theaker J, Gatter K, Evans D, McGee J. Giant cell myocarditis: evidence for the macrophage origin of the giant cells. *J Clin Pathol* 1985;**38**:160–4.

Thierfelder L, Watkins H, MacRae C. Alpha-tropomyosin and cardiac troponin T mutations cause familial hypertrophic cardiomyopathy: a disease of the sarcomere. *Cell* 1994;**77**:1–20.

Valentine H, McKenna W, Mihoyannopoulos P. Sarcoidosis: a pattern of clinical and morphological presentation. *Br Heart J* 1987;**57**:256–63.

Valiathan M, Somers K, Chandrasekharan Kartha C (eds). *Endomyocardial fibrosis*. Delhi: Oxford University Press, 1993;1–302.

Van der Laarse A, Hollaar L, Vliegen H. Myocardial (iso) enzyme activities. DNA concentration and nuclear polyploidy in hearts of patients operated upon for congenital heart disease, and in normal and hypertrophic adult human hearts at autopsy. *Eur J Clin Invest* 1989;**19**:192–200.

van der Linde M, de Koning J, Hoogkamp-Korstanje J *et al*. Range of atrioventricular conduction disturbances in Lyme borreliosis: a report of four cases and review of other published reports. *Br Heart J* 1990;**63**:162–8.

Vliegen H, van der Laarse A, Cornelisse C, Eulderink F. Myocardial changes in pressure overload-induced left ventricular hypertrophy. A study on tissue composition, polyploidization and multinucleation. *Eur Heart J* 1991;**12**:488–94.

Watkins H, Rosenzweig A, Hwang D, *et al*. Characteristics and prognostic implications of myosin missense mutations in familial hypertrophy cardiomyopathy. *N Engl J Med* 1992;**326**:1108–14.

Weber K, Brilla C. Pathological hypertrophy and cardiac interstitium – fibrosis and renin-angiotensin-aldosterone system. *Circulation* 1991;**83**:1849–65.

Williams R. Molecular mimicry and rheumatic fever. *Clin Rheum Dis* 1985;**11**:573–91.

Zimmer G, Zimmermann R, Hess O. Decreased concentration of myofibrils and myofiber hypertrophy are structural determinants of impaired left ventricular function in patients with chronic heart diseases: a multiple logistic regression analysis. *J Am Coll Cardiol* 1992;**20**:1135–42

SIX

TUMOURS OF THE HEART

Primary tumours of the heart and pericardium are rare, with an incidence of between 0.0017% and 0.028% in collective autopsy series (Burke and Virmani 1996); most primary cardiac tumours are benign, over 50% in adults being atrial myxomas. In purely surgical series myxomas form 80% of cardiac tumours (Blondeau 1990). Other primary or secondary tumours in the heart in life are often initially misdiagnosed by echocardiography or at surgery as myxomas. The fact that myxomas are the commonest intracavity tumour often leads to the unwarranted assumption that all tumours protruding into the chamber are myxomas. In a series of cardiac sarcomas diagnosed at the Armed Forces Institute of Pathology (AFIP), nearly 50% of those arising in the left atrium were clinically considered to be myxomas (Burke and Virmani 1996). It is mandatory to examine histologically all cardiac tumours which are surgically excised.

PRIMARY BENIGN TUMOURS

Cardiac myxomas

This is the most frequent primary tumour of the heart and arises from the endocardium as a polypoid, often pedunculated, mass extending into an atrial chamber. The great majority of myxomas are attached to the atrial septum in the region of the foramen ovale (Figs 6.1–6.3), and of these 90% protrude into the left atrium. The most common clinical presentation is of systemic emboli. All surgeons should send peripheral arterial emboli for histological examination to rule out the possibility of myxoma. The second most common symptom is of congestive heart failure due to mitral valve obstruction with murmurs and atrial arrhythmias. The widespread use of echocardiography to screen subjects for heart disease has led to increasing recognition of myxomas as incidental findings. Constitutional upsets are common and may lead to confusion clinically with bacterial endocarditis. There is often episodic low-grade fever, a raised erythrocyte sedimentation rate (ESR), an elevated γ globulin level in the blood, anaemia and weight loss. In a small minority of patients these may be the presenting features. The systemic disorder is thought to be due to the release of inflammatory mediators such as IL-6 from the myxoma (Jourdan et al. 1990).

The majority of patients are usually in the 30–60 year age group. There is an equal sex distribution in most series, but a female predominance has been reported. Most myxomas occur as single tumours, but multiple tumours have been reported in families. The acronyms LAMB (lentiginosis, atrial myxoma, mucocutaneous myxomas, blue naevi) or NAME (naevi, atrial myxoma, mucocutaneous myxoma, eptiledes) have been used to describe an association with multiple cardiac myxomas (Rhodes et al. 1984; Gordon et al. 1985). Carney (1985) and others (Manthos et al. 1993) described their association with additional features such as fibroadenomas of breast, pituitary and cortical adenomas and testicular Sertoli cell tumours (Vidaillet 1988; Vidaillet et al. 1987), to which psammomatous melanotic

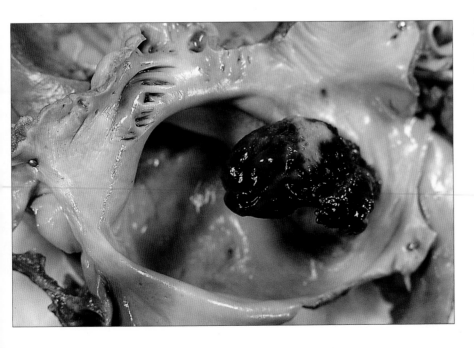

Figure 6.1
Left atrial myxoma. The myxoma is a lobulated smooth dark red glistening mass attached to the edge of the foramen ovale on a broad base.

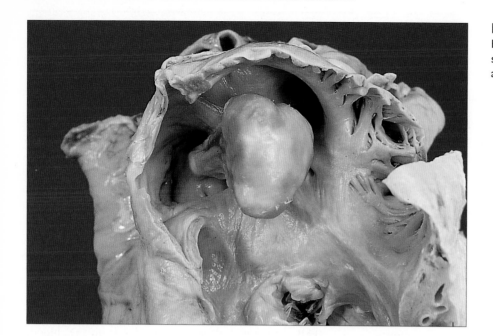

Figure 6.2
Right atrial myxoma. The myxoma is a smooth, round mass attached to a stalk arising from the edge of the foramen ovale.

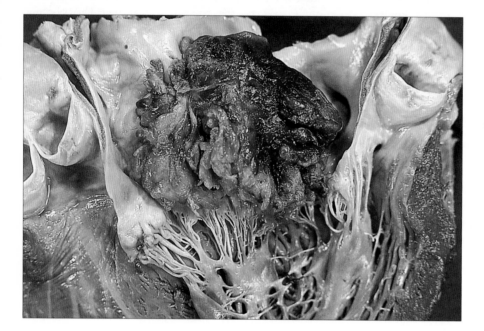

Figure 6.3
Left atrial myxoma. The tumour is very large and attached to the foramen ovale on a broad base. This myxoma has a papillary and fronded appearance and protrudes down into the mitral valve orifice. The anterior cusp of the mitral valve is thickened due to mechanical trauma by the myxoma.

schwannoma has been added (Utiger and Headington 1993). Family studies suggest an autosomal dominant gene with a variable phenotype. In contrast to the more usual non-familial myxomas, patients with this gene are more likely to be young and to have multiple myxomas which are not necessarily attached to the foramen ovale. It has been recommended that all asymptomatic relatives of a patient with an unusually sited myxoma be screened for cardiac myxomas by echocardiography.

Macroscopic findings

Myxomas are located mainly in the atria and are usually attached to the atrial septum in the region of the rim of the fossa ovalis (Figs 6.1–6.3). However, some atrial myxomas are described to originate from sites other than the septum, the most common being the posterior left atrial wall, followed by the anterior wall,

and the atrial appendage. In the AFIP series of myxomas, of 83 in the left atrium, 10 (13%) were not related to the foramen ovale (Burke and Virmani 1996). However, this is likely to be an overestimate since the more typical myxomas which have no unusual features are not necessarily referred for opinions. Such unusual sites need rigorous consideration of whether the tumour really is a myxoma. Myxomas do not usually arise from a cardiac valve; any tumour arising from a valve must be histologically investigated thoroughly to rule out other tumours such as fibroelastoma or myxoid fibrosarcomas.

Macroscopically myxomas have a range of appearances (Figs 6.1–6.4). They may be pedunculated or sessile. Some are smooth and round with a broad attachment. Flat sessile myxomas are rare and are believed to result from embolisation, leaving only the broad base of the

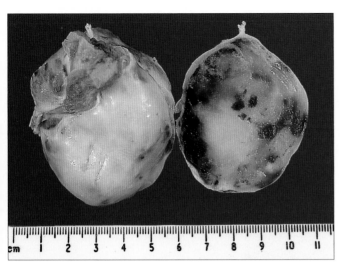

Figure 6.4
Surgical excision of left atrial myxoma. This is the most common type of myxoma which is excised. It is a lobulated mass 5 cm across varying in colour from red to yellow to white with a smooth surface. A cuff of atrial muscle is included on the surgical specimen.

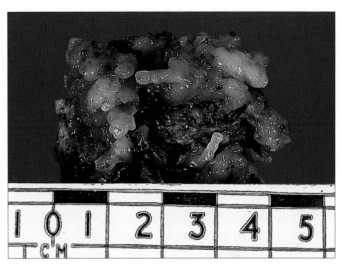

Figure 6.5
Surgical excision of left atrial myxoma. This excised myxoma, 4 cm in diameter, has a number of blunt finger-like protrusions and was very friable. The clinical presentation was of cerebral embolus after which cardiac ECHO showed a left atrial mass.

previously polypoid tumour attached to the endocardium. One distinct variation is to have multiple finger like papillary projections (Figs 6.3–6.5). Myxomas are soft and gelatinous, almost mucoid in appearance, and grey to grey-white, often with areas of haemorrhage or thrombus. Their size varies enormously from 1–15 cm, although the majority are in the 5–6 cm size. The villous or papillary type consists of multiple friable polypoid fronds with a distinctive mucoid or gelatinous appearance; these are extremely friable and embolise frequently. Myxomas often reach such proportions that they fill the atria and project through the valve into the ventricular cavity (Fig. 6.3). If the tumour is smooth and lobulated, a distinctive groove at the distal end may be made by the valve. On cross-sectioning, the broad base of attachment of the myxoma to the atrial septum is obvious. The tumours can calcify which can be seen on radiography and can be felt as hard gritty masses on sectioning.

The rare myxomas which arise in the ventricular cavities are equally divided between the right and left ventricles, and unlike the atria are not usually attached to the ventricular septum. They become moulded in appearance and frequently obstruct the ventricular valves. The finding of either a myxoma situated in the ventricle or multiple myxomas, should always lead to consideration of the familial form of the tumour. At least some of the isolated non-familial myxomas described in the literature as occurring in the ventricle are more likely to have been low-grade sarcomas or be part of the myxoma syndrome. Myxomas which are either not attached to the foramen ovale or occur in the ventricles do appear to have a different behaviour pattern. In the AFIP series of 114 cases, in the 22 not related to the foramen ovale, five recurred. In the 92 attached to the foramen ovale, none recurred.

Microscopic appearance

Myxomas are given that name because of the extensive myxoid matrix composed of acid mucopolysaccharides within which are embedded polygonal cells (lepidic cells) with scanty eosinophilic cytoplasm (Fig. 6.6). These cells have round nuclei with open chromatin pattern and small nucleoli. The cytoplasm is abundant and eosinophilic, but cell borders are indistinct (Fig. 6.7). They are arranged singly often assuming a stellate shape and in small nests. They may on occasion be multi-nucleate. Within the tumour mass, cells cluster several layers thick around capillaries. Throughout the myxoid stroma there are variable amounts of collagen and elastin and there are often large numbers of plasma cells, basophils and eosinophils present. Large thick-walled blood vessels enter the base of the tumour from the site of attachment in the sub-endocardium. Smooth muscle cells accompany the vessels which enter the base of the myxoma. Foci of extra-medullary haemopoiesis are occasionally found. Microscopic calcification is present in 10% of myxomas and areas of bone formation complete with haemopoietic tissue occasionally occur. Haemorrhage with thrombosis, haemosiderin-laden macrophages and fibrosis may be widespread. The tumour is attached and incorporated into the endocardium, but does not extend into the underlying myocardium. Nests of lepidic cells can be found in the adjacent endocardium and wide local excision is therefore needed to ensure that the myxoma does not recur. Complete excision of the atrial septum at the site of attachment is therefore an important fact to establish by the pathologist and great care must be taken to localise the site of attachment of the tumour to the atrial wall, which should be marked by a suture during removal for easy identification. Rarely, glandular inclusions lined by mucin (PASD) positive cells which show

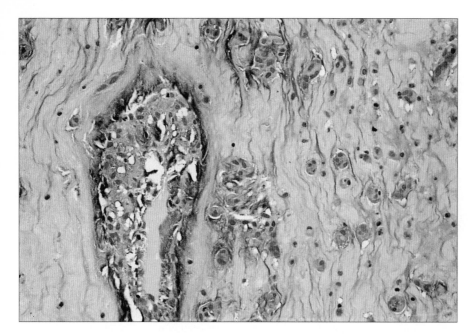

Figure 6.6
Atrial myxoma – histology. There is a eosinophilic myxoid stroma within which there is a large mass of lepidic cells surrounding a space. There are also small clumps of lepidic cells isolated within the stroma. In the immediate vicinity of the lepidic cells the stroma is basophilic (H&E ×56).

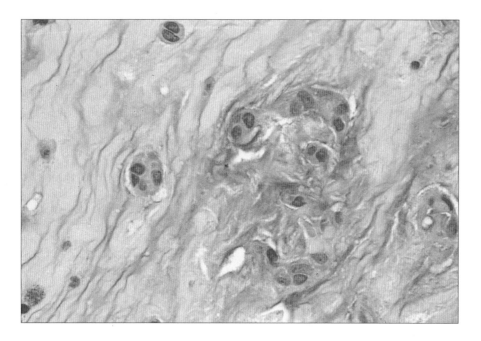

Figure 6.7
Atrial myxoma lepidic cells. The clumps of lepidic cells which have eosinophilic cytoplasm and round nuclei are embedded in myxoid stroma which is basophilic in the areas adjacent to the lepidic cell clumps (H&E ×140).

no atypia or mitoses have been reported (Goldman *et al.* 1987; Johansson 1989). It is important not to misinterpret these as adenocarcinoma. Myxomas vary greatly in the rate at which they grow. An occasional myxoma shows a considerable number of normal mitotic figures in the lepidic cells.

The essential histological feature of myxomas is that of islands and strands of lepidic cells which often surround a central small vascular space lined by endothelial cells. This organised pattern (Figs 6.6–6.8) must be present to diagnose a myxoma. A myxoid stroma in which there are embedded isolated stellate cells can be found in areas of all myxomas, but when this pattern is uniform throughout the tumour, a low-grade myxosarcoma is the more likely diagnosis. The surface of myxomas which have a papillary structure is covered by lepidic cells (Fig. 6.9). Each strand often has isolated myxoma cells embedded in the stroma – these are usually single and not arranged into the clusters seen in the deeper parts of the tumour. Myxosarcomas may mimic this pattern closely, as can any sarcoma projecting into the left atrium. In sarcomas, however, there is far greater cellularity and even in the depths of the tumour no organised clusters of lepid cells occur. There is also far greater variation in cell size with mitoses and atypia. An occasional myxoma will show normal mitosis in lepidic cells. Some myxomas appear to have been present for years and are recognised by echocardiography very late in life. These tumours may have a lot of calcification and degeneration with iron-encrusted elastic fibrils (Gamna bodies); multiple blocks have to be taken to find an area with typical myxoma histology.

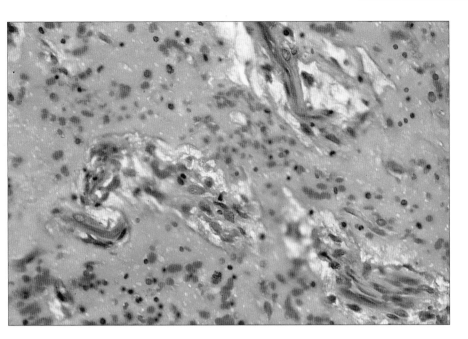

Figure 6.8
Atrial myxoma – histology. Large masses of lepidic cells surround spaces and are themselves surrounded by a clear area with basophilia. The majority of the stroma is eosinophilic and contains numerous red cells and some iron pigment (H&E ×87.5).

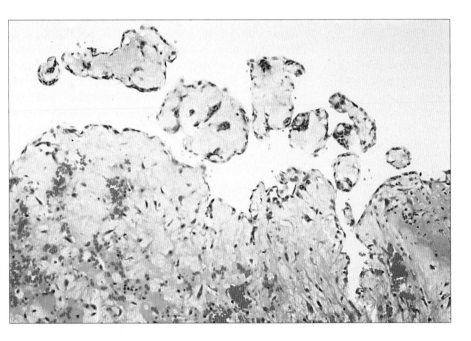

Figure 6.9
Atrial myxoma – histology. The papillary varieties of atrial myxomas show projections covered by lepidic cells. Within the projections isolated lepidic cells are present but the organised clumps of cells seen in the deeper parts of the tumour are absent (H&E ×35).

Histogenesis of cardiac myxomas

Arguments concerning the origin of myxomas continue. They were originally believed to be thrombotic in origin and still are by some workers (Salyer *et al.* 1975) but more recently it has become accepted that they are true neoplasms. DNA analysis of myxomas (Seidman *et al.* 1991; Kotylo *et al.* 1991) has shown most to be diploid and 13% aneuploid. Thrombi are frequent in patients with underlying valve disease, while underlying cardiac disease is rare in myxomas. The myxomatous stroma is rich in proteoglycans with a predominant component of chondroitin sulphate. Hyaluronic acid is also present in large amounts producing the characteristic gelatinous consistency of myxomas (Hendin *et al.* 1990). This type of stroma is not seen in organising thrombi.

When fragments of myxomas are grown *in vitro* in organ culture, a polygonal cell not unlike the lepid cell proliferates (Tanimura *et al.* 1988). This is totally unlike the fibroblastic-like cells which grow from organising thrombi.

The cell of origin giving rise to the tumour known as a myxoma remains contentious. Ultrastructural studies suggest the tumour cells are most like primitive multi-potential mesenchymal cells (Lie 1989; Zhang *et al.* 1989). The concept that this cell is capable of a wide range of phenotypic differentiation is supported by the reported expression of a wide range of antigens (Boxer 1984; Burke and Virmani 1993; Curschellas *et al.* 1991; Govoni *et al.* 1988; Johansson 1989; Krikler *et al.* 1992; Landon *et al.* 1986; McComb 1984; Morales *et al.* 1981; Schuger *et al.* 1987; Tanimura *et al.* 1988).

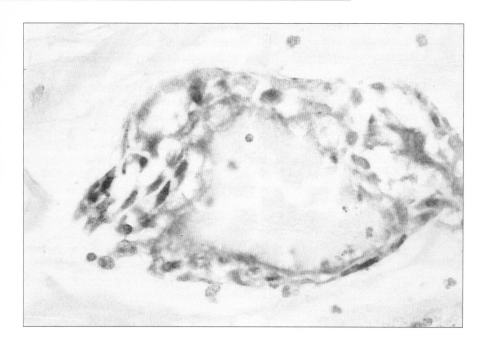

Figure 6.10
Atrial myxoma – immunohistochemistry. The cells lining the central space are stained positively for EN4 on endothelial marker. The cuff of lepidic cells surrounding the space are neurone specific enolase positive.

The lepidic tumour cells often cluster around cells marking as endothelial cells (Fig. 6.10), but whether these are just a supporting stroma or an integral part of the tumour is unclear. Cytokeratin is negative unless there is the glandular pattern of differentiation. Vimentin is usually positive in the tumour cells. Desmin is most frequently described as negative, but some reports find smooth muscle actin in the myxoma cells. Neurone-specific enolase, S-100 and synaptophysin have all been reported as variably positive (Fig. 6.10). Histiocytic/macrophage markers are negative. The cells of the embryonic endocardial cushions resemble myxoma cells and a widely held view is that nests of such cells persist in the endocardium, particularly in the region of the foramen ovale where they can give rise to myxomas (Lie 1989; Markwald *et al.* 1977).

Emboli from cardiac myxomas

Emboli from cardiac myxomas are a frequent occurrence and consist of both fragments of tumour and thrombus from the surface of the tumour. These emboli cause infarction in a number of sites including the brain, spleen gastrointestinal tract and limbs. Embolectomy specimens should always be examined at several levels to exclude a fragment of myxoma being embedded in the embolus.

Behaviour of cardiac myxomas

Myxomas are benign tumours. However, if not completely excised, they will recur at the same site and the incidence is reported at about 2%. Sometimes they recur at intra-cardiac sites distant from the original resection, but this is usually in the familial form of the disease where it is likely to be multiple primary tumours rather than recurrence of the original tumour. Where metastases have been reported, detailed histological review shows that many of these are examples of malignant tumours, i.e. liposarcomas or rhabdomyosarcoma with extensive areas of myxoid degeneration (Attum *et al.* 1987; Rupp *et al.* 1989). There is no evidence to

suggest that a benign atrial myxoma has the capacity to progress to a malignant myxosarcoma. Great care must be taken in examining a tumour mass labelled as myxoma by the surgeon, to avoid missing a malignant tumour. Multiple sections must be taken and any atypia, mitotic activity, chondroid or osteoid stroma points to another diagnosis. Reports of metastases of true myxomas to the brain probably represent local growth of embolised material (Budzilovich *et al.* 1979; Todo *et al.* 1992); pulmonary, bone and skin lesions (Reed *et al.* 1989) have also been described. Localised aneurysms may occur at the site of myxoma emboli (Damasio *et al.* 1975). Embolic myxomas do not possess malignant histological features, and do not give rise to deposits in other internal organs or lymph nodes.

Fibroma

In surgical series including all age groups, fibromas are the second most common benign primary cardiac tumour after myxoma (Feldman and Meyer 1976; Burke *et al.* 1994; Chan *et al.* 1985; Blondeau 1990). In children and infants the most common cardiac tumour after the rhabdomyoma is a fibroma, yet its rarity is emphasised by the fact that fewer than 200 cases are reported in the literature. They are associated with Gorlin's syndrome in which patients develop odontogenic cysts, epidermal cysts, multiple naevi and basal cell carcinomas of the skin. Fibromas of the heart are connective tissue tumours derived from fibroblasts and are very similar to soft tissue fibromas. These tumours occur at all ages and in both sexes, although they are more frequent in childhood with one third of cases being under one year of age. The symptoms depend on the location of the tumour with either sudden death or cardiac failure developing. Some are diagnosed as intracavity tumours by routine echocardiography. The majority of tumours causing sudden death are in the ventricular septum and impinge on the conduction system.

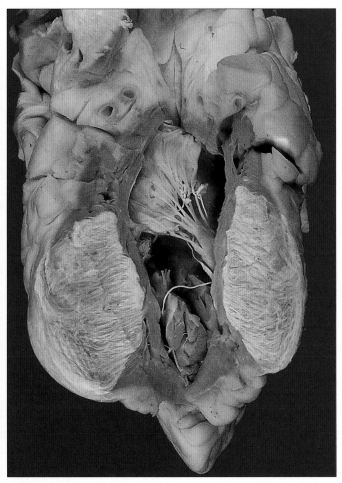

Figure 6.11
Myocardial fibroma. There is a discrete white tumour mass with a whorled appearance on the cut surface in the ventricular myocardium.

Macroscopic description

Fibromas are almost always single and located in the ventricular myocardium, frequently in the ventricular septum (Fig. 6.11). Atrial fibromas are rare. The tumours are firm, grey/white with a whorled appearance like a uterine fibroid and often reach a large size sometimes exceeding 10 cm in diameter. Central calcification is frequent and may even be seen on radiography. In contrast, rhabdomyomas rarely calcify.

Microscopic features

These tumours are non-encapsulated and extend into the surrounding myocardium. There may be the impression of satellite nodules, but in fact these nodules connect to the main tumour mass. Central portions of the tumour are composed of hyalinised fibrous tissue, often with multiple foci of calcification and myxoid cystic degeneration. They have a poor blood supply which may explain the degeneration and calcification. Elastic fibres admixed with areas of cellular fibrous tissue at the periphery may be prominent. Mitotic figures are not seen in these cellular fibrous areas, but can occur in tumours in children under the age of 6 months. Normal cardiac muscle cells are frequently entrapped in the growing edge and may at times be found deep within the tumour. These cells degenerate and become vacuolated, but they are not rhabdomyoma cells with which they are frequently confused. The separation of these tumours from rhabdomyomas and myxomas is easy on resection specimens where careful examination will show only the fibroblasts and collagen. No lepidic cells or spider cells are present. The cellular tumours of infancy may be confused with a low grade fibrosarcoma, but in older children there is no histological evidence of malignancy. Solitary fibrous tumours of the pericardium may look similar, but they are usually seen in adults, are attached to the pericardium and do not infiltrate the myocardium. Inflammatory pseudo-tumours can occur in the heart, but are extremely rare and contain a prominent inflammatory and vascular component, while fibromas usually contain only small foci of lymphocytes and plasma cells, usually at the tumour–myocardium interface.

Papillary fibroelastoma

These are the most common benign cardiac tumours arising on valve cusps (Edwards *et al*. 1991). Like myxomas, they arise from the endocardium, but there the similarity ends. They consist of papillary fronds containing fibrous tissue, elastic fibres and smooth muscle cells set in a mucopolysaccharide matrix covered by hyperplastic endocardial cells. The tumour has a wide range of synonyms including papilloma of valve, myxofibroma or fibroma of valve and giant Lambl's excrescence. The papillary structures are avascular, in contrast to myxomas which are richly vascular. In most patients these tumours are incidental findings at autopsy, not associated with cardiac symptoms and the true incidence is difficult to estimate. Less than 50 cases causing symptoms have been reported. The usual symptoms are angina or sudden unexpected death due to the tumour directly impacting into the ostium of a coronary artery or to cerebral, renal or mesenteric embolisation (Valente *et al*. 1992; Mann and Parker 1994).

Macroscopic features

These tumours resemble a sea anemone when viewed under water (Fig. 6.12) with multiple papillary fronds attached to the endocardium by a short pedicle. They are generally smaller than myxomas, usually 1 cm or less and the fronds are longer, thinner and more delicate than those seen in papillary myxomas. Thrombus may obscure the papillary structure, so a careful examination of all tumours, particularly those resected from the valves, must be made to find these delicate structures. Endocarditis can also complicate the appearance with vegetations obscuring the underlying architecture. Papillary fibroelastomas may rise anywhere in the heart, but most frequently are found on the ventricular aspect of the aortic valve or the free edge of the cusp. On the atrioventricular valves they are seen on the atrial aspect along the lines of closure or on the papillary muscles around the chordae. Occasionally they are multiple, being located on the mitral, aortic, pulmonary and tricuspid valves.

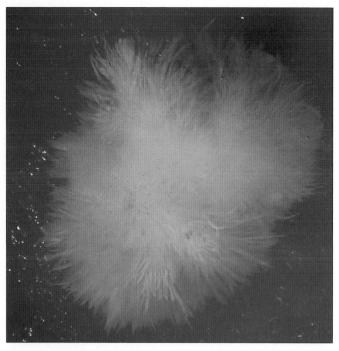

Figure 6.12
Papillary fibroelastoma. This 2 cm tumour was removed surgically from the mitral valve following a cerebral embolus. Viewed under water the very fronded nature of the tumour is obvious. When viewed at open heart surgery or *in situ* in the heart at autopsy the fronds collapse to form a soft mucoid mass often mistaken for a myxoma.

Microscopic appearance

Histologically the papillary fronds consist of a central core of dense connective tissue surrounded by a layer of loose connective tissue and covered by hyperplastic endothelial cells. The layer of loose connective tissue contains collagen and elastic fibres as well as occasional smooth muscle cells. The amount of elastic is variable, but usually a fine mesh work surrounds the central collagen core. Sometimes the entire central core may consist of elastic fibres. The central core is continuous with the underlying connective tissue of the endocardium and appears to be a direct extension of the endocardium. The hyperplastic endocardial cells covering the papillary fronds merge with the endocardium cells.

Origin

Whether the papillary fibroelastoma is a true tumour or a hamartoma is debatable. Microscopically the papillary fronds of these tumours are similar in structure to normal chordae tendineae. This suggests that the papillary fibroelastoma is a true hamartoma and like the chondroid hamartoma of the lung is more frequent in older patients. Many subjects with papillary fibroelastomas have long-standing cardiovascular disease suggesting that the tumours are secondary to mechanical wear and tear. Lambl's excrescences which are small filiform tags occurring especially along the contact surfaces of the heart valves of elderly patients, and are an incidental finding in many autopsies, are most likely related to trauma with minute thrombus formation. Papillary fibroelastoma have been called giant Lambl's excrescences because of this resemblance in appearance and location. The location of both is similar but Lambl's excrescences do not usually occur on the free edge of the aortic valve cusps or on the mural endocardium. Lambl's excrescences have been reported in up to 85% of adult heart valves while papillary fibroelastomas are rare tumours. Lambl's excrescences are multiple in over 90% of patients, whereas papillary fibroelastomas are rarely multiple. In addition Lambl's excrescences consist mainly of fibrin and lack the abundant acid-mucopolysaccharide matrix of fibroelastomas; they do not contain smooth muscle cells.

Rhabdomyoma

Rhabdomyomas are the most common primary benign tumour of the heart in children less than 15 years of age. These tumours are present within the myocardium and are often multiple. They are considered to represent foetal hamartomas (Fenoglio *et al.* 1977; Fenoglio *et al.* 1976). The tumour is derived from myocytes (Burke and Virmani 1991a) although there have been debates whether it might arise from Purkinje cells, i.e conduction tissue myocytes. Approximately half of rhabdomyomas are associated with tuberous sclerosis and if one is found as an incidental finding, the family may need investigation (Byard *et al.* 1991). In patients presenting with tuberous sclerosis, only 60% have a cardiac tumour. Rhabdomyomas often regress as a child grows and many are asymptomatic (Smith *et al.* 1989). Clinically, patients with rhabdomyomas can be divided into three groups.

Neonatal rhabdomyoma

Approximately one-third of patients may be either still-born or die within the first few days of life. 75% of these patients have large intracavity tumours with obstruction of at least one cardiac valve and death is presumed to be secondary to haemodynamic factors. Tuberous sclerosis is difficult to diagnose at this stage. In those who survive into childhood, the tumour may spontaneously regress. Rhabdomyomas can also be seen in children with congenital heart disease, such as hypoplastic left heart, transposition of the great vessels, Ebstein's anomaly, tricuspid and pulmonary atresia.

Cases incidental to tuberous sclerosis

In the second group, again representing about one-third of patients, the majority have clinical evidence of tuberous sclerosis. The rhabdomyomas are incidental findings at autopsy, being small and embedded in the myocardium.

Cardiac cases

The third group of patients present with cardiac symptoms of congestive cardiac failure, cardiac murmurs, arrhythmias and cardiomegaly. The majority of these patients have single large intracavity tumours with marked obstructions of blood flow in at least one cardiac chamber and clinically there is no evidence of

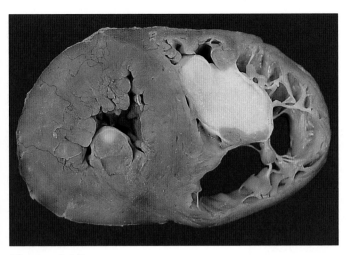

Figure 6.13
Cardiac rhabdomyoma. The tumour is a discrete white mass projecting into the right ventricular cavity. A very much smaller rhabdomyoma is in the posterior papillary muscle of the left ventricle. From an infant with tuberous sclerosis.

tuberous sclerosis. The patients are usually aged under 15 years.

Macroscopic findings

Cardiac rhabdomyomas are usually multiple and occur throughout the heart, but are never found on a cardiac valve. Most frequently they are located in the myocardium of the left and right ventricles including the septum and protrude into the cardiac chamber (Fig. 6.13). The tumours are usually white to yellow/tan in colour and can vary in size from 1 mm to 9 cm.

Microscopic features

The tumours are usually well defined and circumscribed but not encapsulated and are easily distinguished from the surrounding myocardium as nodules of highly cellular tissue. The appearance of the cells are unique to this tumour. These are the 'spider cells' which are pathognomonic of the rhabdomyoma. The typical rhabdomyoma cells are large up to 18 μm in diameter and appear vacuolated being filled with glycogen which can be demonstrated with the periodic acid Schiff reaction (PAS). The spider cells have centrally placed nuclei with elongated cytoplasmic projections of slender myofibrils extending to the periphery of the cell (Fig. 6.14). Often the nucleus and cytoplasmic mass is eccentrically placed against the cell wall and cytoplasmic projections transverse the vacuolated cell. The cells are immunopositive for myoglobin, desmin, actin and vimentin. Microscopic foci of extra-medullary haemopoiesis can be conspicuous.

Histiocytoid cardiomyopathy

This name is inappropriate to this condition which consists of multiple hamartomas (Gelb *et al.* 1993; Malhotra *et al.* 1994) occurring in infants and children resulting in arrhythmias. It is so called because the cells of the hamartoma were considered to resemble histiocytes (Fig. 6.15). The cell of origin is now considered to be either a cardiac myocyte or a Purkinje cell. It is a very rare condition with a female predominance and is confined to early childhood. Cases usually present with cardiac arrhythmias including pre-excitation and there is a significant risk of sudden death (Saffitz *et al.* 1983). Cardiac defects associated with the condition include atrial and ventricular septal defects and hypoplastic left heart syndrome. Other abnormalities include CNS defects, ovarian cysts and generalised oncocytic change in endocrine glands.

Macroscopically the lesions are multiple, yellow raised nodules usually less than 2 mm in diameter situated in the sub-endocardium at the base of the interventricular septum in the left ventricle, but nodules can be found elsewhere.

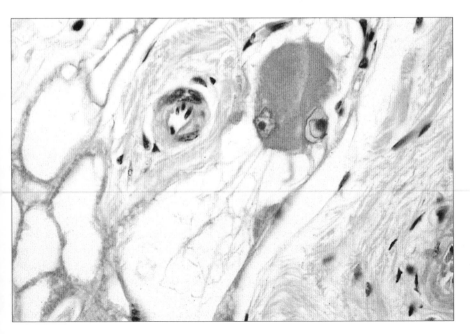

Figure 6.14
Cardiac rhabdomyoma – histology. The tumour is composed of very large almost empty cells. In some of these there is a mass of myofibrillary eosinophilic material containing one or more nuclei with large nucleoli. The nuclei and cytoplasmic material are suspended by strands in the cell leading to the name 'spider web' cells (H&E ×210).

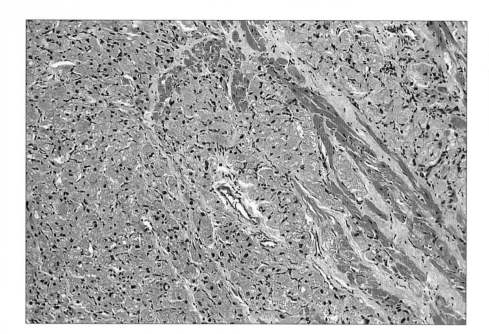

Figure 6.15
Histiocytoid cardiomyopathy. The myocardium is infiltrated by large cells with granular cytoplasm which contrast with the residual normal myocytes which are elongated and eosinophilic. The vacuolated hamartomatous cells contain lipid stainable by oil-red O (H&E ×16).

Microscopically the nodules consist of myocyte converted into large foamy oncocytic cells with eccentric dark nuclei surrounded by collagen. No spider cells are seen. The cytoplasm contains fine droplets of subanophilic material. The cells are weakly positive for desmin, myoglobin and myosin, while they are negative for histiocyte markers.

BENIGN TUMOURS OF ADIPOSE TISSUE

Lipomatous hypertrophy of the atrial septum

The interatrial septum consists largely of an invagination of the atrial roof and contains epicardial fat. This fat is the source of the entity known as lipomatous hypertrophy of the atrial septum, which is in fact a lipoma characterised by excess accumulations of mature adipose tissue forming a recognisable mass which exceeds 2 cm in diameter. This mass may contain and trap the cardiac muscle cells, fibrous tissue, blood vessels and foetal fat cells.

The histogenesis of the massive deposition of adipose tissue in the atrial septum is uncertain. On the one hand fatty tissue is a normal component of the atrial septum and an increase in the number of adipose tissue cells has been regarded as a metabolic disturbance associated with obesity, increasing age, starvation or anaemia. On the other hand the condition is regarded as a benign proliferation or hamartoma of adipocytes (Shirani and Roberts 1993). Many cases are coincidental findings at autopsy and there is a very ill-defined borderline between age-related fatty infiltration of the atria and lipomatous hypertrophy of the septum; for this reason its true incidence is difficult to determine. In cases which are designated as lipomatous hypertrophy, there

is a high frequency of atrial arrhythmias and complete heart block. The latter is the result of isolation of the AV node from its atrial connections. Recognition of massive enlargement of the atrial septum in patients with atrial fibrillation or complete AV block is now possible by magnetic resonance imaging or transoesophageal echocardiography, allowing the diagnosis of lipomatous hypertrophy to be made in life (Rokey *et al.* 1989; Pochis *et al.* 1992).

Macroscopic description

The lipomatous mass is located in the atrial septum and bulges from beneath the atrial endocardium, most frequently into the right atrium. It may protrude so much into the atrial cavity that a differential diagnosis with myxoma has to be considered. The atrial septum measures between 2 and 8 cm in thickness. The main lipomatous mass is often located anterior to the foramen ovale, but may extend into the region of the AV node so it is not surprising that they are associated with arrhythmias. The mass is non-encapsulated but circumscribed and differs in colour and consistency from the epicardial fat, being usually brown and firm in consistency.

Microscopic appearances

The tumours consist of varying proportions of mature adipose tissue and granular/vacuolated foetal fat cells. Fat droplets are usually demonstrated in the mature fat cells and in the granular cells with oil-red O stains. The presence of foetal fat cells is a hallmark of lipomatous hypertrophy of the atrial septum, and occasionally these interatrial masses consist almost entirely of foetal fat. Myocardial cells are usually trapped within the mass, especially at the periphery and these can show bizarre, hypertrophic or degenerative changes, but classic spider cells are never found. Areas of fibrosis and foci of chronic inflammatory cells are frequently present.

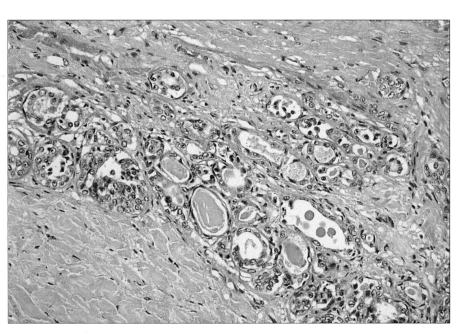

Figure 6.16
Cystic tumour of the AV node. The region of the AV node adjacent to the central fibrous body is replaced by cystic tissue. The cysts contain granular debris and are lined by epithelial-like cells (H&E ×140).

Lipoma

Lipomas are most frequent just beneath the visceral and parietal pericardium (Burke and Virmani 1996). The tumours are usually not associated with cardiac symptoms unless they project into the pericardial sac when they can cause effusions. Parietal pericardial lipomas are often mistaken clinically for pericardial cysts. Multiple myocardial lipomas have been described in tuberous sclerosis; the lipomas can occur anywhere and have been reported on cardiac valves and the endocardium. The pericardial and intracavity lipomas are bosselated and may reach up to 10 cm in diameter. Grossly and microscopically they are identical in appearance to adult fat or lipomas elsewhere in the body.

OTHER BENIGN CARDIAC TUMOURS

Heterotopia and ectopic tissue tumours

Teratoma

These are often intrapericardial masses attached to the root of the pulmonary artery or aorta. They occur usually in young children with a female predominance and may be a cause of sudden death. The tumour is distinctly rare, the largest series being that from the AFIP with 14 cases (McAllister and Fenoglio 1978). The tumours may be up to 15 cm in diameter and usually contain numerous multiloculated cysts with intervening solid areas. Microscopically intrapericardial teratomas resemble benign cystic teratomas of the ovary. The cysts are lined by ciliated columnar epithelium, stratified squamous epithelium or pseudo-stratified mucin secreting columnar epithelium. Within the solid areas, foci of neural tissue are frequent and collection of acinar structures replicating thyroid or pancreas are common. Smooth muscle cells and strap

cells can be seen in the stroma. Cartilage and bone may occasionally be present. They are benign, but must be carefully sampled to rule out a malignant component.

Cystic tumour of the atrioventricular node

There are approximately 70 cases of this rare tumour reported; most are single case reports of sudden death. The tumour is situated in the region of the atrioventricular node and is composed of nests of cells which were in the past considered to be of mesothelial origin and led to the term mesothelioma of the atrioventricular node. The majority of these patients have partial or complete atrioventricular heart block, usually of long duration (Evans and Stovin 1986; Subramanian *et al.* 1989). This tumour has been referred to as the smallest tumour that can cause sudden death. The patients can range in age from 11 months to 70 years with an average age of 38 years. There is a female predominance.

Cystic tumours of the AV node are usually poorly-circumscribed, slightly elevated nodules located in the atrial septum just above the septal leaflet of the tricuspid valve in the region of the AV node (Fig. 6.16). On cross section they are small and multicystic with the cysts ranging in size from 2–20 mm.

The cysts (Fig. 6.16) are lined by a cuboidal cell layer with underlying transitional cells, giving a multi-layered appearance. Between the large cysts are multiple nests of cells of varying size, some with a central lumen while others appear solid. In many areas especially in the smaller nests, the cells are often squamoid in appearance with sebaceous and transitional cells also. Many of the nuclei are ovoid and have a cleft-like longitudinal indentation, resembling so-called coffee-bean nuclei. There is no pleomorphism or mitoses which differentiates this tumour from metastatic adenocarcinoma. The PAS and the alcian blue stain will demonstrate foci of positive staining within the lumen of these cysts and they can occasionally calcify. The cellular nests and cystic structure are set in a dense tissue stroma. Collagen and elastic fibres are abundant. The tumour replaces part or all of the AV node and may extend upwards into the atrial septum and downwards into the AV bundle, but does not extend into the myocardium or into the tricuspid valve. No metastases from the tumour have been reported. The cells are keratin, EMA, CEA and B72.3 positive which favours an epithelial rather than a mesothelial origin (Burke *et al.* 1990). Endocrine cells positive for serotonin and calcitonin have been reported in the lining cells of these cysts (Fine and Raja 1987).

Benign cysts and tumours of pericardium

Both angiomas and lipomas often occur on the epicardial surface as raised nodules. On the parietal pericardium, ectopic thyroid tissue (McAllister and Fenoglio 1978) may produce a nodule. Ectopic thyroid tissue may also rarely be found in the myocardium (Richard *et al.* 1990). Thymomas may also arise in the pericardium without any mediastinal involvement (McAllister and Fenoglio 1978).

The commonest pericardial masses, provided secondary deposits of a malignant tumour elsewhere are excluded, are simple mesothelial cysts. Most are coincidental findings on chest X-ray and this requires excision to exclude something more sinister. Modern computed tomography (CT) and magnetic resonance (MR) scans can, however, diagnose them accurately. The cyst may be unilocular or multiloculated and is lined by a single layer of mesothelial cells (Feigin *et al.* 1977). Positive staining of the cells with antibodies to cytokeratin distinguishes the entity from a lymphangioma which may be macroscopically rather similar.

Small localised proliferations of mesothelial cells on the serosal surface of the pericardium are common. These may be found at surgery and often are dislodged to become free; they then present a conundrum to the surgeon over their identity. These local proliferations are also occasionally seen in cardiac biopsies that have reached the pericardial surface. They should not be over interpreted as secondary tumours. The rather striking name MICE (mesothelial incidental cardiac excrescences) has been applied to this phenomenon (Courtice *et al.* 1994).

Benign vascular tumours of the heart

Blood cysts

A blood cyst (Zimmerman *et al.* 1983) is a separation or cleft between endocardial cells, or between the supporting stroma and endocardial cells, creating a channel containing blood and it is not a tumour, even though it may mimic one. They are found on the endocardium, particularly the valvar endocardium in the new-born and infants. The cysts are usually lined by normal endocardial cells and the lining cells are delimited from surrounding endocardial cells by a basement membrane. Occasionally the blood cyst is not lined by endocardial cells but consists of the endocardial stroma. They are multiple, found along the line of closure of the valve, and are the result of invaginations of the lining endothelium into the underlying connective tissue which fill with blood. Haemosiderin-laden macrophages with fibrosis and lymphocytes can be seen in the surrounding tissue. They are usually found in infants under 2 months of age and rarely after the age of 2 years. They are presumed to result from trauma to the closure line, but are not usually associated with valvar abnormalities or bleeding disorders.

Varix

These are dilated blood vessels in the sub-endocardium, and are frequently mistaken for haemangiomas. They may occur anywhere in the heart, but are common in the right atrium in the inferior rim of the fossa ovalis, where they arise from small veins and consist of a single or cluster of normally-formed vascular channels which are dilated and frequently thrombosed. They are cardiac 'haemorrhoids". They are usually an incidental finding at autopsy with an incidence of 0.07%. Why they arise is unknown and they do not cause symptoms (Rose 1979).

Haemangioma

Haemangiomas consist of benign proliferations of endothelial cells usually forming channels containing blood. They most commonly occur on the epicardial surface of the atria or ventricles (Fig. 6.17). Haemangiomas are largely asymptomatic, and are coincidental autopsy findings at any age from infants to 80 years of age. Symptomatic haemangiomas are rare with only 75 reported cases in the literature (Burke *et*

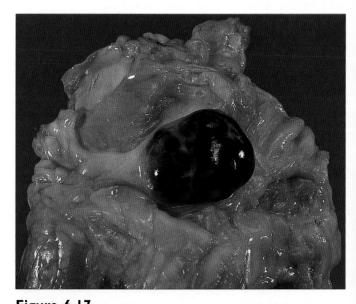

Figure 6.17
Benign haemangioma. This haemangioma is in a typical subpericardial position on the posterior wall of the heart and was a coincidental finding at autopsy.

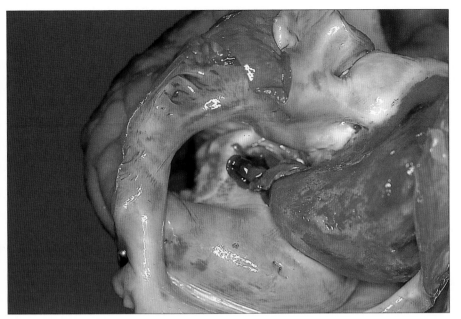

(a)

Figure 6.18 a,b
Angiosarcoma. (a) A large haemorrhagic mass protrudes into the cavity of the left atrium from the septum. Tumour also protruded into the right atrium. (b) Pericardial involvement as a sheet of tumour over the anterior wall of the left ventricle in the same case.

al. 1991). Symptoms are dependent on the location of the tumour and include arrhythmias, pericardial effusions and obstruction to valves or outflows. Characteristically, haemangiomas appear red and haemorrhagic. Capillary haemangiomas consist of haphazardly arranged closely-packed capillary structures, lined by flattened endothelial cells with minimal stroma. Cavernous haemangiomas consist of widely dilated vascular channels lined by flattened endothelial cells with focal, abundant connective tissue between the channels. Some cavernous angiomas are recognised when they become filled with contrast media at coronary angiography.

MALIGNANT TUMOURS OF THE HEART

Angiosarcoma

These malignant tumours originating from vascular endothelium are the most frequently occurring primary malignant cardiac tumour, being about 40% of all primary cardiac sarcomas. Patients are usually adult, ranging in age from 15 to 76 years. Angiosarcomas are found more frequently in men than in women. Most appear to originate in the right atrium, often spread to the epicardial surface (Fig. 6.18) and have early metastases to the lung and elsewhere. The tumours are usually large bulky lesions infiltrating the right atrium and filling the cavity. Invasion into the venae cavae and tricuspid valve is common. Presenting clinical features are usually either due to haemorrhagic pericardial effusions, or due to tumour encroaching on the right atrial cavity, or obstructing the pulmonary outflow.

Histology

Microscopically there is great variation in the appearance of angiosarcomas both between and within the same tumour. Basically angiosarcomas are composed of malignant cells forming vascular channels (Fig. 6.19).

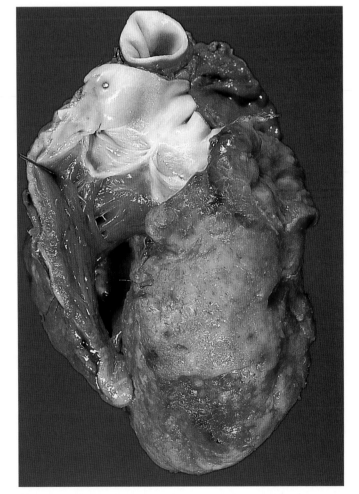

(b)

There may be also solid areas of spindle cells and sheets of anaplastic round cells. A reticulum stain is useful in demonstrating a vascular pattern. The vascular channels vary greatly in size and shape, frequently forming multiple anastomosing channels lined by swollen multi-layered endothelial cells. Pleomorphism is marked, and mitoses are frequent. Spindle cell areas frequently merge

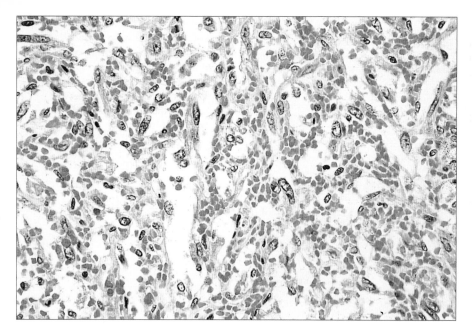

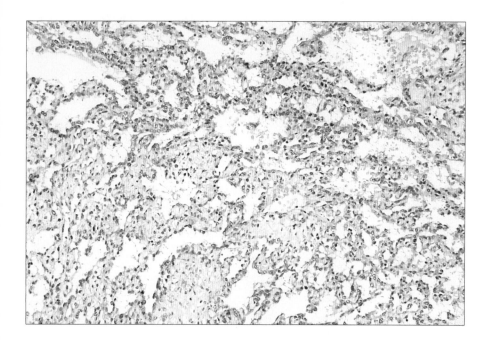

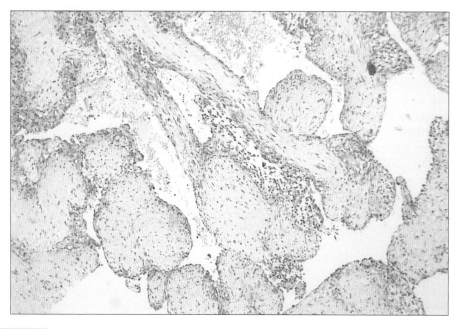

Figure 6.19 a,b,c

Haemangiosarcoma – histology. In (a) the sarcoma is clearly forming well-defined vascular spaces, but the endothelial cells are large pleomorphic and with many mitotic figures. (H&E ×56). In (b) the tumour is forming spaces but these are not blood containing and there are more solid areas of tumour cells (H&E ×56). In (c) the tumour is papillary with the centres of the fronds showing some myxoid material. No angiomatous differentiation is present (H&E ×56). Most haemangiosarcomas show a very wide range of differentiation patterns making diagnosis on biopsy difficult. A myxoid stroma and papillary growth can occur in any cardiac sarcoma whatever its basic differentiation pattern.

with vascular and solid areas of the tumour. Many tumours can have large undifferentiated areas so that extensive sampling of the tumour is important to see more diagnostic areas. Extravasated red blood cells within vacuoles point to the diagnosis. Equally, many angiosarcomas have areas which appear 'benign' with vascular spaces lined by a single layer of endothelium. This variation in pattern makes diagnosis in biopsies sometimes difficult. Biopsies are most frequently encountered when the pericardium is explored to elucidate the cause of a haemorrhagic pericarditis or to relieve tamponade. The tumours are usually unresectable because of extensive pericardial involvement. Endothelial markers may be positive, but are often weak and focal in these tumours.

Differential diagnosis from other sarcomas may be difficult when the tumour contains largely undifferentiated areas. Kaposi's sarcoma may be difficult to distinguish, but these patients are usually HIV positive with skin and other lesions elsewhere. The lesions of Kaposi's sarcoma are usually nodules on the surface of the pericardium with minimal myocardial involvement.

The prognosis of angiosarcomas is poor; radiotherapy and chemotherapy may offer temporary relief but mean survival is only 3 months (Burke and Virmani 1996). Distant metastases occur, particularly to the lung and central nervous system, and local spread is also extensive.

Other sarcomas of the heart

Cardiac sarcomas which are not angiomatous show a very wide range of differentiation patterns including striated muscle, smooth muscle, fibroblastic neural, osteogenic, myxoid and liposarcoma (Table 6.1). In the majority of the sarcomas, the predominant pattern is that of an undifferentiated sarcoma and many histological blocks have to be taken to recognise a particular phenotypic expression. Some sarcomas show more than one differentiation pattern. Immunohistochemistry may be of some but limited help. Desmin expression

suggests myoid differentiation; vimentin marks virtually every sarcoma and is non-discriminatory as is smooth muscle actin. S-100 will identify rhabdomyosarcomas, but care has to be taken to avoid over-interpreting degenerate cardiac muscle entrapped by the tumour as it spreads (Burke and Virmani 1996).

Rhabdomyosarcoma

Between four and seven per cent of primary cardiac malignant tumours are rhabdomyosarcomas (Burke and Virmani 1996). The patients range in age from 3 months to 80 years of age, but they are rare in the paediatric age group. The mean age at presentation is in the second or third decade which is earlier than with other cardiac sarcomas. They occur throughout the myocardium and have no propensity to arise in any one cardiac chamber. The pericardium is usually involved by direct extension of the tumour from the myocardium. Diffuse pericardial involvement which can typically be seen in angiosarcomas is not a feature of rhabdomyosarcomas. The tumours are usually nodular, soft and centrally necrotic. They can look gelatinous, mimicking myxomas or more solid but extensive infiltration of the atrial wall and valves point to the true diagnosis (Fig. 6.20). Metastases occur early to the lungs and other organs.

Microscopically, both embryonal or alveolar and adult forms occur with the adult form being much more frequent (Fig. 6.21). Diagnosis is made by finding a convincing rhabdomyoblast which can be extremely difficult. The rhabdomyoblast includes strap-shaped cells with two or more nuclei, racket-shaped cells and rounded cells. The cytoplasm is often eosinophilic and granular. Cross striations may be seen as high magnifications in phosphotungstic-acid-haematoxylin (PTAH) stains. However, cross striations can be identified in only 20 to 30% of these tumours and electron microscopy may be more useful in delineating cross striations in up to 90% of cases. Identification of these cells is made easier with immunocytochemistry. They

Table 6.1

Differentiation patterns and site of origin of cardiac sarcomas

Patterns	Frequency (% malignant tumours)	Left atrium	Right atrium	Other sites
Angiosarcoma	37%	10%	90%	–
Malignant fibrous histiocytoma	24%	86%	→ pericardium	14%
Leiomyosarcoma	9%	80%	–	20%
Rhabdomyosarcoma	7%	50%	25%	25%
Unclassifiable	7%	66%	33%	–
Fibromyxosarcoma	6%	66%	33%	–
Myxomsarcoma	4%	100%	–	–
Fibrosarcoma	3%	–	–	100%
Osteosarcoma	3%	–	–	100%

After Burke and Virmani (1996)

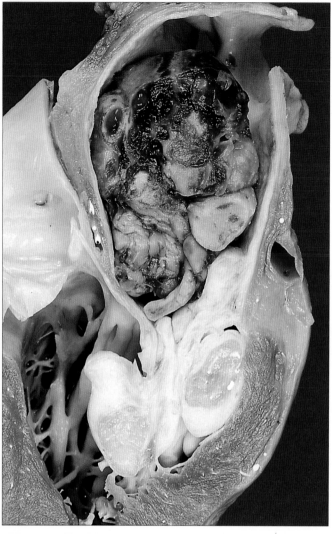

Figure 6.20
Rhabdomyosarcoma. Long axis view through the left atrium and ventricle. The tumour arose in the left atrium and rapidly spread through the mitral valve into the left ventricle. Within the atria the tumour is rather lobulated and myxoid. In the ventricle the tumour is far more solid and white.

stain positive for desmin, myoglobin (Fig. 6.22), troponin T and actin. Myxoid areas, spindle cell areas and solid cellular areas are often found within the same tumour. Microscopic foci of necrosis and haemorrhage are often noted. Areas of alveolar and embryonal rhabdomyosarcomas are common, even in so-called adult rhabdomyosarcomas. Tremendous variation in the microscopic appearance of rhabdomyosarcomas is one clue to its diagnosis.

Osteosarcoma/chondrosarcoma/octeoclastoma

Between three and nine per cent of cardiac sarcomas can be classified as osteosarcomas due to the presence of osteoid in a sarcomatous stroma (Fig. 6.23). The tumours are macroscopically similar to any other type of cardiac sarcoma with the majority being located in the left atrium. Microscopically, the tumours consist of obvious sarcomatous areas producing osteoid (Burke and Virmani 1991b). Multi-nucleated giant cells and pleomorphic cells surround the foci of osteoid. All the tumours also possess fibrosarcomatous areas, often enclosed in association with the areas of osteoid and malignant osteoblasts. Many of the tumours can have mixed foci of chondrosarcoma with an obvious chondroid matrix. Tumours can contain large numbers of giant cells resembling osteoclasts.

Malignant fibrous histiocytoma and fibrosarcoma

The tumours may be nodular or infiltrating, but they are usually firm and white in colour. Necrosis and calcification can occur. They infiltrate the myocardium and can involve cardiac valves.

Microscopically they are composed of spindle-shaped cells with elongated nuclei and tapering cytoplasm. Pleomorphism may be minimal, but mitosis is frequent. The spindle cells are arranged in broad bundles of fascicles. The malignant fibrohistiocytoma has similar

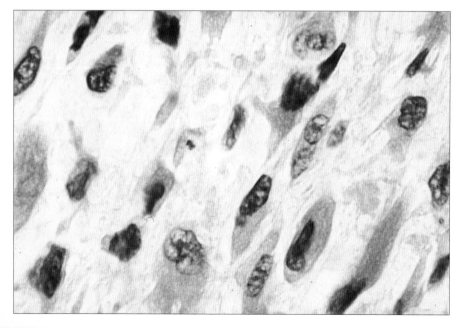

Figure 6.21
Rhabdomyosarcoma. The commonest pattern of differentiation is elongated spindle and strap-shaped cells with eosinophilic cytoplasm. The nuclei are large with prominent nuceoli (H&E ×140).

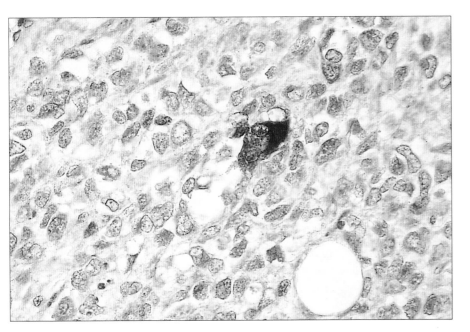

Figure 6.22
Osteogenic sarcoma – immunohistochemistry. In this cardiac sarcoma one tumour cell is strongly positive (peroxidase method) for myoglobin. It is however often difficult to be certain that such positivity is not a normal myocyte isolated within the tumour. Here the positive cell is deep within the mass and looks like a tumour giant cell.

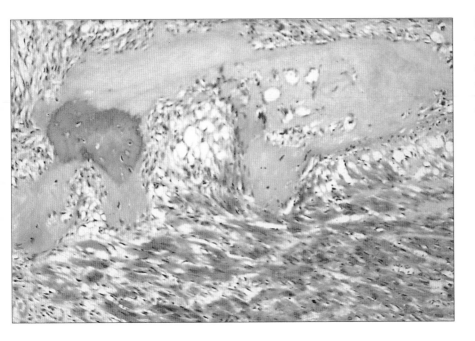

Figure 6.23
Osteogenic sarcoma of heart. The junction of the tumour with normal myocardium is shown. At this junction the sarcoma is comprised of pleomorphic spindle cells while deeper there is osteoid and bone formation (H&E ×56).

features, but a storiform or whorled pattern of the spindle cells and the presence of giant cells differentiate malignant fibrohistiocytoma from fibrosarcoma (Fig. 6.24). The histologic type, be it storiform, pleomorphic, myxoid, giant cell, inflammatory or angiomatoid, does not seem to affect outcome. A high mitotic rate and necrosis indicate a high-grade tumour, and most patients die of their disease within 2 years. Left-sided tumours, a low mitotic rate and absence of necrosis do better, but most patients die within 5 years. These tumours are negative for keratin, myoglobin, desmin, and S-100, HMB-45 and express vimentin, smooth muscle actin and muscle actin, all of which can be found in mesenchymal neoplasms. Differentiation from other tumours depends on clinical history and immunohistochemical markers, but distinction from

rhabdomyosarcoma or fibrosarcoma is seldom clear-cut and opinions on individual tumours may vary.

Leiomyosarcomas, myxosarcomas, liposarcomas and malignant nerve sheath tumours

Sarcomas which show a predominant smooth muscle cell differentiation arise both in the left atrium and pulmonary veins. The histological appearances show compact bundles of spindle-shaped cells, with oval blunt nuclei. The cytoplasm is often vacuolated and desmin staining is often positive. Myxoid areas and more pleomorphic tumour cells are also present.

Myxoid areas, that is a mucoid stroma rich in proteoglycans within which are embedded stellate tumour cells, occur in all cardiac sarcomas, but the term

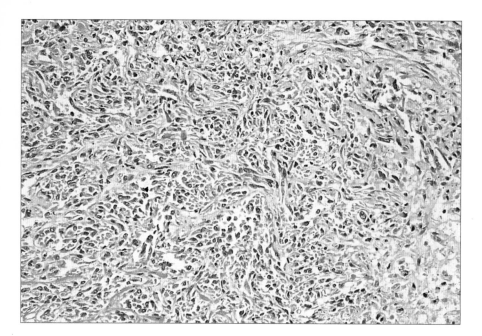

Figure 6.24 a,b
Malignant fibrous histiocytoma of heart. The tumour at low power consists of spindle cells arranged in a storiform pattern. Other areas shown at higher power ($\times$140) contained bizarre multi-nucleated cells but still with a suggestion of a storiform arrangement.

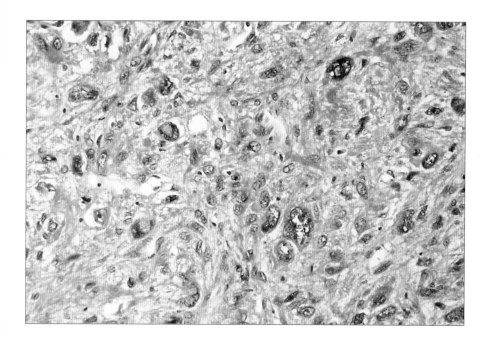

myxosarcoma is best reserved for those tumours in which this is the sole differentiation pattern. The left atrium is the commonest site and the tumour, particularly if it is low grade, may be confused with an atrial myxoma. No link exists between the benign atrial myxoma and the myxosarcoma. The two entities have never been convincingly shown to occur together. Liposarcomas arise in either atria and the slimy cut surface may resemble myxomas. The tumour shows differentiation toward lipoblasts with many vacuolated cells containing lipid droplets. Areas of myxoid or spindle cell differentiation are also present.

Malignant schwannomas show a predominant pattern of neurofibrosarcomatous differentiation, are rare, and best distinguished from the more common fibrosarcoma by S-100 positivity.

Synovial sarcoma

This is extremely rare with only four cases reported. It is a biphasic tumour with mixed spindle and epithelial areas. The epithelial and spindle cell areas stain for keratin, EMA, HBMEA1 and BER-EP4. The spindle areas can be positive for vimentin and occasional cells are S-100 positive.

Distinguishing this from mesothelioma can be difficult. Cytogenetic studies show a translocation X;18 in synovial sarcoma.

Malignant teratoma

Only four cases have been reported, all in children ranging age from one to four years. All four patients had cardiomegaly, three of the tumours were primarily

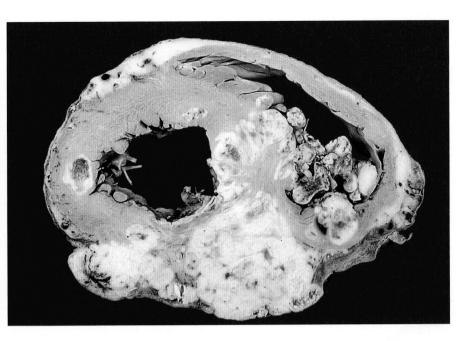

Figure 6.25
Secondary carcinoma of heart. This secondary carcinoma shows all the patterns of cardiac involvement. There are intramyocardial tumour masses, pericardial nodules and tumour projecting into the cavity of the right ventricle.

intrapericardial, attached to the root of the aorta and pulmonary artery. Metastasis to lung and mediastinum with extensive invasion of the myocardium is seen. The malignant portion of the teratoma was identified as embryonal carcinoma in two patients and a squamous cell carcinoma in a third. Malignant areas in another tumour included both embryonal carcinoma and choriocarcinoma. Remnants of benign teratoma may be found at the periphery.

Other malignant tumours can occur in the heart such as thymoma, leiomyosarcoma, liposarcoma and schwannoma. They are very rare, but must always be considered in the differential of a malignant cardiac tumour.

Lymphomas of the heart

Only seven primary malignant lymphomas of the heart have been reported in the AFIP series, with 38 further documented cases. The patients range in age from 14 months to 84 years. The terms 'primary' and 'metastatic' lymphoma of the heart are not entirely meaningful, because the site of origin of multi-focal or extra-nodal lymphoma is not generally possible to determine. If the bulk of lymphoma is confined within the pericardium, and the patient presents with cardiac disease, the term primary lymphoma of the heart is used. The tumours appear to be mainly B-cell lymphomas

In immunosuppressed patients, the development of lymphoproliferative lesions is on the increase in the heart, leading to high-grade lymphomas, usually of the B-cell type.

METASTATIC TUMOURS OF THE HEART

Metastatic tumours are much more frequent than primary cardiac tumours (Abraham *et al.* 1990; Weiss

1992; MacGee 1991). Tumour deposits may occur within the myocardium, project into the cavity of an atrium or ventricle or be pericardial masses (Fig. 6.25). Tumour metastases to the heart are seen in approximately 15% of autopsies of patients with disseminated cancer. Although there are exceptions, epithelial malignancies typically spread to the heart by lymphatics. Lymphatic dissemination in the heart is often the result of retrograde lymphatic spread secondary to blocked mediastinal or hilar lymphatics. The majority of lymph flow in the heart is efferent, which explains the low incidence of cardiac metastases. The lymphatic spread of metastasis is associated with a high incidence of malignant pericardial effusions, in contrast to hematogenous spread, which is associated with myocardial metastases. Melanoma, sarcomas, leukaemia, and renal cell carcinoma metastasise to the heart by the hematogenous route, while lymphomas may involve the heart by virtually any path. Lung carcinoma, thymoma and oesophageal carcinoma involve the heart by direct extension. Renal tumours including Wilms' tumour and renal cell carcinoma, adrenal tumours, liver tumours, and uterine stromal tumours are the most frequent intracavity tumours and reach the right atrium by spreading along the lumen of the vena cava (Fig. 6.26).

Some uncommon tumours, particularly melanoma, germ cell tumours and thymomas have a high rate of metastasis to the heart. The most likely carcinomas to spread to the heart are not surprisingly from the lung and breast. Tumours that have a low rate of cardiac metastasis include carcinoma of the stomach, liver, ovary, colon, and rectum. The frequency of cardiac metastasis in patients with metastatic epithelial malignancies ranges from 4.2% to approximately 30%. The frequency depends in part on the primary neoplasm: lung, breast, thyroid, and kidney cancers have the highest rates of spread to the heart. Much of the reported variation between series, however, may be due to whether cardiac metastases were identified by

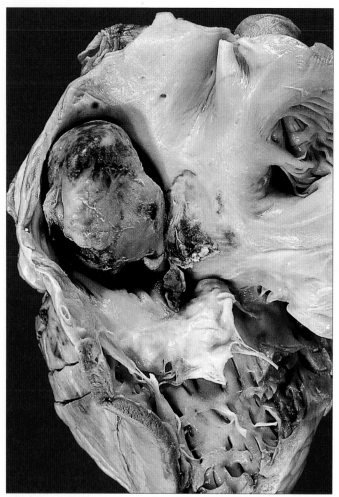

Figure 6.26
Secondary carcinoma of heart. Tumour has spread along the lumen of the inferior vena cava from the liver. Tumour protrudes out into the right atrium.

macroscopic examination alone, or by taking multiple histological blocks in hearts where there was no macroscopic tumour.

Haematological malignancies are especially prone to involve the heart, especially the myocardium. Approximately 35–40% of patients with leukaemia had cardiac involvement at autopsy. Metastatic melanoma is the malignancy most likely to spread to the heart: up to 64% of patients who died of melanoma had cardiac involvement at autopsy. The heart is affected in 8–25% of patients with metastatic soft-tissue or skeletal sarcoma. In a series of childhood autopsies, only 1.6% of children with solid malignancies had evidence of cardiac involvement at autopsy. Tumours metastatic to the heart in children, in order of decreasing frequency, are non-Hodgkin's lymphoma, Wilms' tumour, neuroblastoma, rhabdomyosarcoma, undifferentiated sarcoma, hepatoma, and adrenal cortical carcinoma. In patients with acquired immunodeficiency syndrome (AIDS), Kaposi's sarcoma is the most common neoplasm involving the heart, occurring in about 5% of autopsy cases.

MALIGNANT TUMOURS OF THE PERICARDIUM

Malignant mesothelioma of the pericardium

These are very rare. The age range is from 17 to 83 years. Most mesotheliomas of the pericardium are diffuse and cover the visceral and parietal surfaces. The mesothelioma grows by direct extension to surrounding surfaces. The epicardial myocardium may be focally invaded, but the tumour does not extend to the endocardium or cardiac chamber, which is an important feature distinguishing this tumour from primary cardiac sarcomas. The definition of primary pericardial mesothelioma stipulates that there is no tumour present outside the pericardium, with the exception of lymph node metastases. Because of the relative rarity of pericardial mesotheliomas, it has been difficult to establish a link between them and asbestos exposure. However, there have been increasing reports of pericardial mesothelioma arising in patients with known exposure to asbestos. Over 200 cases have been reported world-wide, but many of these are poorly documented. Of 49 cases reported at the AFIP (Burke and Virmani 1996), 39 were men and 20 were women. The male to female ratio of nearly 2 to 1 is lower than the ratio of 3.5 to 1 for mesotheliomas of the pleura. The higher proportion of women suggests that the link with asbestos exposure is weaker for pericardial than for pleural mesothelioma.

Macroscopically, the tumour forms a bulky nodule that may fill the pericardial cavity, often encircling the heart. Multiple satellite nodules are commonly found along the diaphragmatic and pleural surfaces. Pericardial mesotheliomas often encircle the great vessels and may obstruct the vena cava. The tumour itself is firm and white but haemorrhagic, cystic, and necrotic areas may be present. However, metastatic carcinoma to the pericardium may result also in a bulky, infiltrating tumour, even if the primary tumour is small or occult.

Light microscopic

Malignant mesotheliomas of the pericardium resemble their pleural counterparts with epithelial, mixed (biphasic), and sarcomatoid types on the basis of histologic growth patterns. The epithelial component forms tubules, papillary structures, and cords of infiltrating cells that can incite a fibroblastic stromal response. In biphasic tumours, there is both an epithelial and spindle cell component. The epithelial and spindle cell areas usually merge imperceptibly, and the nuclear features of the spindle cells are often similar to those of the epithelial cells. Over 75% of pericardial mesotheliomas are of the biphasic variety. Sometimes it may be difficult to separate reactive fibroblasts from the malignant spindle cell component of the tumour. Sarcomatoid mesothelioma may focally resemble malignant fibrous histiocytoma or undifferentiated sarcoma, but the cells have large oval nuclei, prominent nucleoli, and abundant cytoplasm, and there is usually a subpopulation of cells with a rounded contour hinting at the epithelial component of the tumour. In the AFIP files, six pericardial mesothelial tumours had spindled and epithelial areas, one was predominantly sarcomatoid, and one was predominantly epithelial with a tubulopapillary pattern.

The presence of hyaluronic acid in mesothelioma has been classically used in the past for diagnosis. Mesothelioma contains both cellular and extracellular hyaluronic acid and chondroitin sulphate which are positive for colloidal iron and Alcian blue at pH 2.5 which disappears with hyaluronidase, but only 50% of tumours stain. It is also a very capricious stain which can be difficult to interpret, so many laboratories do not use it for routine diagnosis of mesothelioma.

The diagnosis is usually made on the basis of ultrastructural and immunohistochemical evaluation of the tumour. Immunohistochemically, virtually 100% of pleural mesotheliomas express cytokeratin, primarily in its high molecular weight form, in epithelioid areas; sarcomatoid cells express cytokeratin in about 75% of cases, often focally. Vimentin is preferentially expressed in the spindle cell areas of mesothelioma, but less often than cytokeratin. Epithelial membrane antigen is frequently present in the epithelial areas of mesothelioma, although expression of this antigen appears inconsistent. Mesotheliomas, in general, do not express carcinoembryonic antigen, B72.3 antigen, and LeuMl.

Differentiating mesothelioma and adenocarcinoma is facilitated by histochemical, ultrastructural, and immunohistological studies. In general, a definitive diagnosis is rendered only after a panel of stains has been performed. The simplest histochemical stain that identifies adenocarcinoma is the periodic acid-Schiff (PAS) after diastase pretreatment. Intracytoplasmic PASD positive vacuoles are never present in mesotheliomas, but are present in 46–61% of adenocarcinomas of all types and 52% of adenocarcinomas of the lung. Carcinoembryonic antigen is expressed in 77–95% of adenocarcinomas and in 0–22% of mesotheliomas. Polyclonal antisera should be absorbed against splenic tissues to remove antibodies that cross-react with nonspecific glycoproteins. Monoclonal antibodies are generally more specific than polyclonal antisera, and are less often positive in mesothelioma; a positive reaction with carcinoembryonic antigen is very useful in excluding malignant mesothelioma.

LeuMl, a cell membrane-associated glycoprotein, is present in 0–8% of mesotheliomas, but in 80–100% of adenocarcinomas of the lung, and 42–60% of carcinomas of all types. B72.3 antigen, BER-EP4, and MOC-31 are markers of adenocarcinoma that are also rarely, if ever, expressed by mesothelioma.

The mean survival of patients with pericardial mesotheliomas is shorter than that of patients with pleural and peritoneal mesotheliomas.

Reactive mesothelial hyperplasia

It can be extremely difficult to distinguish reactive mesothelial proliferations from malignant mesothelioma. Benign mesothelial proliferations occasionally result in recurrent pericardial effusions that suggest malignancy. In general, malignant mesotheliomas infiltrate the underlying fibrous and fatty tissue or myocardium, and have spindle malignant sarcomatoid areas, all features lacking in reactive mesothelial processes. Immunohistochemical stains are of no use in separating malignant from benign mesothelial reactions.

Malignant fibrous tumour of the pericardium

Solitary fibrous tumours of the pericardium are rare and most are benign: some may have cellular areas with pleomorphism and mitotic figures indicating that they are malignant fibrous tumours which may recur and infiltrate surrounding structures. In contrast to sarcomatoid mesotheliomas, solitary fibrous tumours are composed of relatively bland spindled cells similar to fibrosarcoma. There is no expression of epithelial markers and the cells are CD34 positive.

References

Abraham KP, Reddy V, Gattuso P. Neoplasms metastatic to the heart: a review of 3314 consecutive autopsies. *Am J Cardiovasc Pathol* 1990;13:195–8.

Attum AA, Johnson GS, Masri Z, Girardet R, Lansing AM. Malignant clinical behaviour of cardiac myxomas and myxoid imitators. *Ann Thorac Surg* 1987;44:217–22.

Blondeau P. Primary cardiac tumours-French studies of 533 cases. *Thorac Cardiovasc Surg* 1990;38:192–5.

Boxer ME. Cardiac myxoma: an immunoperoxidase study of histogenesis. *Histopathology* 1984;8:861–72.

Budzilovich G, Aleksic S, Greco A, Fernandez J, Harris J, Finegold M. Malignant cardiac myxoma with cerebral metastases. *Surg Neurol* 1979;11:461–9.

Burke AP, Anderson PG, Virmani R, James TN, Herera GA, Ceballos R. Tumors of the atrioventricular nodal region. A clinical and immunohistochemical study. *Arch Pathol Lab Med* 1990;114:1057–62.

Burke AP, Johns J, Virmani R. Hemangiomas of the heart: a clinicopathologic study of 10 cases. *Am J Cardiovasc Pathol* 1991;13:283–90.

Burke AP, Virmani R. Cardiac rhabdomyoma: a clinical pathological study. *Mod Pathol* 1991a;4:70–4.

Burke AP, Virmani R. Osteosarcomas of the heart. *Am J Surg Pathol* 1991b;15:289–95.

Burke AP, Virmani R. Cardiac myxomas. A clinicopathologic study. *Am J Clin Pathol* 1993;100:671–80.

Burke AP, Rosado-de-Christenson M, Templeton PA, Virmani R. Cardiac fibroma: clinicopathologic correlates and surgical treatment. *J Thor Cardiovasc Surg* 1994;108:862–70.

Burke AP, Virmani R. *Tumours of heart and great*

vessels. *Atlas of tumour pathology*, 3rd series, fascicle 16. Washington DC: Armed Forces Institute of Pathology, 1996.

Byard RW, Smith NM, Bourne AJ. Incidental cardiac rhabdomyomas: a significant finding necessitating additional investigation at the time of autopsy. *J Forensic Sci* 1991;36:1229–33.

Carney JA. Differences between non-familial and familial cardiac myxoma. *Am J Surg Pathol* 1985;9:53–5.

Chan HSD, Sonley MJ, Moes CA, Daneman A, Smith CR, Martin DJ. Primary and secondary tumors of childhood involving the heart, pericardium and great vessels. A report of 75 cases and review of the literature. *Cancer* 1985;56:825–36.

Courtice RW, Stimson WA, Walley VM. Tissue fragments recovered at cardiac surgery masquerading as tumoural proliferations. Evidence suggesting iatrogenic or artefactual origin and common occurrence. *Am J Surg Pathol* 1994;18:167–74.

Curschellas E, Toia D, Borner M, Mihatsch MJ, Gudat F. Cardiac myxomas: immunohistochemical study of benign and malignant variants. *Virchows Arch* 1991;418:485–91.

Damasio H, Seabra-Gomes R, da Silva JP, Damasio AR, Antunes JL, Multiple cerebral aneurysms and cardiac myxoma. *Arch Neurol* 1975;32:269–70.

Evans DW, Stovin PGI. Fatal heart block due to mesothelioma of the atrioventricular node. *Br Heart J* 1986;56:572–4.

Edwards FH, Hale D, Cohen A, Thompson L, Pezzella AT, Virmani R. Primary cardiac valve tumours. *Ann Thorac Surg* 1991;52:1127–31.

Feigin DS, Fenoglio JJ, McAllister HA, Madewell JE. Pericardial cysts. A radiologic-pathologic correlation and review. *Radiology* 1977;125:15–20.

Feldman PS, Meyer MW. Fibroelastic hamartoma (fibroma) of the heart. *Cancer* 1976;38:314–23.

Fenoglio JJ Jr, Diana DJ, Bowen TE, McAllister HA, Ferrans VJ. Ultrastructure of a cardiac rhabdomyoma. *Hum Pathol* 1977;8:700–6.

Fenoglio JJ, McAllister HA, Ferrans VJ. Cardiac rhabdomyoma: a clinicopathologic and electron microscopic study. *Am J Cardiol* 1976;38:241–51.

Fine G, Raju U. Congenital polycystic tumour of atrioventricular node (endodermal heterotopia mesothelioma) a histogenic appraisal with evidence of its endodermal origin. *Hum Pathol* 1987;18:791–5.

Gelb AB, van Meter SH, Billingham ME, Berry GJ, Rouse RV. Infantile histiocytoid cardiomyopathy myocardial or conduction system hamartoma: what is the cell type involved? *Hum Pathol* 1993;24:1226–31.

Goldman BI, Frydman C, Harpaz N, Ryan SF, Loiterman D. Glandular cardiac myxomas. *Cancer* 1987;59:1767–75.

Gordon H, Carpenter PC, Shenoy BV, Go VL. The complex of myxomas, spotty pigmentation and endocrine overactivity. *Med Baltimore* 1985;64:270–83.

Govoni E, Severi B, Cenacchi G *et al.* Ultrastructural and immunohistochemical contribution to the histo-genesis of human cardiac myxoma. *Ultrastruc Pathol* 1988;12:22–33.

Hendin BN, Longaker MT, Finkbeiner WE, Roberts LJ, Stern R. Hyaluronic acid deposition in cardiac myxomas: localization using a hyaluronate-specific binding protein. *Am J Cardiovasc Pathol* 1990;3:209–15.

Johansson L. Histogenesis of cardiac myxomas. An immunohistochemical study of 19 cases, including one with glandular structures, and review of the literature. *Arch Pathol Lab Med* 1989;113:735–41.

Jourdan M, Bataille R, Seguin J, Zhang XG, Chaptal PA, Klein B. Constitutive production of interleukin-6 and immunologic features in cardiac myxomas. *Arthritis Rheum* 1990;33:398–402.

Krikler DM, Rode J, Davies MJ, Woolf N, Moss E. Atrial myxoma: a tumour in search of its origins. *Br Heart J* 1992;67:89–91.

Kotylo PK, Kennedy JE, Waller BF, Sample RB. DNA analysis of cardiac myxomas. *Chest* 1991;99:1203–7.

Landon G, Ordonez NG, Guarda LA. Cardiac myxomas. An immunohistochemical study using endothelial, histiocytic and smooth muscle cell markers. *Arch Pathol Lab Med* 1986;110:116–20.

Lie JT. The identity and histogenesis of cardiac myxoma. A controversy put to rest. *Arch Pathol Lab Med* 1989;113:724–26.

MacGee W. Metastatic and invasive tumour involving the heart in a geriatric population: a necropsy study. *Virchow Archiv Pathol Anat* 1991;419:183–9.

Malhotra V, Ferrans VJ, Virmani R. Infantile histiocytoid cardiomyopathy: report of three cases and review of literature. *Am Heart J* 1994;128:1009–21.

Mann J, Parker DJ. Papillary fibroelastoma of the mitral valve: a rare cause of transient neurological defects. *Br Heart J* 1994;71:76-7.

Manthos CL, Sutherland RS, Sims JE, Perloff JJ. Carney's complex in a patient with hormone-producing sertoli cell tumour of the testicle. *J Urol* 1993;150:1511–12.

Markwald RR, Fitzharris TP, Manmasek FJ. Structural development of endocardial cushions. *Am J Anat* 1977;148:85–119.

McAllister HA, Ferrans VJ. Cardiac rhabdomyoma: A clinicopathological and electron microscopic study. *Am J Cardiol* 1976;38:241–51.

McAllister HA, Fenoglio JJ Jr. *Tumors of the cardiovascular system. Atlas of tumor pathology*, 2nd series, fascicle 15. Washington DC: Armed Forces Institute of Pathology, 1978;62–3.

McComb RD. Heterogeneous expression of factor VIII/von Willebrand factor by cardiac myxoma cells. *Am J Surg Pathol* 1984;8:539–44.

Morales AR, Fine G, Castro A, Madji M. Cardiac myxomas (endocardioma). An immunocytochemical assessment of histogenesis. *Hum Pathol* 1981;12:896–9.

Pochis WT, Saeian K, Sagar KB. Usefulness of transesophageal echocardiography in diagnosing lipomatous hypertrophy of the atrial septum with comparison to transthoracic echocardiography. *Am J Cardiol* 1992;70:396–8.

Reed RJ, Utz MP, Terezakis N. Embolic and metastatic cardiac myxomas. *Am J Dermatopathol* 1989;**11**:157–65.

Rhodes AR, Silverman RA, Harrist TJ, Perez-Atayde Ar. Mucocutaneous lentigines, cardiomucocutaneous myxomas and multiple blue naevi. The 'LAMB' syndrome. *J Am Acad Dermatol* 1984;**10**:72–82.

Richard I, Whittaker JS, Deiraniya AK, Hassan R. Intracardiac ectopic thyroid: a case report and review of published ones. *Thorax* 1990;**45**:293–4.

Rokey R, Mulvagh SL, Chierif K, Mattox KL, Johnston DL. Lipomatous encasement and compression of the heart: antemortem diagnosis by cardiac nuclear magnetic resonance imaging and catheterisation. *Am Heart J* 1989;**117**:952–3.

Rose AG. Venous malformation of the heart. *Arch Pathol Lab Med* 1979;**103**:18–20.

Rupp GM, Heyman RA, Martinez AJ, Sekhar LN, Jungreis CA. The pathology of metastatic cardiac myxomas. *Am J Clin Pathol* 1989;**91**:221–7.

Saffitz JM, Ferrans V, Rodriquez E, Lewis F, Roberts W. Histiocytoid cardiomyopathy: a cause of sudden death in apparently healthy infants. *Am J Cardiol* 1983;**52**:215–6.

Salyer WR, Page DSL, Hutchins GM. The development of cardiac myxomas and papillary endocardial lesions from mural thrombus. *Am Heart J* 1975;**89**:4–17.

Schuger L, Ron N, Rosenmann E. Cardiac myxoma: a retrospective immunohistochemical study. *Pathol Res Pract* 1987;**182**:63–6.

Seidman JD, Berman JJ, Hitchcock CL, Becker RL, Merner W, Moore GW, Virmani R, Yetter RA. DNA analysis of cardiomyxomas. *Hum Pathol* 1991;**22**:494–500.

Shirani J, Roberts WC. Clinical electrocardiographic and morphologic features of massive fatty deposits (lipomatous hypertrophy) in the atrial septum. *J Am Coll Cardiol* 1993;**22**:226–38.

Smith HC, Watson GH, Patel RG, Super M. Cardiac rhabdomyomata in tuberous sclerosis: their course and diagnostic value. *Arch Dis Child* 1989;**64**:196–200.

Subramanian R, Flygenring B. Mesothelioma of the atrioventricular node and congenital complete heart block. *Clin Cardiol* 1989;**12**:3469–72.

Tanimura A, Kitazono M, Nagayama K, Tanaka S, Kosuga K. Cardiac myxoma: morphological histochemical and tissue culture studies. *Hum Pathol* 1988;**19**:316–22.

Todo T, Usui M, Nagashima K. Cerebral metastasis of malignant cardiac myxoma. *Surg Neurol* 1992;**37**:374–9.

Utiger CA, Headington JT. Psammomatous melanotic schwannoma. A new cutaneous marked for Carney's complex. *Arch Dermatol* 1993;**129**:202–4.

Valente M, Basso C, Thiene G *et al*. Fibroelastic papilloma: a not so benign cardiac tumour. *Cardiovasc Pathol* 1992;**1**:61–6.

Vidaillet HJ, Seward JB, Fyke FE, Su WPD, Tajik AJ. 'Syndrome myxoma': a subset of patients with cardiac myxoma associated with pigmented skin lesions and peripheral and endocrine neoplasms. *Br Heart J* 1987;**57**:247–55.

Vidaillet HJ. Cardiac tumors associated with hereditary syndromes. *Am J Cardiol* 1988;**22**:89–98.

Weiss L. An analysis of the incidence of myocardial metastasis from solid cancers. *Br Heart J* 1992;**68**:501–4.

Zhang P, Jones JW, Anderson WR. Cardiac myxomas – correlative study by light, transmission and scanning electron microscopy. *Am J Cardiovasc Pathol* 1989;**2**:295–300.

Zimmerman KG, Paplanus SH, Dong S, Nagle RB. Congenital blood cysts of the heart valves. *Hum Pathol* 1983;**14**:699–703.

SEVEN

DISEASES OF THE AORTA

THE NORMAL AORTA

The aorta arises from the aortic sinuses which contain the aortic valve and then continues up and over to the left as the ascending aorta. The aortic arch passes over the hilum of the left lung and the descending thoracic and abdominal aorta. Just distal to the left subclavian artery, there is often a puckered or depressed area visible on the intima which is the site of the closed ductus.

The ventriculo-aortic junction is characterised by three sinuses (sinuses of Valsalva) which support the semilunar attachments of the aortic valve. Each sinus is the area of the aorta above the attachment of the semilunar leaflets, extending up to a ridge encircling the aorta at the commissures known as the supra-aortic ridge or sinu-tubular ridge. Two of the sinuses usually give rise to the coronary arteries (*see* Chapters 1 and 2). The sinus portion of the aorta is 1.5 times wider than the proximal tubular aorta, a fact that is appreciated more easily during life with angiography, and at autopsy only if the aorta is fixed by pressure perfusion.

The normal aorta (Figs 7.1, 7.2) has a thin intima lined by endothelium, a prominent media containing parallel elastic lamellae separated by smooth muscle cells, some

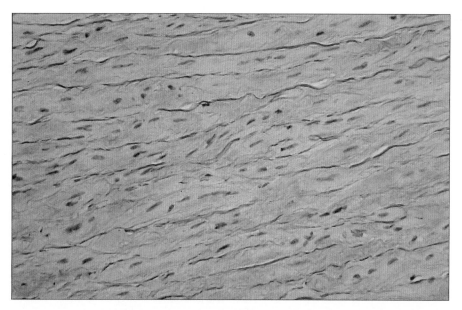

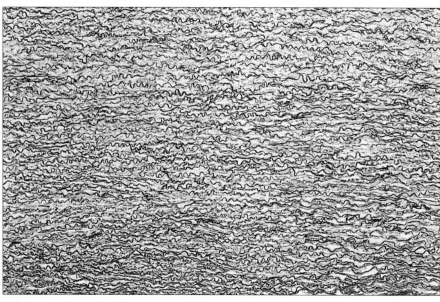

Figure 7.1 a,b
Normal adult aorta – histology. In (a) H&E staining shows (×10) the media to contain collagen and smooth muscle cells as well as a blue staining proteoglycans. This degree of basophilia is normal and it does not indicate an abnormality unless there is destruction of elastic laminae. (b) Elastic staining (×10) shows the parallel lamellae with collagen and smooth muscle cells interspersed.

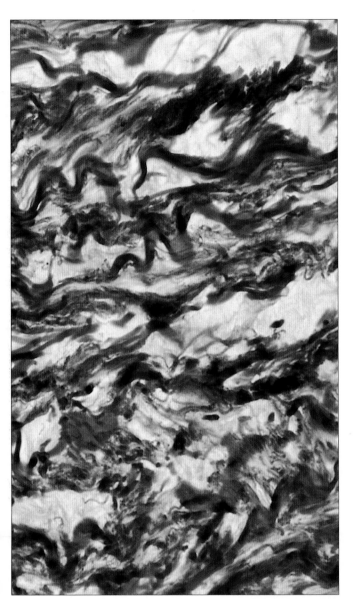

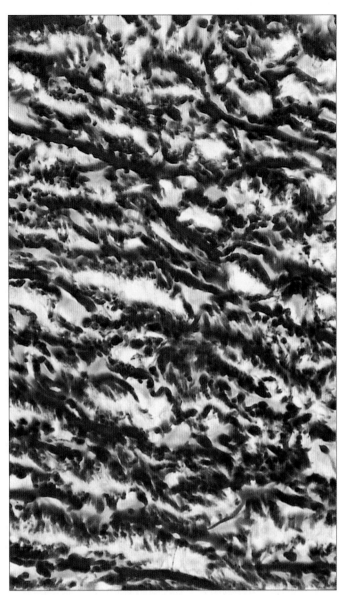

Figure 7.2
Normal aorta (Elastic van Gieson). The aortic media in children (left picture) compared with adults (right picture) shows fewer elastic laminae, more smooth muscle and less collagen.

collagen fibres and a mucoid ground substance rich in proteoglycans. Each lamella and the adjacent zone containing the smooth muscle cells, which synthesise the connective tissue matrix, is a lamellar unit (Clark and Glagov 1985). The parallel elastic lamellae are more numerous in the ascending aorta, usually 55 units while the descending aorta has up to 28 units. The media should not be regarded as a static structure. The number of lamellae is only 35 at birth; by adult life it is 55. After middle age the actual number of lamellae is difficult to count because each unit has reduplicated finer elastic lamellae alongside the major one. Small vessels penetrate into the outer fifth of the media from the adventitia and form a capillary arcade. The inner four-fifths of the aortic media is avascular. With increasing age the elastic lamellae reduplicate and in small foci fragment. The number of smooth muscle cells decreases, the mucoid ground substance becomes more prominent, and the number of collagen fibres increases. These medial changes alter the compliance of the aortic

wall and result in dilatation (Bouissou *et al*. 1987) with elongation, a process known as aortic ectasia. In the ascending aorta the dilatation leads to 'unfolding' of the aorta as seen in a chest X-ray. The increase in rigidity of the aorta leads to the widening of the pulse pressure in old age. With advancing age the intima thickens and develops fine elastic laminae which make a clear distinction of intima from the media far from easy histologically (Bouissou *et al*. 1987). The aortic sinus area contains predominantly fibrous tissue without elastic, explaining why the sinuses bulge in systole.

DISEASES OF THE AORTA – INTRODUCTION

Aortic disease is dominated by aneurysms of various types. All aneurysms mean that an underlying medial disease is present which has destroyed the capacity of

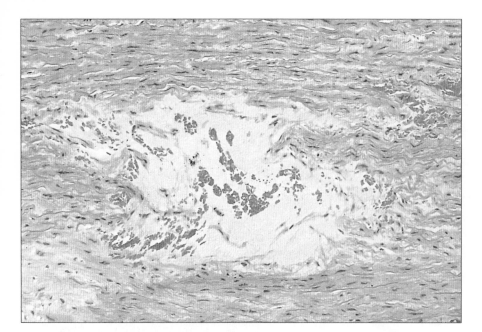

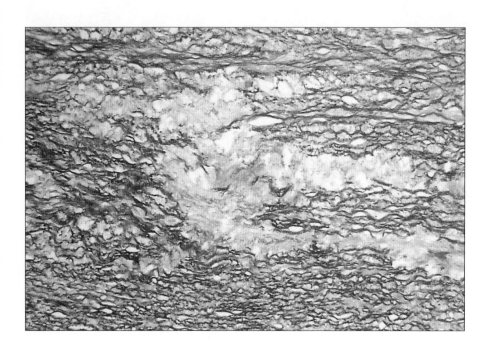

Figure 7.3 a,b
Cystic medial change in aorta. (a) There is a focal cystic area filled with basophilic ground substance (H&E ×35). (b) In the section stained by elastic Van Gieson, the cystic areas displace the elastic lamellae but the degree of disruption and fragmentation is mild. This degree of change can be found in elderly subjects with senile aortic dilatation.

the tissue to resist the haemodynamic force exerted in systole. Three disease processes can destroy the media. First atherosclerosis, although an intimal disease, is associated with widespread medial atrophy. Second, there are non-inflammatory 'degenerations' of the media (aortopathy), and finally there is inflammatory aortitis of the media and adventitia.

Histological changes in the aortic media

There are two broad categories of aortic medial response. One is non-inflammatory and associated with elastic lamina disruption, accumulation of cystic collections of proteoglycans, and acid connective tissue mucopolysaccharides. The other is inflammatory (aorti-

tis) with medial destruction associated with a lymphocytic and plasma cell infiltrate extending into the media along the vasa vasorum from the adventitia.

Non-inflammatory medial disease

The aortic media undergoes very significant histological changes with increasing age. These changes are so common that it is very difficult to say with any certainty that the media is normal or abnormal for any particular individual, or that the changes are specific for any particular disease. The complex changes in the media involve permutations of:

1. Smooth muscle cell loss – the elastic laminae lie closer together and appear straighter than usual. The normal young aortic media when stained for connec-

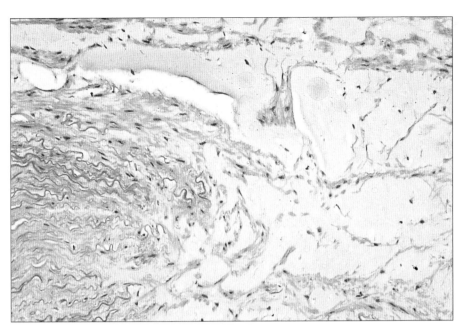

Figure 7.4 a,b,c

Severe cystic medial change in aorta. (a) There is major replacement of the medial structure by cystic spaces containing basophilic material (H&E ×35). (b) In the elastic Van Gieson stained section the extreme degree of fragmentation of the elastic lamellae can be seen (×35). (c) When stains such as Alcian blue are used the accumulation of acid mucopolysaccharide can be shown. Acid mucopolysaccharides are, however, very abundant in even the normal aortic media and the mere presence of Alcian blue positive material in the absence of elastic lamellae fragmentation must be interpreted as normal (×35).

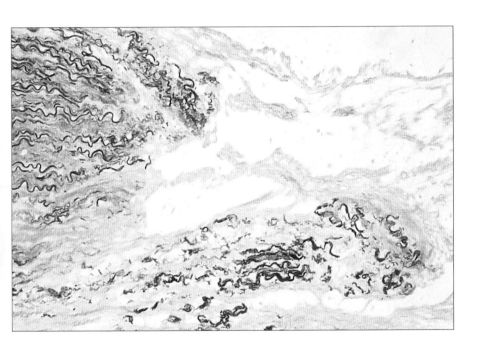

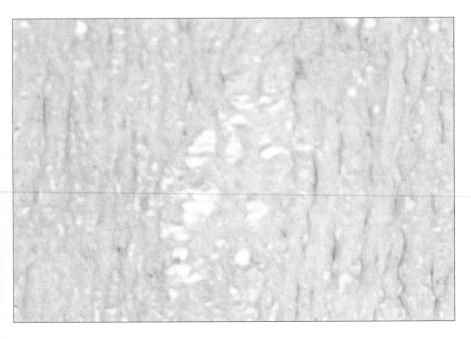

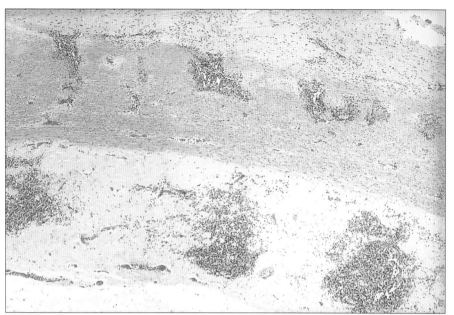

(a)

Figure 7.5 a,b,c
Aortitis due to syphilis. At low power (a) the focal accumulation of chronic inflammatory cells can be seen in both the adventitia and the media. At higher power (b and c) the focal aggregates of chronic inflammatory cells are seen to be associated with marked local destruction of the elastic lamellae (a) H&E ×8.75. (b) H&E, elastic Van Gieson ×82). (c) H&E ×82.

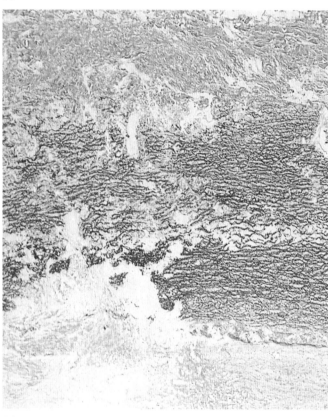

(b)

(c)

tive tissue by the elastic-Van Gieson or a trichrome method shows relatively little collagen. This increases in amount as smooth muscle cell loss develops. Smooth muscle cell loss may be zonal, occurring in the mid third of the media and in extreme cases the media become totally acellular but the elastic lamellae are intact.

2. Elastic fragmentation.
3. Cystic change – there are focal areas of elastic lamina disruption associated with pools of connective tissue mucin. In its extreme form where there are many areas of cystic change, the name cystic medial necrosis is often applied. The name Erdheim is attached

to this appearance. It is far from clear which cells or tissue have undergone necrosis, and histologically, although the areas adjacent to cystic areas are often acellular without smooth muscle nuclei, there is no real evidence that this loss was by necrosis. The acellular areas do not invoke an inflammatory response. Medial smooth muscle cells have a low expression of FAS constitutively; this can be upregulated very easily to invoke apoptosis which may be the mechanism involved in smooth muscle loss.

Because this spectrum of histological change including cystic transformation occurs to some degree in any

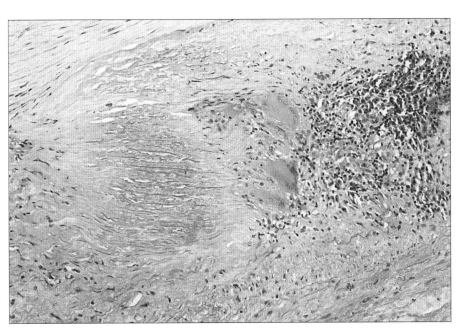

Figure 7.6
Giant cell aortitis. The media has an area of acellular eosinophilic change in which the elastic laminae are still intact. At the margins of this area there are giant cells and a heavy chronic inflammatory cell infiltrate. As the disease activity wanes the media becomes less infiltrated by chronic inflammatory cells, leaving areas in the media without nuclei and eosinophilic elastic fibres. When many histological blocks are taken, however, some residual giant cells are often found allowing the diagnosis to be made (H&E ×56).

aorta which is undergoing age-related dilatation, the histology has been regarded as non-specific (Schlatmann and Becker 1977) and not a direct cause of either dissection or aneurysms. More extreme degrees of all these changes (Figs 7.3, 7.4) are found in genetic diseases of connective tissue synthesis such as Marfan's disease. Severe medial degenerative cystic change is also found in the aortic root dilatation responsible for a high proportion of cases of isolated aortic regurgitation (see Chapter 3), and in some aortic aneurysms. Overall, the medial changes will alter the patterns of circumferential and shear stress distribution in systole and predispose to both aneurysm and dissection (*see* Pathogenesis of aortic dissection, p. 179).

Inflammatory medial disease

The archetypal cause of inflammatory medial disease is syphilis. There are round focal areas of medial destruction in which the elastic laminae are absent, and in these areas are aggregates of lymphocytes and plasma cells. The inflammatory process extends in from the adventitia along the vasa vasorum which show marked endarteritis obliterans (Fig. 7.5). The areas of destruction in the media do not show cystic change, and ultimately are converted to fibrous scars. The overlying intima develops irregular thickening due to smooth muscle proliferation. Although the overall thickness of the vessel wall thins, the adventitia is inflamed and thickened. In very acute syphilis small microgummata with small giant cells and central necrosis occur, but it is far more usual to see the later more chronic stages of the aortitis in which they are absent. Very occasionally microorganisms can be found (Virmani and McCallister 1986). The chronic stage of syphilitic aortitis can be taken as the essential histopathology of a chronic aortitis. Very similar changes can occur in anklyosing spondylitis, rheumatoid arthritis, Behçet's disease and rarely in any of the systemic vasculitis/collagen diseases. One specific variant of aortitis has distinguishing histological features (Fig. 7.6). In giant cell

aortitis there are plates of totally acellular medial tissue in which giant cells appear to be in relation to the ends of broken elastic laminae. There is also a generalised non-specific aortitis. Giant cell aortitis occurs in elderly women with a raised ESR, a systemic pyrexial disease and is often associated with polymyalgia rheumatica.

AORTIC ANEURYSMS – TYPES AND DEFINITIONS

Aneurysms can be defined as external bulges of a blood-containing structure which expand in systole. All aneurysms have the risk of external rupture. In true aortic aneurysms, the wall is made up of all the constituents of the aortic wall, i.e. intima, media and adventitia. In what are called false aneurysms the external bulge has a wall consisting of adventitia or periaortic tissue only (Fig. 7.7). The aneurysm sac communicates with the lumen via a narrow defect in the media. True aneurysms may be confined to a short segment of the aorta and bulge out to one side – these are saccular in type. In contrast, diffuse aneurysms involve the whole circumference of the aorta and often extend over a long distance. Diffuse aneurysms of the ascending aorta are almost always associated with aortic regurgitation, due to dilatation of the aortic root at the level of the supra-aortic ridge. Dissecting aneurysms of the aorta (better termed aortic dissections) are very different. Here there is an intimal tear which allows blood to enter the media and form a track which extends both proximally and distally. The dissection track is in the outer third of the media, in the plane of the capillary arcade. The blood in the tract will pulsate when viewed from outside, hence the dissecting process is termed an aneurysm. The majority of dissection tracks ultimately break outward and rupture through the adventitia. However, the intimal tear and the external exit point are often widely separated.

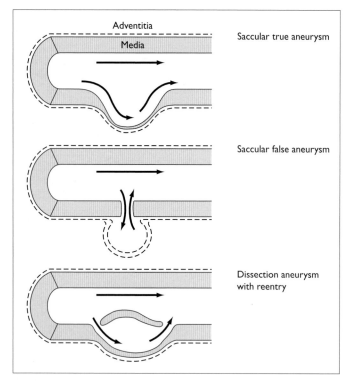

Figure 7.7

Diagrammatic representation of true, false and dissecting aneurysms. In true aneurysms the wall is derived from all the elements of the aortic wall. In false aneurysms there is a narrow entry point and the external sac is made up of adventitia alone. In dissection with re-entry the external bulge is made up of adventitia and some media.

Aortic false aneurysms are virtually always due to either penetrating trauma such as knife wounds or closed chest trauma (Table 7.1). Dissecting aneurysms are caused by non-inflammatory medial disease. True aneurysms are caused by atherosclerosis or aortitis or non-inflammatory medial disease.

Aortic dissection

All aortic dissections are characterised by a separation of the media with tracking of blood longitudinally. An intimal tear is identified in the majority of cases. In over 60% of patients the tear marking the beginning of the dissection is in the ascending aorta (Fig. 7.8), usually about 2 cm above the aortic valve. The majority of tears are transverse, although they may be T-shaped or vertical. The intimal tear is located in the aortic arch in about 10% of cases, where it is more liable to be longitudinal (Fig. 7.9). The tear is in the descending aorta in 25% of cases and rarely in the abdominal aorta (3% of cases) (Roberts 1991; Doroghazi and Slater 1983). A careful search of the intima is necessary in all cases of medial dissection to find the entrance tear. Proximal extension of the dissection is much less frequent than distal propagation. The intramedial haematoma so formed, progresses distally as far as branching points and often involves the head and neck vessels. The development of this haematoma results in a false lumen with expansion and weakening of the aortic wall resulting in aneurysm formation.

Table 7.1

Aortic aneurysms.

Type of aortic aneurysm	Cause
False saccular aneurysm	Trauma
True diffuse and saccular aneurysms	Connective tissue genetic disorders Non-inflammatory medial disease Aortitis Atherosclerosis
Dissecting aneurysms	Connective tissue genetic disorders Non-inflammatory medial disease

There is some contention over whether it is possible to find at autopsy aortic dissection without an intimal tear. The authors have never seen such a case, but they are reported in the literature. The incidence of dissection without an intimal tear was 4% in 505 cases in one series (Hirst *et al.* 1958).

Various types of classification of dissection of the aorta have been made, largely to allow comparison of different surgical repair techniques and series to be carried out while ensuring that like was being considered with like. The basic classification (DeBakey *et al.* 1965) distinguishes Type I – confined to ascending aorta; Type II – arch of aorta; Type III – distal to left subclavian artery with distal dissection. Further refinement of Type III is often made into non-communicating and communicating where the track has re-entered the aortic lumen either distally or proximally (Erbel *et al.* 1993) (Fig. 7.10). It should be emphasised that these classifications are purely for description relative to surgical treatment and do not imply any basic pathogenetic differences.

An intimal-medial tear with the formation of an intramedial haematoma can have several consequences:

1. External rupture of the intramedial haematoma occurs. This is common in dissection of the ascending aorta because the external wall is very thin consisting mainly of adventitia with just a thin layer of outer media. This rupture results in massive haemorrhage into the mediastinum, pleural cavities or pericardium resulting in the sudden onset of chest pain and rapid death (Figs 7.8, 7.9).

With improved imaging and the use of non-invasive transoesophageal echocardiography, early diagnosis of dissecting aneurysm is possible and surgery can be undertaken immediately which is pivotal to survival. In patients with dissection affecting the ascending aorta, immediate operation is essential while with uncomplicated dissection sparing the ascending aorta, initial management is medical with control of blood pressure and bed rest. Improvements in

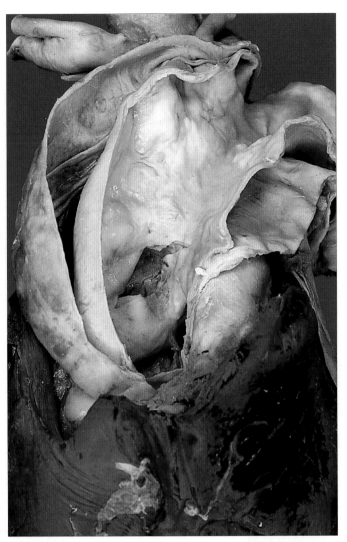

Figure 7.8
Dissection of aorta. There is a transverse tear in the intima of the ascending aorta which communicates with a large dissection track passing up to the arch. Death by haemopericardium – hypertension in life.

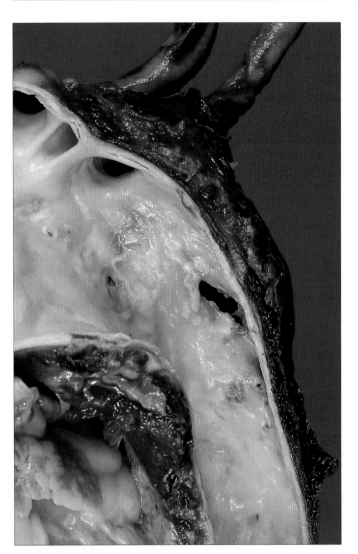

Figure 7.9
Dissection of aorta. There is a vertical intimal tear in this descending thoracic aortic dissection.

imaging and surgical techniques have reduced the mortality from thoracic dissection.

2. A re-entry tear may develop in the intima distal to the primary intimal tear leading to two aortic lumens. The frequency of external rupture in the ascending aorta means at this site re-entry is rare; about 10% of dissections on the abdominal aorta, however, develop a re-entry intimal tear (Fig. 7.10).

3. The development of a chronic aneurysm with thrombus formation in the track which is still communicating with the lumen to some extent (Fig. 7.11).

4. A small localised dissection may heal leaving a transverse or longitudinal U-shaped depression in the intima and media (Fig. 7.12).

5. Dissecting aneurysm may produce stenosis of branches of the aorta (Fig. 7.13) due to extension of the haematoma into the media with occlusion of the vessel lumen and distal ischaemia.

6. Finally about 10% of all acute aortic dissections will progress to a chronic or healed phase (Fig. 7.14). Many of these cases have a re-entry site in the abdominal aorta (De Bakey type 3 or distal dissections). The double-barrel aorta has a false channel that is often larger than the true lumen, so that the term aneurysm is more appropriate here than in acute dissections where there is often little dilatation. The lining of the false channel shows fibro-muscular thickening. Mural thrombi in the channel may become organised, forming thrombo-atherosclerotic plaques. Calcification may become prominent in the wall of the false channel, and sometimes the lumen may be completely occluded by thrombus. Healed dissections can be compatible with long survival and are occasionally discovered in patients as coincidental findings at autopsy, indicating that an acute dissection may be silent.

The pathogenesis of aortic dissection

The pathogenesis of aortic dissection is extremely complex.

Risk factors for aortic dissection

Epidemiological studies using case control methods and family studies clearly show that the risk of dissection is greatly increased in a number of circumstances (Table

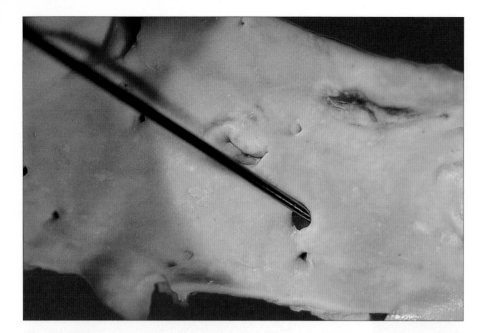

Figure 7.10
Dissection of aorta. There is an intimal re-entry tear in the iliac artery.

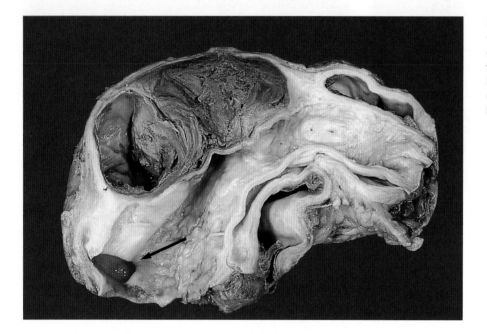

Figure 7.11
Chronic dissection aneurysm. This chronic dissection aneurysm was surgically excised from the thoracic aorta in a patient with Marfan's disease. There is an intimal tear (arrow) and a dissection track filled with laminated thrombus.

7.2). Contrary to popular misconception atherosclerosis and inflammatory aortitis do not cause dissection. The means by which these risk factors operate is only partially understood. Hypertension presumably operates by increasing the mechanical forces which are imposed on the aorta. The normal aorta is, however, an extremely strong structure resisting very high distending pressures, as well as being able to withstand considerable shear stress when fluids are injected directly into the media in an attempt to separate the layers. This suggests that hypertension only operates as a potentiating factor on an aorta with some prior medial abnormality (Davies *et al.* 1996). The higher risk of aortic dissection in association with bicuspid aortic valves is well established (Larson and Edwards 1984; Lindsay 1988). It has often been postulated that asymmetric high velocity jets through bicuspid valves might alter stress distribution in the first part of the

Table 7.2
Factors increasing risk of aortic dissection.

Hypertension
Coarctation of aorta
Bicuspid aortic valves
Marfan's disease
Other genetic defects of connective tissue synthesis
Family history – no stigmata of Marfan's

ascending aorta. Echocardiographic studies (Hahn *et al.* 1992) show no relation between aortic dilatation and the degree of disturbance of vascular flow in bicuspid valves. This suggests that there is a primary defect in the development of the aorta and cusps in bicuspid valves which is either at a structural or molecular level.

Taking dissecting aneurysms of the aorta overall, more than 80% occur over the age of 60 years and hypertension is the only discernible risk factor (Erbel 1996). In patients under 40 years, dissection is strongly related to genetic defects of connective tissue synthesis such as Marfan's disease.

Pathogenesis of dissection

The aorta is subject to huge circumferential wall stress in systole as well as shear stresses which exert forces trying to separate the layers of the wall. In the normal aorta, the structures are symmetric and distribute the stresses equally across the vessel wall. Hypertension elevates these stresses. Once any dyshomogeneity of the media develops, stresses become unevenly distributed. The amount of stress cannot be reduced in total, therefore a portion of the aortic wall will be subject to both elevated circumferential and shear stress. This means that any age-related disease process which creates dyshomogeneity will be progressive and this has been highlighted by Schlatmann and Becker (1977) in their description of the aortic medial changes being 'non-specific'. Dissection in Marfan's disease is not difficult to explain in that part of the role of fibrillin is in promoting the adhesion of elastin fibrils. Abnormal fibrillin would enhance the sensitivity of the aorta to shear forces, i.e. those which allow the medial layers to be separated when they slide relative to each other. The current controversy over the pathogenesis of dissection is whether the initial event is an intramedial haematoma due to bleeding from the vasa vasorum which separates the elastic laminae, and then ruptures into the lumen by an intimal tear, or whether the intimal tear is the initial event allowing blood to enter the media and separate the tissue layers. The data supporting the concept that an intramedial haematoma is the initiating event comes entirely from clinical echocardiography and magnetic resonance imaging. In patients whose sudden onset of chest or back pain suggested aortic dissection, the initial images show an intramural aortic haematoma with no connection with the lumen. Over the next few days a

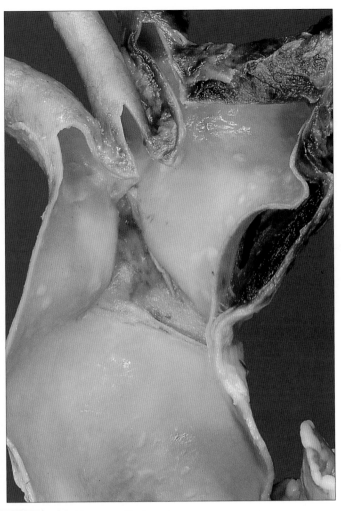

Figure 7.12
Healed chronic aortic dissection. There is a depressed U-shaped scar on the intima at the site of healing of a localised dissection tear.

The concept that there is a molecular defect responsible for aortic dissection is most strongly supported by Marfan's disease, in which the risk is very high and 80% of subjects will ultimately die of cardiac disease.

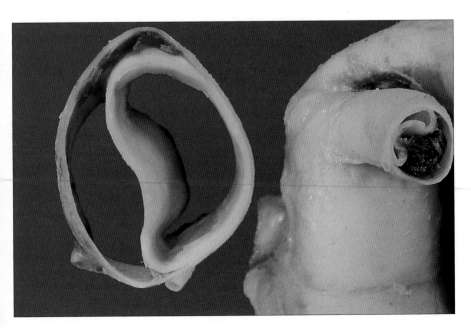

Figure 7.13
Acute aortic dissection. A cross-section of the ascending aorta shows the dissection track which extends into the subclavian artery. The thrombus in the dissection track compresses the true arterial lumen.

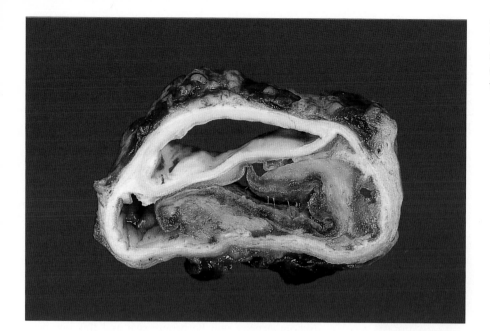

Figure 7.14
Chronic aortic dissection. A transverse section of the aorta shows chronic dissection with a false lumen filled with thrombus.

very high proportion of these cases then develop an entry point to the aortic lumen (Mohr-Kahaly *et al.* 1991). The initial event is regarded as due to shear forces rupturing small medial vessels. The view is entirely dependent on the imaging modality being sufficiently sensitive to detect small intimal tears, and therefore its being able to exclude their presence. The alternative and more established view that the intimal tear is the most common initiating event is supported by pathology studies and other clinical series using ECHO and MR. Whatever the initial event, haemodynamic forces in the aortic media would favour extension of the haematoma distally in systole and proximally due to recoil in diastole. The presence of a haematoma would shift stress on to the inner zone of the media, which would then be subject to both increased circumferential and longitudinal forces leading to rupture.

Marfan's disease

Marfan's disease is an autosomal dominant genetic disorder of connective tissue. The genetic basis of the condition has recently become clarified with mutations of the fibrillin genes being responsible for most cases. The phenotypic expressions of the fibrillin gene disorders are very wide with mixtures of cardiac, skeletal and ocular abnormalities (Table 7.3).

Fibrillin is a 350 Kd glycoprotein that is the major component of the 12 mm extracellular microfibrils which act as a network for elastin deposition and is a constituent of the elastic fibre.

Abnormal production of fibrillin in these patients results in abnormal elastic fibres which lead to the skeletal and cardiovascular abnormalities in this syndrome. Aortic disease is the most serious cardiovascular manifestation in individuals with Marfan's disease, and represents its most lethal complication.

Table 7.3
Phenotype spectrum in fibrillin gene defects.

Chromosome 15   Fibrillin-1 gene
Marfan's disease   – Eye dominant
– Skeletal dominant
– CVS dominant
Neonatal Marfan's diseases
Ectopia lentis
Isolated familial aortic root dilatation/aortic dissection
MASS phenotype   – Mitral prolapse
– Aortic root dilatation
– Skeletal abnormality
– Skin involvement
Marfanoid craniosynostosis
Chromosome 5   Fibrillin-2 gene
Congenital contractual arachnodactyly

Aortic root dilatation can be the initial aortic abnormality, consisting of dilatation of the sinuses of Valsalva as well as expansion of the sinutubular junction and the aortic annulus leading to progressive aortic regurgitation (Chapter 3). There is usually coexistent mitral regurgitation. In Marfan's disease the left ventricle dilates to a disproportionate degree, suggesting that the cardiac interstitial connective tissue is abnormal. Aortic dissection may be the initial cardiac presentation of patients with Marfan's syndrome and it can occur without aortic dilatation. A keystone of the management of patients with Marfan's disease is anticipation of the complications of aortic root dilatation and dissection. Echocardiography is used to track the size of the aortic root to detect progressive enlargement and forestall complications by a prophylactic replacement of the aortic root. A cut-off point of 5.5 cm in diameter is taken as the point at which replacement is advised. The operation is major and carries an operative risk, but the risk of the complications such as dissection carries a mortality risk of well over 50% (Treasure 1993; Pasic *et al.* 1992; Hwa *et al.* 1993). It must be re-emphasised, however, that in Marfan's disease dissection can occur in the absence of any dilatation or even histological abnormality emphasising that the defect is at molecular level.

In Marfan's patients with acute or chronic type II and III dissections, therapy is also aggressive because of the risk of progressive aortic dilatation, further dissection, and/or possible rupture. Early operation using a Dacron graft replacement is used for acute type B dissection, a large localised false aneurysm or refractory hypertension. The substantial incidence of late complications is because of the susceptibility to other serious aortic and cardiac problems.

The fibrillin gene on chromosome 15 responsible for cardiac defects is very large. The gene abnormalities include a wide range of point mutations, repeats, deletions, premature stop codons etc. The complexity is so great that each Marfan family is virtually unique. The gene abnormalities produce a wide range of results ranging from virtually all the fibrillin being the mutant type to families in whom the amount of mutant fibrillin produced is less than 10%, the rest being the wild type, due to the normal gene inherited from the normal parent (Pereira *et al.* 1994). The result is a huge phenotypic range of severity which includes fully developed severe skeletal and cardiac disease through the MAAS syndrome (mild aortic and mitral regurgitation with minimal skeletal abnormality) to familial aortic dissection without any skeletal manifestations.

Marfan's disease in infancy has a particularly sinister prognosis. The main cause of death is progressive mitral and tricuspid regurgitation rather than the aortic disease which predominates in adults (Geva *et al.* 1990).

Medial structure in Marfan's disease

One stated view is that medial degeneration, in the form of cystic medial necrosis, is an essential prerequisite for dissection in Marfan's. Our own experience in a centre where a considerable amount of aortic surgery for Marfan's patients is carried out is that this is an oversimplification. If the aorta is dilated, medial histological changes are usually easily found; where dissection has occurred in an aorta which is not dilated the media may look histologically normal apart from the dissection track. The medial changes recognised histologically in Marfan's disease are also very patchy and require taking a number of histological blocks from as many separate areas of media as is possible. The practice of sending a specimen of an aorta to a histopathologist and asking the question whether cystic medial necrosis is present with a view to establishing a diagnosis of Marfan's disease is misguided. Cystic medial change in some cases is a late morphological expression of the molecular abnormality. It may not be present if aortic dissection occurs early. Cystic medial

change is also not specific for abnormalities of the fibrillin gene, and can occur in the other genes associated with different components of the connective tissue.

TRAUMATIC ANEURYSMS OF THE AORTA

Complete aortic transections are becoming more common due to high velocity impact injuries and account for up to a fifth of the mortality in vehicle accidents. The great majority of these complete full thickness transverse tears are just distal to the left subclavian artery at the isthmus of the aorta. About 20% are in the ascending aorta. Multiple tears are also common. A very small proportion of traumatic aortic tears, perhaps 2% in all (Erbel 1996), are partial and lead to a subadventitial haematoma. This then passes into an aneurysm of the 'false' type. Such aneurysms develop by about 3 months after the trauma and may persist for years. Most will ultimately rupture to cause death, unless treated surgically (Erbel 1996).

These late post-traumatic aneurysms are often very discrete and saccular in type. The operative specimen should be examined histologically in blocks which pass from the normal aorta through the edge of the aneurysm sac. The characteristic appearance is of a normal media with a very abrupt change to the fibrous wall of the aneurysm which contains no elastic tissue. The abrupt line of medial loss is the original site of the tear. Aortitis or aortopathy are absent in the adjacent normal media.

SACCULAR AND DIFFUSE TRUE ANEURYSMS

There are many causes of these aneurysms, encompassing either aortopathy or aortitis. In addition atherosclerosis and direct infection can cause such aneurysms. The site of the aneurysm and the state of the rest of the aorta will give macroscopic clues on the pathogenesis which is then followed by histological examination. Histological blocks should be taken from the edges of the aneurysm sac as it passes into more normal aortic wall. Such sections should indicate whether the aneurysm is due to aortitis, non-inflammatory aortopathy, or atherosclerosis. Elucidation of the pathogenesis of aortic aneurysms will often need additional information such as the human lymphocyte antigen (HLA) status, the erythrocyte sedimentation rate (ESR) and other immunological tests, as well as serology for syphilis. A family history of any other aneurysms is also needed. While it is usually possible to categorise aneurysms as inflammatory or non-inflammatory, even this may be easy. Burnt-out aortitis is particularly difficult in this regard and leaves a thin-walled aorta with diffuse fibrous medial replacement with a few residual inflammatory cells present in the adventitia alone.

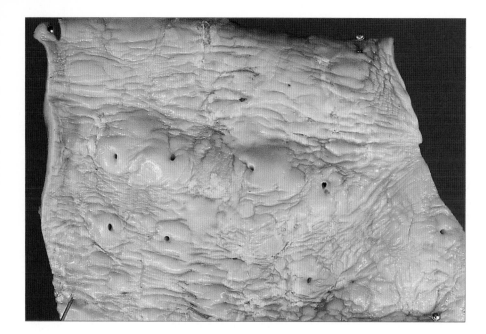

Figure 7.15
Intimal scarring in aortitis. The intima of the thoracic aorta shows wrinkling with longitudinal furrows and there are white hyaline plaques around the orifices of the intercostal arteries. This tree-bark scarring is commonest in aortitis but has no specificity for the different causes of aortitis. Tree-bark scarring can also occur in non-inflammatory medial disease.

The great majority of atherosclerotic aneurysms are in the abdomen below the renal artery. The majority of aneurysms due to aortitis and aortopathy are thoracic.

Aneurysms due to aortitis

Syphilis

About one-third of patients with untreated primary syphilis will develop tertiary disease, amongst whom 80% will have cardiovascular manifestations (Jackman and Radolf 1989). Syphilitic aortitis tends to affect a discrete segment of the aorta – a band just above the aortic valve is the most common site. At this site it causes aortic regurgitation and may be associated with coronary ostial stenosis. Discrete bands of aortitis at other sites in the aorta (Fig. 7.15) can be recognised by the wrinkled tree-bark scarring of the intima and are often coincidental findings at autopsy. 10–40% of patients who develop localised aortitis will go on to develop localised saccular aneurysms (Jackman and Radolf 1989). Most syphilitic aneurysms occur in the ascending aorta and arch and can compress or rupture into the right bronchus, the superior vena cava or the right pulmonary artery. Erosion into the back of the sternum was common in the last century and specimens illustrating this can be found in many pathology museums. Syphilitic descending thoracic aneurysms compress or rupture into the oesophagus or trachea. Syphilitic abdominal aneurysms are very rare, but popliteal aneurysms are a classic site described by John Hunter in the eighteenth century.

Non-syphilitic infective aortic aneurysms

Tuberculous aortic aneurysms are very rare when it is considered that only 100 cases were reported up to 1965 (Silbergleit *et al.* 1965). The majority of examples were direct spread from tuberculosis in the vertebral column, but some were direct infection of the media in miliary tuberculosis (Felson *et al.* 1977). Mycotic aortic

aneurysms follow an episode of bacterial endocarditis or septicaemia. They are usually discrete, eccentric, saccular aneurysms with well-defined edges in an aorta which is otherwise normal. *Staphylococcus aureus*, pneumococci and even *Salmonella typhi* can cause such aneurysms. They have a high risk of rupture unless surgically treated. The exact pathogenesis of this type of aneurysm is unclear. The amount of tissue destruction suggests that direct medial implantation of viable organisms occurs via the vasa vasorum. Immune reactions to the antigens of the infective agent may play a role in the tissue damage (Bennett 1967).

Rheumatoid arthritis

Rheumatoid nodules may occur in the aorta with a central area of necrosis surrounded by palisading histiocytes or a non-specific panaortitis indistinguishable from syphilis, ankylosing spondylitis and scleroderma. The inflammatory process most frequently involves the ascending aorta and aortic valve leading to aortic incompetence (Chapter 3). Only rarely is the thoracic or abdominal aorta involved with aneurysm formation. The severity of aortitis is related to the severity of the joint disease.

Ankylosing spondylitis

This is a connective tissue disease mainly affecting the sacroiliac joints. Aortic disease occurs in 1–10% of patients (Bulkley and Roberts 1973) and is related to the duration of the disease, but occasionally predates the joint disease. It can be distinguished from syphilis by the localised nature of the aortic involvement (*see* Chapter 3). The sinuses of Valsalva are mainly involved at the level of the semi-lunar cusps and the disease usually only extends up a few centimetres into the ascending aorta. It is a disease with a male predominance and patients are HLA-B27 positive in up to 95% of cases and 50% of their first-degree relatives, indicating a genetic basis for the disease.

Giant cell aortitis

This is usually a disease of the elderly with an incidence of 15–30 cases per 100 000 persons over the age of 50 years. It is more common in women and black people. The aetiology is unknown, but has been considered to be autoimmune in nature. In temporal giant cell arteritis, extracranial arteritis and aortitis occurs in 10–15% of patients and has been underestimated in the past. The aorta can look exactly similar to the tree-bark effect seen in the intima in syphilis. The aorta may dilate leading to aneurysm formation and incompetence of the aortic valve. In the media, there is a particular pattern of inflammation in which a band of elastic is surrounded by inflammatory cells, which are mainly lymphocytes, epithelioid cells and multinucleate giant cells at the edge of this band. Elastic Van Gieson stain reveals that this band is an area of elastic which has been digested by the giant cells and is a typical histological pattern in giant cell aortitis (Fig. 7.6). Nonspecific chronic inflammatory cells including lymphocytes and plasma cells at the medial/adventitial junction may be seen in the chronic healing stage and make the appearance indistinguishable from other causes of aortitis. Renal artery involvement is rare.

Atherosclerotic aortic aneurysms

All pathologists who carry out autopsies are well aware that the aorta is a primary site for the development of atherosclerosis. Examination of the intimal surface shows the full range of plaques from fatty streaks to ulcerated plaques covered by thrombus (Fig. 7.16). The extent of intimal involvement by plaques has been studied in a number of epidemiological autopsy studies. These show that the number of aortic plaques on a population basis is an indicator of the risk of ischaemic heart disease in that geographic population. Risk factors such as diabetes, hypertension and smoking are associated with a greater number of aortic plaques when compared to control subjects. The size of the lumen of the aorta is, however, such that thrombosis occurring over plaques is not a common cause of clinical symptoms. Plaque thrombosis in the aorta is initiated by loss of the cap over a lipid rich plaque. This exposes the lipid core and a polyploid mass of lipid and thrombus forms over the plaque. Ultimately the thrombus is lysed or embolises downstream leaving shallow depressed areas in the intima which become recovered by endothelium.

Pathological studies of the development of aortic atherosclerosis, looking at different age groups from infancy onward, show that atherosclerosis first develops in the abdominal aorta and is always present there to a greater degree than in the rest of the aorta.

Saccular and diffuse abdominal aortic aneurysms virtually always occur in the segment between the renal artery orifices and the aortic bifurcation (Fig. 7.17). Indeed this is the commonest site of aortic aneurysms overall.

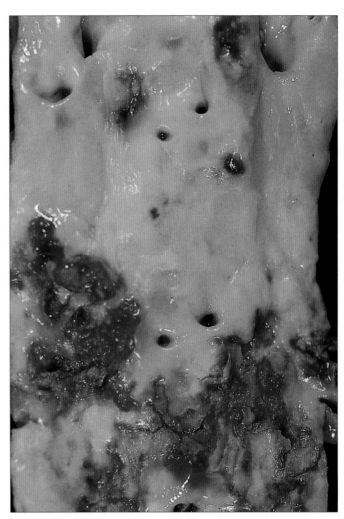

Figure 7.16
Aortic atherosclerosis. The intimal surface shows plaques at all stages but many have ulcerated, leaving a surface covered by a mixture of lipid debris from the core and thrombus.

Frequency of aortic aneurysms

True aneurysms in the lower abdominal aorta below the renal arteries are a relatively common autopsy finding both as a cause of death and coincidental to another cause. Comparison of series is not easy, because opinions differ on how much the aorta has to be enlarged for it to be termed an aneurysm, but estimates of 2–4% of autopsies revealing an aneurysm of the aorta in adults are credible (Erbel 1996). Three-quarters of all aortic aneurysms are in the abdominal aorta below the renal arteries. About a quarter of all the abdominal aneurysms found in autopsies are the cause of death; this implies that a large proportion are coincidental findings. It also implies that there is a considerable number of undiagnosed aortic aneurysms in the general community. In contrast, aortic dissection has a very high mortality and it is not found as a coincidence.

Pathogenesis of atherosclerotic aortic aneurysms

The concordance of the aneurysm with the maximal site of atherosclerosis is the strongest indicator that there is a causal relation. Atherosclerosis is known to induce medial atrophy in a wide range of arteries of different

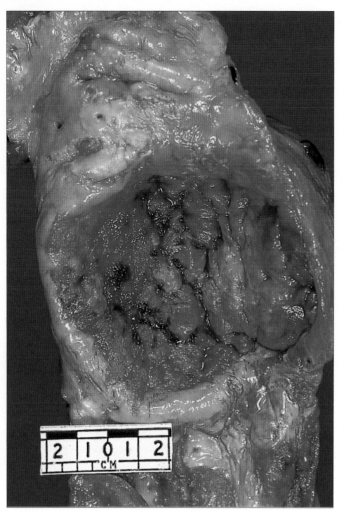

Figure 7.17
Aortic atherosclerotic aneurysm. There is a large saccular aneurysm below the renal arteries. The aneurysm sac contains a large amount of thrombus.

sizes. The mechanism is unclear but may be in part due to hypoxia as the medial smooth muscle cells are normally dependent on oxygen diffusion from the lumen. The abdominal aorta is, however, the only site at which atherosclerosis causes aneurysms and other complementary factors must be involved. The risk factors for abdominal aortic aneurysms are somewhat different than for atherosclerosis in general. Atherosclerotic aneurysms are nine times more common in men than women, are strongly related to smoking and hypertension, but less strongly to hyperlipidaemia than coronary artery disease. Abdominal aortic aneurysms in males are very clearly familial.

For an index case there is a 15% chance of an offspring developing an abdominal aortic aneurysm and up to a 30% chance in siblings (Collin and Walton 1989; Fine 1993) set against a risk of 2–5% prevalence in the general population (Auerbach and Garfunkel 1980; Fine 1993). While the genetics are far from clear, one 'aneurysm' gene has been located on chromosome 16, but the gene function is as yet undetermined. Polymorphisms of the haptoglobin gene at this site have been linked to increased degradation of elastin.

Enhanced proteolytic activity has also been identified at the site of abdominal aortic aneurysms (Dietz 1995). There seems therefore to be a primary role for atherosclerosis with an additional role played by another genetic mechanism, perhaps involving connective tissue degradation by macrophages.

Atherosclerotic abdominal aortic aneurysms are usually fusiform and involve the whole circumference of the aorta. The aneurysm may however be asymmetric, and bulge more to one side than the other. The diameter can be anything from 7 to 30 cm. The wall consists of dense hyaline fibrous tissue with a lining of laminated old and recent thrombus. Abundant lipid-filled macrophages are mixed with the thrombus and the adjacent aorta shows extensive atherosclerosis. It is usually very difficult to find any residual elastic tissue in the aneurysm wall. The natural history of abdominal aortic aneurysms is to expand and the rate is accelerated by hypertension. Routine echocardiography of the abdominal aorta shows that dilatation of more than 5 cm occurs in up to 5% of healthy individuals over 50 years of age.

These subjects, who are usually male, need annual checks to follow the expansion to forestall rupture by surgery. A rate of increase of more than 0.5 cm per annum or a value of 7 cm is an indication for prophylactic surgery.

Aortic periaortitis and aneurysms

The concept of chronic periaortitis is that there is a large adventitial component of inflammation in some cases of aortic atherosclerosis with intimal proliferation, medial thinning and adventitial fibrosis (Parums 1990). The total aortic wall thickness may be markedly increased. The histological features are like those of conventional atherosclerotic aneurysms with the addition of large amounts of hyaline periaortic fibrous tissue within which are a large number of plasma cells and often lymphoid follicle with germinal centres. The fibrous tissue may be very cellular in areas with a whorled pattern. On computerised tomography there is a large abdominal periaortic fibrotic mass with or without aortic dilatation. The inflammation is presumed to be secondary to atherosclerosis which is often severe and advanced.

Periaortitis has also been linked to retroperitoneal fibrosis in which there is a retroperitoneal mass with ureteric obstruction. There is a view that the abdominal aortic aneurysm with this degree of periadventitial inflammation is primarily inflammatory, with atherosclerosis as a secondary phenomenon. Studies have shown shrinkage of the periaortic mass in response to steroid therapy in idiopathic retroperitoneal fibrosis and in aneurysms as well as spontaneous shrinkage with time. Routine autopsy histology suggests that 40% of the population over the age of 50 years will have some degree of periarterial and periaortic inflammation representing subclinical periaortitis and the clinical incidence may be in the order of 0.4%. The current view is that these

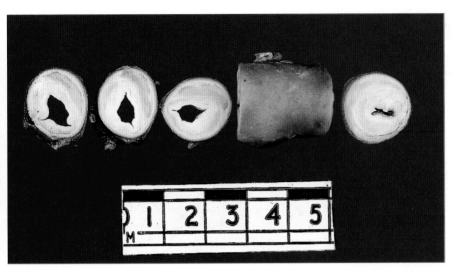

Figure 7.18
Takayasu's disease of aorta. A resection specimen of a stenotic segment of the descending aorta is shown. There is dense intimal fibrosis with a little yellow lipid which narrows the lumen of the aorta to a severe degree. The narrow segment was 6 cm in length. The intimal lesions often contain a small amount of lipid but the dense fibrosis and the extreme narrowing of the lumen indicate that this is not aortic atherosclerotic disease.

periaortitis or inflammatory atherosclerotic aneurysms are part of the overall spectrum of atherosclerosis in which there is a local immune response to oxidised low density lipoprotein (LDL) reaching out of the atherosclerotic tissue. This form of thick-walled aneurysm may comprise up to 10% of lower abdominal aortic aneurysms and, apart from a slightly lower risk of rupture and the risk of ureteric obstruction coupled with a greater difficulty at surgery, behave very little different from the more typical thin-walled atherosclerotic aneurysms.

Saccular aneurysms due to non-inflammatory disease

Saccular aneurysms are encountered in which the media has cystic change with elastic disruption but no evidence of dissection or aortitis. In a minority there is a family history and a number of genetic defects in connective tissue synthesis are known. In general, Marfan's disease and defects of the fibrillin gene interfere with the adhesion of connective tissue and predispose to dissection. However, saccular or diffuse aneurysms do also occur. Abdominal aortic aneurysms at a young age are a feature of certain rare Marfan families. Collagen is the main matrix protein resisting expansile pressure in the aorta. Defects in the synthesis of type I collagen lead to osteogenesis imperfecta in which there is often generalised aortic dilatation with diffuse calcification. Type IV Ehlers–Danlos syndrome, which has a defect in type III collagen, has aneurysm formation and spontaneous rupture in the aorta and other large arteries. A number of groups have now identified gene defects in type III collagen which are predominantly expressed as aortic aneurysm formation with minimal or no systemic abnormalities (Dietz 1995). At the present time, however, the majority of aneurysms due to non-inflammatory disease are of unknown cause. The consensus view is that these patients have an arterial wall that is predisposed to dilate in the presence of normal or moderately elevated haemodynamic stress – this predisposition is even further unmasked as age-related changes occur in the media.

Takayasu's disease

Takayasu's disease is characterised by aortic occlusion rather than by dilatation and aneurysms (Fig. 7.18). Takayasu's arteritis is known by a variety of other names pointing to the clinical spectrum of disease, including pulseless disease and aortic arch syndrome. It is a chronic occlusive inflammatory disease that affects the aorta and its brachiocephalic branches. It is characterised by marked cicatrization of all layers of the involved arteries and by dense bands of inflammatory cells in the media. Eventually the vessels have the appearance of very thick-walled rigid tubes with marked narrowing and ultimate obliteration of the lumen due to superimposed thrombosis leading to obstructive lesions of the innominate, subclavian and common carotid arteries. There is a predilection for involvement of vessels at their point of origin from the aorta. Multi-segmental involvement with normal areas in between are typical. Aortic aneurysms occurring proximal to very narrow segments have been emphasised in some reports. There are three components to the disease: intimal fibrosis; medial elastic destruction with fibrosis; inflammation and adventitial fibrosis in the vessel wall. Extensive necrosis of the media is apparent with a dense cellular infiltrate of lymphocytes, plasma cells and a few polymorphonuclear cells. Giant cells may be seen and can make the lesions appear similar to giant cell aortitis. The inflammatory changes are more pronounced in the early stages of the disease with fibrosis in the later stages. Immunosuppressive therapy is therefore useful in the early stages while surgical bypass procedures are used for the later stages. The natural history of the disease is slowly progressive

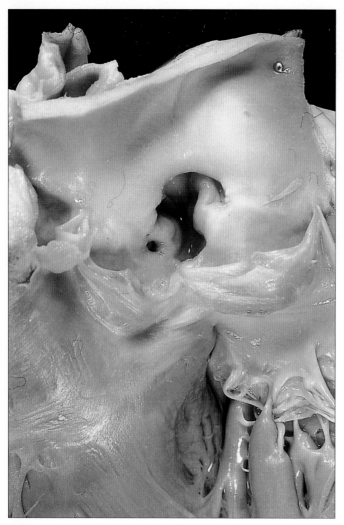

Figure 7.19
Sinus of Valsalva aneurysm. There is a saccular aneurysm just above the aortic valve cusp adjacent to the right coronary artery orifice.

The name Takayasu should not be applied to an aortitis in which there is no aortic or large artery narrowing. There is a confusing tendency, which should be discouraged, to apply the name to aortitis with aneurysms in all subjects who come from the Middle East. This misclassification is often also made when giant cells are present. Giant cells are not specific for Takayasu aortitis and their presence in association with a saccular aneurysm alone is not diagnostic. If Takayasu is used in an indiscriminate way, progress on elucidating the pathogenesis will be delayed. It is a fact that a high proportion of saccular aneurysms in the aorta in the orient, from the Middle East to China, are due to an aortitis which is non-specific and whose cause is unknown.

The aetiology of Takayasu's disease is unknown and the source of much speculation (Hall *et al.* 1985; Nakao *et al.* 1967). There is a higher incidence of HLA-B5 antigen expression in cases compared with controls. Patients can be anti-nuclear and rheumatoid factor-positive suggesting Takayasu's disease is in the spectrum of rheumatic–rheumatoid disorders, while others believe that it is a connective tissue disease linked to autoimmunity. The simultaneous occurrence of glomerulonephritis and Takayasu's disease suggest a common immunologic basis for both lesions. There is also an association between Takayasu's disease and two other chronic sclerosing disorders, retroperitoneal fibrosis and Riedel's thyroiditis. The frequent occurrence of tuberculosis in patients with Takayasu's disease has led some authors to consider that the aortic lesions may be a type of tuberculous angiitis where they postulate an allergic reaction to the tuberculous focus elsewhere in the body (Gajaraj and Victor 1981). In any event, 'a hypersensitivity type of mesenchymal vascular response is seen as the underlying mechanism.

Sinus of Valsalva aneurysms

Sinus of Valsalva aneurysms due to infective endocarditis are described in Chapter 4. Rupture of a congenital sinus of Valsalva (Fig. 7.19) usually occurs in middle age, and can be a cause of sudden death or of intractable cardiac failure. Therefore detailed examination of all the aortic sinuses is essential in any patient dying suddenly, both to examine the coronary artery ostia and the sinuses themselves. The lesion is caused by a congenital separation of the sinus from the media of the root of the aorta with formation of an aneurysm at the point where the aortic cusp is attached to the aorta itself. There is no relation to Marfan's syndrome and no abnormality of collagen or other blood vessels has been detected in these patients. Wide-mouthed openings can be seen with ballooning in patients being investigated for other conditions, but the lesion is rare, only forming 0.2% of abnormalities in a specialist referral centre. The majority (66% of cases) arise from the right coronary sinus, 25% from the non-coronary sinus and the remainder from the left sinus. Because of the central position of the aorta the aneurysm can rupture into any cardiac chamber, but particularly the right

over months to years. It is more prevalent in females of oriental origin in the 15–45 year age bracket. Although it occurs most frequently in the orient, cases of Takayasu's disease have been reported from many countries around the world. Involvement of the coronary arteries occurs in 15–25% of cases with ostial stenosis, and aortic root dilatation can lead to aortic regurgitation. There are no specific laboratory tests, although the ESR and acute phase proteins are elevated.

Takayasu's disease has been classified into four types based upon the findings at aortography. Type 1 involves the aortic arch and its branches only, type 2 has involvement of the thoracic and abdominal aorta only. With abdominal aorta involvement, one can get renal artery occlusion and hypertension, both in children and adults. Type 3 has involvement of the arch with thoracic and abdominal aorta and is the most frequent in autopsy series, while type 4 has extensive involvement of the whole length of the aorta as well as the pulmonary arteries (Lupi-Herrera 1977).

ventricular outflow tract and right atrium. Often the clinical presentation may mimic an acquired ventricular septal defect with left to right shunting.

TUMOURS OF THE AORTA

These are extremely rare and occur in elderly males. Only 31 cases have been described since 1973; most have been malignant fibrous histiocytomas (Erbel 1996). Angiographically the tumour may present as a thoracic or abdominal aortic aneurysm or there may be obstruction of a branch due to ingrowth of the tumour. Tumours arising in the media usually invade locally while intimal lesions grow along the lumen and give rise to thromboemboli in peripheral vessels. Aortic intimal sarcomas have arisen in relation to Dacron grafts.

References

Auerbach O, Garfinkel L. Atherosclerosis and aneurysms of aorta in relation to smoking habits and age. *Chest* 1980;**78**:805–9.

Bennett D. Primary mycotic aneurysms of the aorta. Report of case and review of the literature. *Arch Surg* 1967;**94**:758–65.

Bouissou H, Pieraggi M, Julian M. Age-Related Morphological Changes of the Arterial Wall. In: Camilleri J-P, Berry C, Fiessinger J-N, Bariety J (eds). *Diseases of the arterial wall*. London: Springer-Verlag, 1987; 71–8.

Bulkley B, Roberts W. Ankylosing spondylitis and aortic regurgitation. Description of the characteristic cardiovascular lesion from study of eight necropsy patients. *Circulation* 1973;**48**:1014–27.

Clark JM, Glagov S. Transmural organization of the aortic media: the lamellar unit revised. *Arteriosclerosis* 1985;**5**:19–34.

Collin J, Walton J. Is abdominal aortic aneurysm a familial disease? *Br Med J* 1989;**299**:918–9.

Davies M, Treasure T, Richardson P. The pathogenesis of spontaneous arterial dissection. *Heart* 1996;**75**:434–5.

De Bakey M, Walter S, Cooley D. Dissecting aneurysms of aorta. *J Thorac Surg* 1965;**49**:130–49.

Dietz HC. New insights into the genetic basis of aortic aneurysms. In: Schoen FJ, Gimbrone MA (eds). *Cardiovascular pathology: clinicopathologic correlations and pathogenetic mechanisms*. Baltimore: Williams and Wilkins, 1995;144–55.

Doroghazi R, Slater E. *Aortic dissection*. New York: McGraw-Hill, 1983;133–64.

Erbel R, Oelert H, Meyer J. Influence of medical and surgical therapy on aortic dissection evaluated by transesophageal echocardiography. *Circulation* 1993;**87**:1604–15.

Erbel R. Disease of the aorta. In: Julian DG, Camm A, Fox K, Hall R, Poole-Wilson P (eds). *Diseases of the heart*, 2nd edn. London: WB Saunders, 1996; 1299–330.

Felson B, Akers P, Hall G. Mycotic tuberculous aneurysm of the thoracic aorta. *JAMA* 1977;**237**: 1104–8.

Fine LG. Abdominal aortic aneurysm: report of a meeting of physicians and scientists. University College London Medical School. *Lancet* 1993;**341**: 215–20.

Gajaraj A, Victor S. Tuberculous aortoarteritis. *Clin Radiol* 1981;**32**:461–6.

Geva T, Sanders S, Diogenes M, Rockenmacher S, Van Praagh R. Two-dimensional and Doppler echocardiographic and pathologic characteristics of the infantile Marfan syndrome. *Am J Cardiol* 1990;**65**: 1230–7.

Hahn RT, Roman MJ, Mogtader AH, Devereux RB. Association of aortic dilatation with regurgitation, stenotic and functionally normal bicuspid aortic valves. *Am J Coll Cardiol* 1992;**19**:283–8.

Hall S, Barr W, Lie J. Takayasu arteritis. A study of 32 North American patients. *Medicine* 1985;**64**:89–99.

Hirst AJ, Johns VJ, Kime SJ. Dissecting aneurysm of the aorta: a review of 505 cases. *Medicine* 1958;**37**: 217–97.

Hwa J, Richards J, Huang G *et al*. The natural history of aortic root dilatation in Marfan syndrome. *Med J Aust* 1993;**158**:558–62.

Jackman J, Radolf J. Cardiovascular syphilis. *Am J Med* 1989;**87**:425–33.

Larson E, Edwards W. Risk factors for aortic dissection: a necropsy study of 161 cases. *Am J Cardiol* 1984;**53**:849–55.

Lindsay J Jr. Coarctation of the aorta, bicuspid aortic valve and abnormal ascending aortic wall. *Am J Cardiol* 1988;**61**:182–4.

Lupi-Herrera E. Takayasu's arteritis. Clinical study of 107 cases. *Am Heart J* 1977;**93**:94–103.

Mohr-Kahaly S, Erbel R, Puth M, Zotz R, Meyer J. Aortic intramural hematoma visualised by transesophageal echocardiography. Follow-up and prognostic implications. *Circulation* 1991;**84**: II–128A.

Nakao K, Ikeda M, Kimata S. Takayasu's arteritis. Clinical report of eighty-four cases and immunological studies of seven cases. *Circulation* 1967; **35**:1141–55.

Parums D. The spectrum of chronic periaortitis. *Histopathology* 1990;**16**:423–31.

Pasic M, von Segesser L, Carrel T, Laske A, Bauer E, Turnina M. Surgical treatment of cardiovascular complications in Marfan syndrome: a 27 year experience. *Eur J Cardiothorac Surg* 1992;**6**:149–55.

Pereira L, Levran O, Ramirez F, Lynch JR, Sykes B, Pyretiz RE, Dietz HC. A molecular approach to the stratification of cardiovascular risk in families with Marfan's syndrome. *N Engl J Med* 1994;**331**: 148–53.

Roberts W. Aortic dissection: anatomy, consequences and causes. *Am Heart J* 1991;**101**:195–214.

Schlatmann T, Becker A. Pathogenesis of dissecting aneurysms of aorta. Comparative histopathologic study of significance of medial changes. *Am J Cardiol* 1977;**39**:21–6.

Silbergleit A, Arbulu A, Defever B, Nedwicki E. Tuberculous aortitis – surgical resection of ruptured abdominal false aneurysm. *JAMA* 1965;**193**:333–5.

Treasure T. Elective replacement of the aortic root in Marfan's syndrome. *Br Heart J* 1993;**69**:101–3.

Virmani R, McCallister HJ. Pathology of the aorta and major arteries. In: Lande A, Berkmen Y, McAllister H (eds). *Aortitis: clinical, pathologic and radiologic aspects*. New York: Raven Press, 1986; 7–53.

EIGHT

INVESTIGATION OF SUDDEN
CARDIAC DEATH

INTRODUCTION

Many pathologists will carry out autopsies for the legal authorities on sudden deaths occurring outside hospital. A sequential approach is needed (Table 8.1).

The first step involves excluding, in as far as possible, unnatural causes of death. The history obtained by the police officers concerning the circumstances of the death is the vital first step. The autopsy should not begin without this history. An experienced Coroner's officer develops a feel for the circumstances and may be more willing to express these verbally than in writing. A major point is whether there is the slightest indication of drug abuse including cocaine, solvent abuse,

'speed' and 'crack'. Once any evidence of external trauma is excluded at the autopsy, non-cardiac causes of sudden death such as ruptured aortic aneurysms, ruptured berry cerebral aneurysms and haemorrhage or perforation of peptic ulcers should be excluded. The next stage is to consider the numerous potential cardiac causes of sudden death. Many can be recognised macroscopically, but some such as acute myocarditis can only be recognised with certainty by microscopy (Liberthson 1996) (Table 8.2).

There will then remain a small group of the order of 5% of cases of sudden death in which no clear structural cause of death is found. In these cases it is mandatory to reconfirm the circumstances of death and to carry out toxicology on stomach contents, urine and blood. Any previous medical history should be taken into account. There is an excess of sudden deaths without a clear structural cardiac cause in epileptic

Table 8.1
The sequential approach to sudden death investigation.

1. Consider unnatural death
Circumstances of death
External examination of body

2. Exclude non-cardiac death
Cerebral haemorrhage
Pulmonary embolism
Perforated GI ulcer
Aortic aneurysm

3. Consider macroscopic cardiac disease
Ischaemic heart disease
Left ventricular hypertrophy
Cardiomyopathy
Myocarditis
Valve disease
Anomalous coronary arteries

4. Consider microscopic finding in myocardium
Confirm cardiomyopathy
Diagnose myocarditis
Diagnose idiopathic fibrosis

5. Reappraise history – toxicology screen
Epilepsy
Alcohol
Psychiatric drugs
Carbon monoxide poisoning
Electrocution
Family history of other sudden death/medical conditions
Prior history syncopal/fainting attacks or palpitations

Table 8.2
Cardiac causes of sudden death.

Ischaemic Heart Disease
With acute myocardial infarction
With coronary thrombosis
With old myocardial infarction
With coronary stenosis alone

Anomalous Coronary Arteries

Left Ventricular Hypertrophy
Hypertension
Athletes
Idiopathic
Aortic stenosis

Floppy Mitral Valve

Cardiomyopathy
Hypertrophic
Right ventricular dysplasia
Myocarditis
Sarcoid
Idiopathic myocardial fibrosis

Macroscopic Normal Heart
Long QT syndrome
Pre-excitation
Brugada syndrome

subjects, in subjects with a fatty liver due to excess alcohol ingestion, and in patients on psychiatric drugs.

In progressing through this sequence, the pathologist should not feel under pressure to provide an answer before histology and toxicology are available. While Coroners are always anxious to avoid delay, cost and distress to relatives, they also take seriously their responsibility to provide an accurate cause of death.

The pathologist must also bear in mind the necessity to provide a cause of death which is as accurate as possible and plausible. Plausibility will mean judgements being made on probability and Coroners will usually be very willing to discuss this aspect with the pathologist in individual cases.

Plausibility will involve a component of whether any structural abnormality found has a known mechanism which could cause death by ventricular arrhythmias. This need can be illustrated by some examples. A left-sided vena cava or a bicuspid non-stenotic aortic valve are found in autopsies on subjects who die of non-cardiac causes. Neither anomaly has a clear mechanistic link to arrhythmias and in isolation cannot be given as a cause of sudden death. In contrast, when both coronary arteries arise in one aortic sinus the literature records many living subjects who develop myocardial ischaemia on emotion or exercise when the misplaced artery crosses from left to right, or vice versa, between the aorta and pulmonary trunk. When this anomaly is found at autopsy, and there is no other cause of death, it is therefore reasonable to say it is the cause.

Definitions of sudden cardiac death

The definition of sudden death varies widely from within minutes (instantaneous), less than 1 hour, less than 6 hours or less than 24 hours of the onset of symptoms in the last episode prior to death. Less than 1 hour is the most widely used; the WHO still uses a definition of less than 24 hours which begins to encompass many non-cardiac respiratory diseases. There is no correct or ideal definition, but some of the differences in causes reported in series are probably due to selection bias introduced by these differing definitions. Also incorporated into the definition is an element of death being unexpected and natural. The term unexpected is also subject to considerable latitude; there is agreement that the subject should be previously well enough to go about his or her every day life, i.e. not be in heart failure. There is however disagreement about whether subjects with a known prior heart condition, such as stable angina or treated hypertension, are included or excluded. These semantic differences do not necessarily matter as long as every study clearly states their particular selection bias allowing like to be compared with like.

Mechanisms of sudden cardiac death

There are now numerous reports of individuals who have died suddenly while wearing Holter ambulatory ECG devices, and reports which record the rhythm present when resuscitation teams first arrive. Three mechanisms for what is called cardiac arrest occur. The most common (80%) is the sudden onset of ventricular fibrillation which may or may not follow a prior complex arrhythmia such as ventricular tachycardia. If not converted back by electroversion, ventricular fibrillation will ultimately lead to asystole. Some patients develop primary asystole in which – although an atrial sinus beat is initiated – no ventricular contractions occur. Another subgroup is electromechanical dissociation in which ventricular electrical activity and a QRS complex occur, but there is no cardiac output. The onset of any of these three arrhythmias will lead rapidly to biological death which is in effect brain death. The odds of surviving an episode of cardiac arrest depend in a linear fashion on the time interval before a ventricular response with a good systemic output is restored. Defibrillation within 1 minute has 80% success; after 10 minutes only 10% success (Holmberg and Chamberlain 1996). These periods can be prolonged if external cardiac massage provides some blood to the brain. There is no clear relation of any of the mechanisms of cardiac arrest to any particular cardiac pathology. In carrying out autopsies on sudden cardiac death, many pathologists like to give a mechanism of death followed by its cause. Some of the words used for the mechanisms have very precise clinical meanings and autopsy reports will be better understood if such meanings are taken into account. Acute cardiac failure to the clinician means pulmonary oedema; the pathologist has an excellent way of recording this by simply weighing each lung. Unless each lung weighs more than 700g, words like acute cardiac failure should not be applied. Cardiogenic shock implies a very low blood pressure and poor peripheral perfusion and can only be recognised by the clinical history of the last hour of life. Where there is no pulmonary oedema it is best to record deaths as cardiac arrest. For example a cause of death given as:

1a. Cardiac arrest
1b. Coronary thrombosis
1c. Coronary atherosclerosis

would mean rapid death without pulmonary oedema or macroscopic evidence of infarction.

1a. Acute cardiac failure
1b. Acute myocardial infarction
1c. Coronary thrombosis and atherosclerosis

would indicate pulmonary oedema was present with a recognisable acute infarct.

Incidence of sudden cardiac death

Up to 50% of all cardiac disease deaths are sudden and of these at least 85% are due to ischaemic heart disease. Overall in the US between 300 000 and 400 000 sudden cardiac deaths occur per year. Of those that die from ischaemic heart disease, sudden death is the presenting feature in 40% – that is the disease had not previously been recognised. The incidence of sudden cardiac death in women is less than a third of that in males (Kannel and Thomas 1982). The necessity for pathologists who carry out autopsies on sudden deaths to have some expertise in examining the heart is self evident.

Cardiac causes of sudden death

Ischaemic heart disease

The largest single cause of sudden cardiac death is coronary atherosclerosis. The ubiquitous presence of plaques in the coronary arteries in subjects in the developed world, however, creates a problem for the pathologist in knowing whether to ascribe death as being due to coronary disease. By considering the pattern of the disease present in the coronary arteries and the myocardium, probabilities can be applied.

The basic facts needed are the presence or absence of coronary thrombus, the severity and extent of the chronic stenotic lesions, and the presence or absence of myocardial scars and/or acute infarction. The practice of regarding the pin-point arterial lumen as being the indicator of more than 75% diameter stenosis, and therefore undoubtedly significant in terms of coronary flow, is discussed in Chapter 2.

The descending plausibility or probability of coronary disease being the cause of death is shown in Table 8.3. Sudden death in coronary atherosclerosis has two main mechanisms. Acute ischaemia causes ventricular arrhythmias which pass into ventricular fibrillation. Ectopic ventricular beats often initiate fibrillation by falling on the previous T wave. In the second mechanism chronic myocardial scarring provides the substrate for a re-entry mediated ventricular tachycardia, which may degenerate into ventricular fibrillation.

It is impossible clearly to define the lower limit at which coronary stenosis without thrombosis or myocardial scarring or infarction is not the cause of death. All that can be said is that, if a single isolated segment of 50% diameter stenosis with a morphologically normal myocardium can cause death, the mechanism is unclear. Mechanisms such as coronary artery spasm would have to be postulated but are impossible to prove by morphological/histological studies. Many living males over 50 years in the general population will have an equivalent degree of disease without it being the cause of death. The problem becomes even more pronounced in older subjects. Cardiac hypertrophy acts both as an adjunct to coronary disease and also predisposes to ventricular arrhythmias even in the absence of coronary disease. This inevitably raises the difficult question of how much hypertrophy in the left ventricle can cause death in its own right. The probability of a causal link to death rises with increasing degrees of hypertrophy. Because of all these difficulties, many series which report the different causes of sudden death define sudden ischaemic death on the basis that at least one segment of a major coronary artery must have more

Table 8.3

Probability of death being due to IHD when no other cause is found at autopsy.

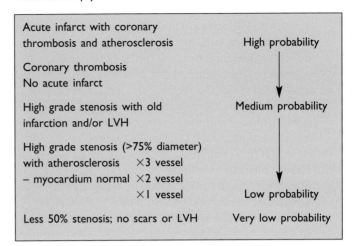

Acute infarct with coronary thrombosis and atherosclerosis	High probability
Coronary thrombosis No acute infarct	
High grade stenosis with old infarction and/or LVH	Medium probability
High grade stenosis (>75% diameter) with atherosclerosis ×3 vessel – myocardium normal ×2 vessel ×1 vessel	Low probability
Less 50% stenosis; no scars or LVH	Very low probability

than 75% diameter stenosis (Davies *et al.* 1989; Warnes and Roberts 1984). Another group has defined the lower limit as 65% stenosis (Virmani *et al.* 1995). The difficulties inherent in making these assessments are discussed more fully in Chapter 2. In practice, in most victims of ischaemic sudden death, all three major coronary arteries have more than 75% stenosis. The figures in three large series ranged from 52 to 61% (Davies *et al.* 1989; Warnes and Roberts 1984; Perper *et al.* 1975). Women and black subjects who die of ischaemic heart disease have higher proportions of single and double vessel disease than Caucasian males in whom triple vessel disease is preponderant (Virmani *et al.* 1995).

When thrombus large enough to be seen with the naked eye is present in a coronary artery it is likely to be the cause of a sudden death. Such thrombi are very rare in 'control' hearts from accidental deaths and even if found in such deaths it is impossible to say that they were not contributing to death. The reported frequency of finding thrombi in sudden coronary death is very wide ranging, from 15 to 75% (Davies *et al.* 1989; Warnes and Roberts 1984). In fact the discrepancy is largely explained by different case selection mixes. Any autopsy series which includes subjects who had a chest pain prodrome before suddenly dying, and subjects without prior stable angina who did not know they had coronary disease, will have high proportions of acute thrombi. Any autopsy series in which prodromal chest pain is used as an exclusion factor and in which patients with known prior ischaemic heart disease are included (and therefore more likely to have myocardial scarring), will have a lower frequency of coronary thrombi at autopsy.

These differences are essentially due to the fact that there are two clear causes of sudden ischaemic death: one is related to new acute ischaemia, the most common precipitator of which is coronary thrombosis, and the other is ventricular arrhythmias arising in a previously scarred myocardium.

In examining the heart in sudden cardiac death due to ischaemic heart disease, the pathologist is looking for any morphological evidence of acute myocardial ischaemia. The most common finding is for a cause of acute ischaemia such as thrombosis to be present, but for the myocardium to be morphologically normal. The normality is not unexpected; it is well-known that acute myocardial infarction requires the subject to survive at least 6–12 hours for recognised histological changes to occur. More sensitive methods of demonstrating myocardial necrosis (Chapter 2) will identify early infarction in a proportion of cases but by no means all. This fact causes confusion to some pathologists who regard sudden ischaemic death as being due to acute myocardial infarction. Indeed many studies trying to validate sensitive methods of demonstrating myocardial infarction use sudden cardiac death with coronary thrombi as the test bed. Clinical studies of patients resuscitated from cardiac arrest due to thrombosis and coronary disease, however, clearly show that only between 25% and 50% develop an infarct by ECG or enzyme rises (Cobb *et al.* 1980). Sudden death with coronary thrombosis is therefore not synonymous with acute myocardial infarction; ventricular fibrillation can be caused by acute myocardial ischaemia which is transient and does not cause cell death. It is always worth examining the myocardium distal to a coronary thrombus for histological evidence of distal platelet emboli which are one mechanism for transient ischaemia (*see* Chapter 2).

One indubitable cause of sudden death due to ischaemic heart disease is haemopericardium due to myocardial rupture. This is responsible for approximately 10% of sudden out-of-hospital ischaemic heart disease deaths. Most of the ruptures are of the type seen early after the onset in which the infarct is barely visible to the naked eye (*see* Chapter 2).

Hypertrophy and sudden death

There is considerable evidence from epidemiological studies such as Framingham that left ventricular hypertrophy is an independent risk factor for sudden death in association with ischaemic heart disease, in relation to other cardiovascular disease and in isolation when hypertension is present (Levy *et al.* 1990; Frohlich 1992). Hypertrophy is associated with arrhythmias. Angina can develop in patients with hypertension or aortic valve stenosis in the absence of any coronary artery disease, suggesting that alterations in intramyocardial blood flow occur and that metabolic demand outstrips oxygen supply particularly in the subendocardial zone (Shapiro and Sugden 1996) where wall stress is highest. The capillary density falls and the amount of interstitial fibrosis in the myocardium rises with pressure-load hypertrophy, particularly in the subendocardial zone. For the pathologist carrying out autopsies on sudden cardiac death, the question is at what degree of left ventricular hypertrophy is the risk of a fatal arrhythmia sufficient that the death can be ascribed to the hypertrophy if no other disease is present. There are

no exact data on this point in relation to total heart weight, but it is reasonable to carry out histology and look for evidence of increased subendocardial fibrosis. This does not usually occur at heart weights of less than 500 g, or total heart weights of less than 30% over the predicted norm for body size.

Non-atherosclerotic coronary artery disease

Coronary artery spasm in the absence of atherosclerosis is a rare but documented clinical entity. The subject, usually a woman, develops unprovoked transient spontaneous attacks of anginal pain associated with very marked ST segment elevation in the ECG. The condition is known as Prinzmetal or variant angina. About 20% of cases develop sufficient spasm to cause acute infarction soon after the onset of the disease. Most cases settle and the symptoms become less severe with time with a very good overall 5-year survival. The spasm is usually confined to one site in the coronary artery tree and may be related to an eccentric plaque causing no, or very mild, stenosis (Scholl *et al.* 1986; Brown *et al.* 1984). Given that there is an appreciable incidence of acute regional infarction following spasm, some sudden deaths will be expected to occur. For the pathologist to recognise the condition, he will need either a clear clinical history of intermittent severe resting chest pain before the final event or evidence of regional myocardial infarction in the absence of thrombosis or dissection or emboli in the subtending artery (Fig. 8.1). Provided that there is a clear history of resting anginal type chest pain in the weeks before death, there is sufficient probability to give coronary spasm as a cause of death, particularly in women. If there is no such history, to ascribe death due to spasm is no more than a possibility. Cocaine abuse causes death by inducing coronary spasm (Karch 1996).

A wide range of psychiatric drugs as well as cocaine (Bauman *et al.* 1994) may act to heighten sympathetic activity under stress or under restraint and precipitate death with a morphologically normal heart.

Sudden death while playing active competitive sport is rare (Hillis *et al.* 1994). The incidence, calculated as two cases per 100 000 subject years, is far too small to discourage such activities in apparently fit individuals. Nevertheless, pathologists will encounter such cases. The most frequent cause over the age of 30 years is coronary artery atherosclerosis. In younger subjects, anomalous coronary arteries, hypertrophic cardiomyopathy, right ventricular dysplasia and the long QT syndrome are all strikingly prone to cause sudden death on exercise rather than at rest or in bed at night. Closed chest trauma of a degree insufficient to cause sternal or rib fractures or to cause contusion to the myocardium or coronary arteries may be associated with sudden death (Maron *et al.* 1995).

Mild to moderate closed chest trauma associated with thrombosis on atherosclerosis in the left anterior descending artery is notoriously difficult to categorise on a cause-and-effect basis. It is conceivable that mild

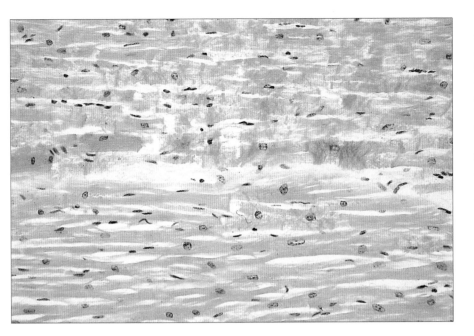

Figure 8.1
Contraction band necrosis. Some small foci of contraction band formation can be found in sudden death from any cause including trauma. In this case a young woman dying suddenly without known cause, with a history of chest pain, there are large areas of contraction band necrosis adjacent to more normal myocardium. The coronary arteries were morphologically normal but spasm is one potential cause of death. The use of cocaine will produce this picture but the drug screen was negative.

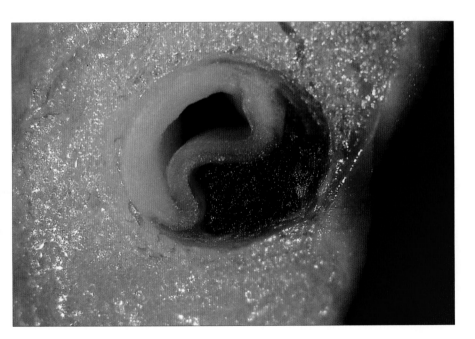

Figure 8.2
Coronary artery dissection. A subadventitial haematoma in the proximal portion of the right coronary artery compresses the lumen. Sudden death in a young male.

trauma or an acute rise in blood pressure due to the stress of an accident will cause plaque disruption. On the other hand, plaque disruption is a very common event in subjects who have not had chest trauma. The ageing of any myocardial infarction present is often needed. If the trauma occurred less than 24 hours before death, yet organisation has begun, the infarct clearly predates the trauma.

Spontaneous coronary artery dissection (*see* Chapter 2) is a cause of sudden death. The subadventitial haematoma compressing the lumen can usually be seen by the naked eye (Fig. 8.2), particularly because the subjects are often young, and atherosclerosis and calcification is absent, making the arteries easy to examine. Anomalous coronary arteries (Chapter 2) are an appreciable cause of sudden death on exercise, often in previously asymptomatic young individuals, and are

frequently not recognised by inexperienced pathologists. There is a large number of variations in coronary anatomy (Chapter 2) but some specific subvarieties are the substrate for sudden death (Roberts 1986; Burke *et al*. 1991). These are: (Taylor *et al*. 1992) the origin of the left main or left anterior descending coronary artery or right coronary artery from the pulmonary trunk (17%) (Fig. 8.3); the left coronary artery arising in the right aortic sinus and crossing between the aorta and pulmonary trunk to reach the anterior wall of the left ventricle (20%); the right and left orifices being in the left aortic sinus with the right crossing between the aorta and pulmonary trunk (25%); single ostium in one aortic sinus (16%); and hypoplastic segments of the main coronary trunks (5%). The figures refer to the relative frequency in the 242 cases referral practice of the Armed Forces Institute of Pathology. The frequency of sudden death was greatest with arteries which

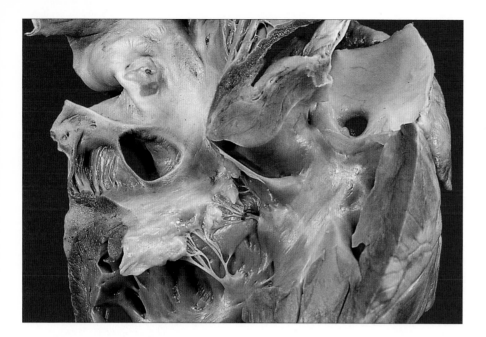

Figure 8.3
Anomalous coronary artery from pulmonary trunk. The right coronary arteries arise from the pulmonary trunk. The coronary sinus is large due to the increased myocardial blood flow due to shunts which develop between the aorta and pulmonary trunk. Female aged 30 years with good exercise tolerance until sudden death.

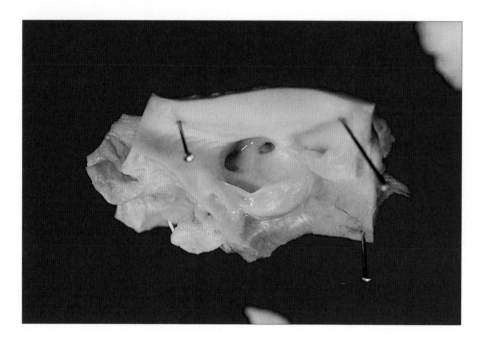

Figure 8.4
Anomalous origin of coronary artery. Both coronary orifices lie in the right aortic sinus. The left coronary artery crossed between the aorta and pulmonary trunk. Child aged 9 years – sudden death.

crossed right to left or vice versa between the aorta and pulmonary trunks (Fig. 8.4) where the coronary is thought to be compressed, have episodes of spasm and finally develop intimal obliterative changes.

The origin of anomalous coronary arteries may have a slit-like orifice also contributing to the risk of sudden death (Cheitlin *et al.* 1974; Virmani *et al.* 1984). Origins in the pulmonary trunk lead to a left to right shunt and the artery opening into the pulmonary trunk becomes large and the artery dilated and tortuous. Subendocardial ischaemia and fibrosis develops. A striking feature is that sudden death occurs at any age up to young adulthood, that exercise tolerance is very good, and many of the subjects play competitive sport before dying suddenly on exercise. A proportion of these subjects have intermittent chest pain on exercise, but this is seldom recognised as being angina.

Hypoplasia of a major segment of a coronary artery (Fig. 8.5) is most frequently seen in infant sudden deaths and involve aplasia of the main left or the proximal; ischaemic fibrosis is usually seen in the area of the missing artery. Coronary artery bridging (Fig. 8.6), where a segment of a major epicardial artery is covered by a layer of myocardial muscle for part of its course, has also been implicated by some authors in sudden death (Corrado *et al.* 1992). Well-established clinical cases where bridges can be seen to constrict the coronary artery to cause angina, which has been relieved by dividing the bridge surgically, are described as individual case reports (Tio *et al.* 1997). Myocardial bridges have also been described as rare causes of acute myocardial infarction (Felman and Baughman 1986). Bridging usually affects the middle portion of the left anterior descending artery and the diagonal and left marginal branches of the circumflex

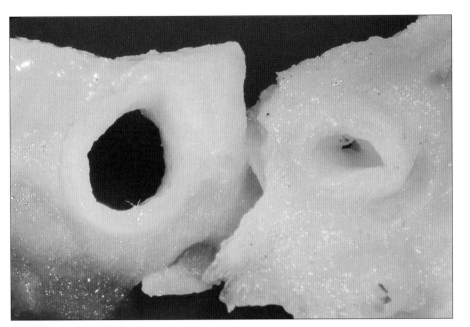

Figure 8.5 a,b
Coronary artery hypoplasia. In this child of 18 months autopsy showed an atretic segment in the proximal left anterior descending artery and no left circumflex artery. The right coronary artery was large and fed the distal left anterior descending coronary artery via a conus branch running across the anterior surface of the right ventricle. Ischaemic fibrosis was present into the anterior-lateral papillary muscle. Sudden death.

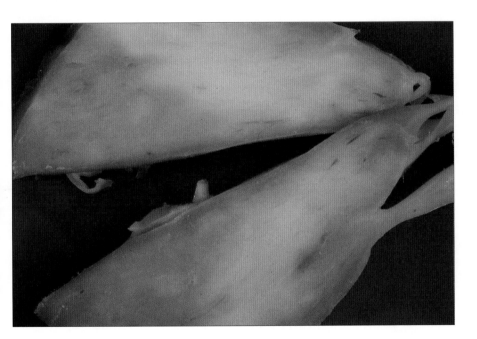

artery. It is a very common phenomenon and can be found in many normal hearts from autopsies where there are clear non-cardiac causes of death (Ishall *et al.* 1986). The frequency of bridging in control hearts is such that it is difficult to be certain of the significance of bridging in a sudden death without a cause. All that can be said is that a causal relation is possible rather than probable. Bridged segments of coronary artery are protected from atheroma, but plaques develop where the artery enters and leaves the tunnel. Protagonists of the view that arterial bridging is a common cause of sudden death argue either that spasm occurs at these entry and exit points, or that in a proportion of bridges the overlying cardiac muscle is disorganised and abnormally innervated, making it likely to hypercontract and compress the artery.

Sudden cardiac death and valve disease

Once severe left ventricular hypertrophy has developed in aortic valve stenosis, sudden death is an appreciable risk whether the patient is symptomatic or asymptomatic (Chizner *et al.* 1980). The relation between mitral valve prolapse and sudden death is much more complex. Mitral valve prolapse is very common in young populations and in a high proportion of such subjects it is physiological. In an unknown but smaller proportion, prolapse is due to the morphological abnormality known as the floppy valve (Chapter 3). The natural history of the subjects who have a floppy valve is, in general, very benign and is associated with mild late systolic regurgitation unless a complication such as chordal rupture, ring dilatation or bacterial endocarditis occurs (Chapter 4). It is this group of complicated floppy valves that develop severe mitral regurgitation

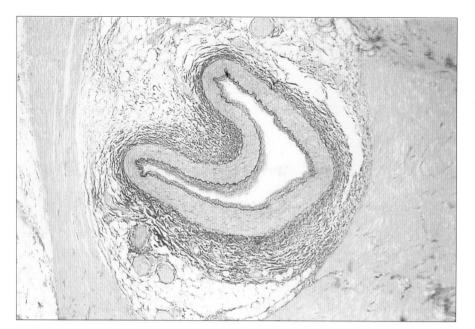

Figure 8.6
Coronary artery bridging. The left anterior descending coronary artery lies within the myocardium and is covered by a subpericardial layer of cardiac muscle. Such bridged arteries appear compressed at autopsy but may not be so in life. Coincidental finding unrelated to death (EVG ×22.4).

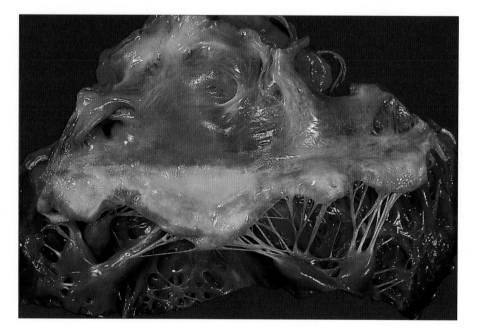

Figure 8.7
Floppy mitral valve – sudden death. A woman of 36 years with a long history of frequent ectopic beats and moderate regurgitation due to a prolapsing mitral valve. Autopsy after sudden death shows the typical opaque expanded cusps of the floppy valve. Chordal rupture was absent, the coronary arteries were normal and myocardial histology normal. In the absence of any other disease, and a clear history of ectopic beats, death was ascribed as being due to the floppy valve.

and develop chronic cardiac failure. A number of patients with floppy mitral valves are troubled by ventricular arrhythmias, in particular repeated ectopic beats; sudden death may occur in this subgroup (Fig. 8.7) but it is a rare phenomenon occurring in perhaps 1–4 per 10 000 patients with significant mitral valve prolapse (Duren *et al.* 1988).

The challenge for the pathologist carrying out autopsies on sudden death is whether a floppy valve is the sole cause of death or just a coincidental finding. A direct causal association with death is likely if there is a clear history of arrhythmia in life, or if there are ruptured chordae or other indications of severe mitral regurgitation. A comparison of the pathological findings in cases of floppy mitral valves, in which there were other clear

causes of death in subjects dying suddenly without other cause, showed significant differences. Floppy valves associated with sudden cardiac death had larger ring circumferences, greater degrees of cusp expansion, and more endocardial thickening, due to the impact of the hypermobile valve and chordae (Farb *et al.* 1992). The mechanism of the ventricular arrhythmias may be the mechanical impact of the chordae on the endocardium, or stretching of the papillary muscles by the cusp hypermobility. In some of the cases of sudden cardiac death due to floppy valves the myocardium is structurally abnormal. The myocardium at the base of the papillary muscles shows myocyte hypertrophy and considerable interstitial fibrosis. The ventricular wall may thicken, particularly on the lateral aspect. It is not clear whether the myocardial changes, which would

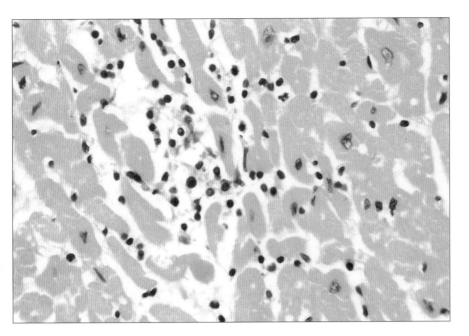

Figure 8.8
Focal myocarditis. This focus of interstitial myocarditis was the only lesion found in this case of sudden death without obvious cause. It cannot be construed as a reasonable cause of death – similar lesions can be found in control hearts if multiple myocardial histology blocks are taken. If, for example, five of ten blocks contain several foci then the relation to death would be more plausible.

clearly predispose to arrhythmias, are purely secondary to the valve abnormality or reflect a separate linked myocardial genetic disease. In Marfan's disease, sudden death and ventricular arrhythmias are also a risk when there is mitral valve involvement. The ventricle often shows more dilatation than would be expected for the degree of valve abnormality, which would further enhance the risk of an arrhythmia.

Myocarditis and sudden cardiac death

All studies of series of sudden cardiac deaths record cases in which very clear and severe cases of acute non-specific myocarditis are present. As emphasised in Chapter 5, acute myocarditis cannot be recognised or excluded without histology. To be considered as a plausible cause of death, myocarditis has to be diffuse or at least multifocal. A single focus of inflammation found after taking a number of histological blocks in a case of unexplained death is not a plausible cause (Fig. 8.8). Previously unsuspected cardiac sarcoidosis is also a cause of sudden death. The pattern of the scarring (Chapter 5) usually makes the diagnosis suspected at the time of autopsy but histological confirmation is needed.

Cardiomyopathy and sudden death

The familial genetic forms of hypertrophic cardiomy-opathy all carry a significant risk of sudden death both in symptomatic and asymptomatic subjects. Sudden death is often the first indication that a family is carry-ing one of the genes. Forms of the disease in which the heart shows marked hypertrophy with increases of total heart weight over 500 g and a thick-walled symmetric or asymmetric left ventricle with a small cavity, are easy to diagnose with the naked eye, although there should always be histological confirmation of disarray. Sudden death becomes an appreciable risk as soon as the adolescent growth phase begins and continues through-out life. Up to 1.5% of subjects who carry one of the hypertrophic cardiomyopathy genes dies suddenly each

year. Donald Teare (1958) first clearly described the asymmetric form of hypertrophic cardiomyopathy while working as a forensic pathologist. Over the succeeding decades family members of his original cases have been shown to have abnormal β heavy chain myosin genes. It was not until ECHO studies of whole families were carried out in life that it was realised the cardiac pheno-type in known gene carriers was very diverse. Pathology studies have now confirmed this diversity. The heart weights are not necessarily increased, the ventricle may not be thick-walled, and a macroscopic appearance close to normal occurs. This relative normality of the macroscopic appearance is a feature of the troponin T mutations. For the pathologist this means it is never wise to be dogmatic about the presence or absence of hypertrophic cardiomyopathy until histological blocks have been taken throughout the left ventricle. The minimum degree of examination is that blocks should be taken to show the full thickness of the septum close to the aortic valve as well as septal, anterior, lateral and posterior blocks at mid-ventricular level.

Dilated cardiomyopathy is a rare cause of sudden cardiac death before the patient is symptomatic with heart failure. Myocardial fibrosis visible macroscopi-cally in the absence of coronary disease, ventricular dilatation or a history of cardiac failure is encountered and is given a number of names – we favour idiopathic fibrosis (IF). There are several patterns of fibrosis associated with sudden death in patients who have had good exercise tolerance in life. One pattern is rather fine and diffuse scarring associated with some hypertrophy (Fig. 8.9); another pattern has circumferential depressed scars in the subpericardial zone of the left ventricle (Fig. 8.10). The pathogenesis of neither form is known. One view is that these cases are due to prior acute myocardi-tis. The increasing recognition of genes which cause myocardial disease, however, raises the possibility that some idiopathic fibrosis is genetic. The pattern of left ventricular disease that occurs in right ventricular

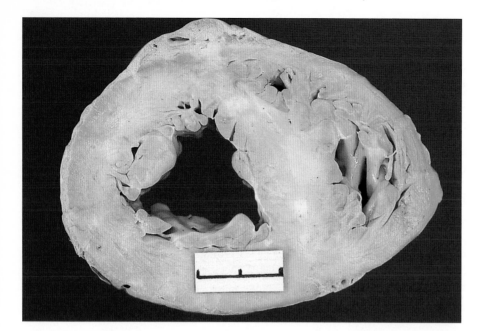

Figure 8.9
Idiopathic myocardial fibrosis. Sudden death in a male of 42 years without a history of hypertension and without coronary disease. There is some ventricular wall thickening and multiple small foci of fibrosis throughout.

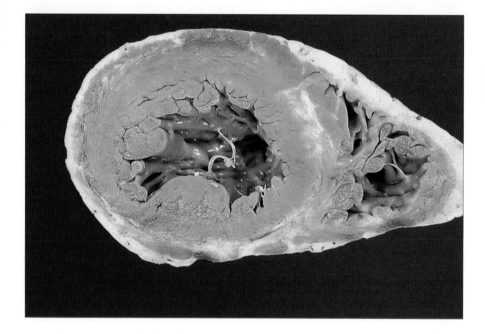

Figure 8.10
Idiopathic myocardial fibrosis. There is a linear depressed scar in the septum and in the posterior wall of the left ventricle. The scar is subepicardial. Male of 26 years – sudden death. No prior disability.

dysplasia and in myotonic dystrophy is very similar to the second form of fibrosis described above. Carriers of the myotonic dystrophy gene (Chapter 5) are at risk of sudden death before the heart is structurally abnormal and pose a problem for the pathologist if the family history is unknown.

Right ventricular dysplasia is another familial cardiomyopathy in which arrhythmias such as ventricular tachycardia and sudden death are a feature in subjects who do not have reduced exercise tolerance and often play active sport. Sudden death usually occurs on exercise. In the UK the disease appears significantly less common than hypertrophic cardiomyopathy, but in other geographic areas the gene seems more prevalent (Thiene *et al.* 1988). The extreme phenotype with either a diffusely dilated right ventricle or localised almost

aneurysmal dilatations particularly in the right ventricular outflow, are readily diagnosed with the naked eye at autopsy. Less pronounced phenotypes are all too easily missed. The localised areas of right ventricular thinning may be very discrete, occupying only 2–3 cm in diameter, and be small out-pouches rather than aneurysms. For the pathologist it is wise always specifically to consider right ventricular dysplasia and examine the right ventricle very closely to detect thin areas in the wall which transmit light, and in which fat and fibrous tissue replace the wall. Family studies of the disease record that sudden deaths can occur in asymptomatic individuals in whom the morphological abnormalities are minimal. While it is important not to miss right ventricular dysplasia, it is also easy to overinterpret the simple fatty infiltration of the right ventricle which is so common in women and is age-related. In true right ventricular dysplasia the wall is thin; in fatty infiltration, it remains thick.

There is a responsibility for pathologists accurately to diagnose cardiomyopathies, because these are familial conditions and other family members carrying the genes are at risk of sudden death. The gene carriers can be detected by non-invasive tests and treatments are available to reduce the risk of sudden death. It is undefined in the UK whose responsibility it is to inform the family practitioner of the index case, but the pathologist is in the position to ensure that his report is made available to the family via the family doctor through the coroner.

SUDDEN DEATH WITHOUT CARDIAC MORPHOLOGICAL ABNORMALITY

There is a significant number of cases of sudden death in which no macroscopic or microscopic structural abnormality is found in the heart, there is no disease of any other organ and toxicology is negative. In such cases the medical history should be reviewed. There are some conditions such as epilepsy and alcoholic liver disease in which there appears to be a small excess of sudden deaths. A prior history of syncopal attacks or fainting episodes may point to a disease of the conduction system (Table 8.4). Some conduction disorder have a morphological substrate, an example being pre-excitation (Wolff–Parkinson–White syndrome), others such as the long QT interval syndrome have no structural basis, being a genetic defect in ion channels. A proportion of patients being investigated for symptoms such as palpitations show short bursts of non-sustained ventricular tachycardia or multiple ventricular ectopics. Where the heart is morphologically normal by echocardiography and electrophysiological studies in life show no pre-excitation, the QT interval is normal and the QRS complex normal, the term 'electrical disease of the heart' is sometimes applied. The prognosis is usually good, but a small number die suddenly. Without a prior cardiological investigations such cases will be undiagnosable at autopsy.

Sudden death in epilepsy

It has become very clear that there is an excess of sudden unexpected death in subjects who have a clinical history of epilepsy and are usually taking anticonvulsant therapy (Nashef and Brown 1996). Understanding and studying the phenomenon is hindered by the marked variation in how these cases are certified. The phenomenon is best certified as sudden death in epilepsy (SUDEP). Implicit in this definition is that the term status epilepticus should be confined to cases of epileptic death where there is a clear history of a grand mal seizure and lacerations of the tongue. Also implicit is the exclusion of any heart disease such as myocarditis by histology. The reason subjects with epilepsy should die suddenly is not yet well-defined. Many of the cases occur at night and the victim is found

Table 8.4

Conduction system abnormalities postulated to be responsible for sudden death.

Structural
Dysplasia of nodal arteries
AV nodal dispersion
Intra-myocardial right bundle branch
Anomalous conduction pathways (pre-excitation, WPW syndrome)
Nodo-ventricular
Fasciculo-ventricular
Atrio-fascicular
AV ring tissue
Dual AV node
Functional
Long QT syndrome
Brugada syndrome
Primary electrical disease

dead. Pulmonary oedema is often present and it is thought that hypoxia due to reduced respiratory drive induces this oedema and then death. EEG monitoring during sleep in epileptics shows that brain activity may suddenly cease for periods and the phenomenon is a brain arrest almost like cardiac arrest. Unless brain activity restarts before hypoxia causes cardiac arrest, death will occur.

Sudden death in alcoholic fatty liver

Many sudden deaths in subjects with alcoholic liver disease are explicable by very high blood alcohol levels, by inhalation of vomit and from ruptured oesophageal varices. In some cases, however, death is sudden and autopsy shows a fatty liver, no other abnormality, and blood alcohol levels well below the lethal level. The phenomenon is recorded in surveys from many parts of the world (Thomas *et al.* 1988) but is not explained in mechanistic terms.

Sudden death in anorexia nervosa

Sudden death without morphological cause has been reported both in subjects undertaking drastic rapid weight loss and in anorexia nervosa (Isner *et al.* 1995). Prolongation of the QT interval due to electrolyte disturbance is a likely cause (Liberthson 1996).

The conduction system in sudden death without macroscopic cardiac abnormality

A number of arrhythmias and conduction disturbances are known clinically to be associated with a risk of sudden death. Normal sinus rhythm is initiated by the pacing P cells of the sinoatrial node. The impulse then passes through atrial muscle which contracts and reaches the AV node where a delay occurs. The impulse then passes rapidly down the penetrating atrioventricular bundle of His to be distributed via the left and right bundle branches to the ventricles. The cells of the sinus node normally control rate by virtue of having the highest rates of discharge. There are cells in the AV node and bundle of His capable of initiating a rhythm, but the rate is low and normally suppressed by the faster sinus rate.

The sinoatrial node is subject to a number of pathological processes which include an age-related loss of the number of P cells, amyloidosis, occlusion of the nodal artery by coronary atherosclerosis, myocarditis etc. With the exception of the age-related change, none of these processes are specific for the node. SA nodal disease leads to sinoatrial block or the sick sinus syndrome. The node intermittently ceases to discharge, causing a syncopal attack; these attacks are, however, very rarely fatal because an escape rhythm is initiated by other pacing cells in the AV nodal area.

Sinoatrial disease does not therefore figure in any consideration of sudden death. In contrast, anatomical disruption or destruction of the AV node and the bundle of His is associated with sudden death. In complete heart block the atria and ventricles contract independently at different rates. The ventricular rate is slow and subject to intermittent cessation, causing syncope (Stokes–Adams attacks). If the ventricle does not restart in minutes, hypoxia will cause ventricular fibrillation and death. The processes which transect the AV nodal area are many and varied. If complete heart block is fully documented in life, it is worth studying the conduction system to elucidate the cause. This is technically time-consuming and requires considerable experience of the normal structure.

The bundle branches connect with a very widespread subendocardial layer of Purkinje cells, which are the finest branches of the conduction system before the impulse for contraction passes into the ordinary myocardium. Purkinje cells have specialised tight junctions for rapid conduction and have scanty myofibrils appearing empty and vacuolated when compared with contractile myocytes. The conduction system down to the peripheral ventricular system is totally isolated from the ordinary myocardium. In the normal heart, the only electrical connection between atria and ventricles is via the bundle of His which is only 2 mm in diameter. In the embryo, conduction tissue develops around the whole circumference of the atrioventricular rings, but is steadily isolated as the connective tissue matrix of the valve rings develop, finally leaving the bundle of His as the only connection. The residual nodal tissue is commonly seen in adult hearts (AV ring tissue) but has no function since it does not join atria to ventricle (Anderson et al. 1974). This ring tissue was originally described by Kent.

Junctional tachycardia and sudden death

Junctional tachycardia arises in the AV node, the bundle of His or the AV ring tissue and cause both tachycardia and sudden death. These junctional arrhythmias are examples of re-entry tachycardia. In these, there is a circle of conducting tissue in which a circus movement of excitation is set up. The circle of conducting tissue uses the normal conduction system as

one limb and anomalous, i.e. extra connections, between atria and ventricle as the other limb. The anomalous pathways used are either in the lateral aspects of the tricuspid and mitral valve rings or in the septum. Patients with these pathways suffer attacks of sudden tachycardia. The anomalous pathway often activates the ventricle, first leading to the term pre-excitation or Wolff–Parkinson–White syndrome. Sudden death is a risk in these attacks (Munger et al. 1993).

Indications for examination of the conduction system

When there is a clear clinical history with documented electrocardiographic changes of complete AV block or pre-excitation, histological examination of the conduction system is a useful exercise in clinicopathological correlation. The ECG will give information on where the histological examination should concentrate. AV block will be nodal or more distal. Pre-excitation will be in either the right or left atrioventricular rings or septal. Knowledge of where the lesion is reduces the amount of technical work to a manageable proportion.

When there are no electrocardiographic data available because the patient has not had syncopal attacks or palpitations, or has not been sufficiently disturbed by them to seek medical advice, it is possible that a sudden cardiac death is the presenting feature of either AV block or pre-excitation. Other than in rare circumstances it is impossible to prove this hypothesis by histological examination of the conduction system and we agree with Virmani and colleagues (1995) that the exercise is not worthwhile. The reasons are that age-related changes and minor anatomical variations are very common in the conduction system in control hearts, and that the anomalous pathways are often very difficult to trace in serial sections. Persistent ring tissue is very common in control hearts and it takes hundreds of serial sections to be able to show that it does not join atria to ventricles.

The exceptions where histological examination is indicated are if there is any macroscopic abnormality in the region of the AV node – a localised nodule may turn out to be a mesothelioma of the AV node; or in sudden death in infants or children. Congenital heart block is a cause of sudden death and is due to absence of the atrial portion of the AV node – histological blocks show only fatty tissue at the site and the first recognisable part of the conduction system is the penetrating bundle buried in a fibrous body which is often hyperplastic with tiny foci of calcification. This form of AV block present at birth is associated with maternal connective tissue disorders particularly lupus erythematosus but also rheumatoid and dematomyositis. Soluble antibodies of the anti-RO and La type cross the placenta to damage the developing heart. It is important to exclude congenital AV block in childhood sudden deaths because other siblings may be at risk.

A number of groups do, however, regularly examine the conduction system in young sudden deaths without apparent cause. A myriad of morphological changes are described in the conduction system and reported very often as case reports without control data. The studies are therefore anecdotal and retrospective – the great majority do not even use case control methodology – making the reports difficult to interpret. Amongst the changes in the conduction system described are those in Table 8.4. A few attempts at case control studies have been made. In 18 cases of unexplained sudden death in S.E. Asian immigrants, where the phenomenon seems unusually common (Kirschner *et al.* 1987), 14 of the hearts had foetal dispersion of the node and 13 accessory conduction connections in the AV nodal area. Similar findings were present in 35 of 124 hearts (28%). In 12 of 27 unexplained deaths (44%) there were abnormalities of the nodal artery compared to one in 17 control accidental deaths (Burke *et al.* 1993). There is a general trend for minor anatomical abnormalities to be more common in unexplained deaths compared with controls, but the overlap with normal hearts is very large; the minor anatomical abnormalities are observations, not proof, of any particular mechanism for sudden death.

The long QT and Brugada syndrome

There has been clinical recognition for many years that a genetic condition existed in which the ECG showed a prolongation of the QT interval, and in which the subject had episodes of ventricular tachycardia and a significant risk of sudden death. The condition is now known to be due to a range of gene defects leading to abnormal sodium and potassium ion channels on the myocyte. The abnormality is physiological and there is no structural abnormality of the heart or conduction system. In Brugada syndrome there is intermittent right bundle branch block with intermittent ST segment elevation and a risk of sudden death. The pathophysiological basis is not known (Brugada and Brugada 1996).

Certification of sudden unexplained death

After detailed autopsy with toxicology, there remains a not insubstantial number of cases in which no cause for death has been revealed. The reported frequency of this phenomenon varies widely and has been reported to be as high as 50% in children, but in adults up to the age of 50 years it is of the order of 4% of cases of sudden death, in whom there are no circumstances to suggest that disease was unnatural (Maron *et al.* 1980; Burke *et al.* 1993; Topaz and Edwards 1985; Thomas *et al.* 1988). In 166 sudden natural deaths in Maryland, in which extra cardiac disease had been excluded, 33 (20%) had morphologically normal hearts (Virmani *et al.* 1995). A recent survey conducted through the Coroner's Society suggests that about 120 cases of unexplained sudden death occur in young adults in England per year.

It is important that the pathological diagnosis is accurate in such cases. Conditions such as hypertrophic cardiomyopathy and right ventricular dysplasia can be easily missed and referral to a specialist cardiovascular pathologist is often helpful. Our personal experience of referred hearts, which were thought to have no abnormality, is that approximately 20% do have an abnormality sufficient to explain death. Where the heart is normal, it is important to consider the needs of the family. They will need counselling and possible screening of first-degree relatives for conditions like the long QT interval. Whether to hold an inquest and arrive at an open verdict, or give a cause of death such as sudden adult death syndrome, will depend on the views of the local coroner.

References

Anderson R, Davies M, Becker A. Atrioventricular ring specialised tissue in the normal heart. *Eur J Cardiol* 1974;2:19–27.

Bauman JL, Grawe JJ, Winecoff AP, Hairman RJ. Cocaine-related sudden cardiac death: a hypothesis correlating basic science and clinical observations. *J Clin Pharmacol* 1994;34:902–11.

Brown B, Bolson E, Dodge H. Dynamic mechanisms in human coronary stenosis. *Circulation* 1984;70:917–22.

Brugada J, Brugada P. What to do in patients with no structural heart disease and sudden arrhythmic death? *Am J Cardiol* 1996;78:69–75.

Burke A, Farb A, Virmani R, Goodwin J, Smialek J. Sports related and non sports related sudden cardiac death in young adults. *Am Heart J* 1991;121:568–75.

Burke A, Subramanian R, Smialek J, Virmani R. Non-atherosclerotic narrowing of the atrioventricular node artery and sudden death. *J Am Coll Cardiol* 1993;21:117–22.

Cheitlin M, DeCastro C, McAllister H. Sudden death as a complication of anomalous left coronary origin from the anterior sinus of Valsalva. *Circulation* 1974; 50:780–7.

Chizner M, Pearle D, deLeon AJ. The natural history of aortic stenosis in adults. *Am Heart J* 1980;99:419–24.

Cobb L, Werner J, Trobaugh G. Sudden cardiac death. A decade's experience with out-of-hospital resuscitation. II. Outcome of resuscitation, management and future directions. *Mod Conc Cardiovasc Dis* 1980; 49:31–42.

Corrado D, Thiene G, Cocco P, Frescura C. Non-atherosclerotic coronary artery disease and sudden death in the young. *Br Heart J* 1992;68:601–7.

Davies M, Bland J, Hangartner J, Angelini A, Thomas A. Factors influencing the presence or absence of acute coronary artery thrombi in sudden ischaemic death. *Eur Heart J* 1989;10:203–8.

Duren D, Becker A, Dunning A. Long term follow up of idiopathic mitral valve prolapse in 300 patients: a prospective study. *J Am Coll Cardiol* 1988;11:42–7.

Farb A, Tang A, Atkinson J, McCarthy W, Virmani R. Comparison of cardiac findings in patients with mitral valve prolapse who die suddenly to those who have congestive heart failure from mitral regurgitation and to those with fatal noncardiac conditions. *Am J Cardiol* 1992;70:234–9.

Felman A, Baughman K. Myocardial infarction association with a myocardial bridge. *Am Heart J* 1986;**111**:784–8.

Frohlich E, Apstein C, Chobanian A. The heart in hypertension. *Am Heart J* 1992;**327**:998–1008.

Hillis WS, McIntyre PD, Maclean J, Goodwin JF, McKenna WJ. ABC of sports medicine. Sudden death in sport. *BMJ* 1994;**309**:657–60.

Holmberg S, Chamberlain D. Cardiac arrest and cardiopulmonary resuscitation. In: Julian D, Camm A, Fox K, Hall R, Poole-Wilson P (eds). *Diseases of the heart*, London: WB Saunders, 1996: 1457–81.

Ishall T, Hosoda Y, Osaka T *et al*. The significance of myocardial bridge upon atherosclerosis in the left anterior descending coronary artery. *J Pathol* 1986; **148**:279–92.

Isner JM, Roberts WC, Heymsfield SB, Yager J. Anorexia nervosa and sudden death. *Ann Intern Med* 1985;**102**:49–52.

Kannel W, Thomas HJ. Sudden coronary death. The Framingham Study. *Ann NY Acad Sci* 1982;**382**: 3–21.

Karch SB. Cardiac arrest in cocaine users. *Am J Emerg Med* 1996;**14**:79–81.

Kirschner R, Echner F, Baron R. The cardiac pathology of sudden unexplained nocturnal death in S.E. Asian refugees. *JAMA* 1987;**256**:2700.

Levy D, Garrison R, Savage D, Kannel W, Castelli W. Prognostic implications of echocardiographically determined left ventricular mass in the Framingham Study. *N Engl J Med* 1990;**322**:1561–6.

Liberthson RR. Sudden death from cardiac causes in children and young adults. *N Engl J Med* 1996;**334**: 1039–44.

Maron BJ, Roberts WC, McAllister HA. Sudden death in young athletes. *Circulation* 1980;**62**:218–29.

Maron BJ, Poliac LC, Kaplan JA, Mueller FO. Blunt impact to the chest leading to sudden death from cardiac arrest during sports activities. *N Engl J Med* 1995;**333**:337–42.

Munger TM, Packer DL, Hammill SC, Feldman BJ, Bailey KR, Ballard DJ, Holmes Dr, Gersh BJ. A population-based study of the natural history of Wolff–Parkinson–White syndrome in Olmstead County, Minnesota, 1953–1989. *Circulation* 1993; **87**:866–73.

Nashef L, Brown S. Epilepsy and sudden death. *Lancet* 1996;**348**:1324–5.

Perper J, Kuller L, Cooper M. Arteriosclerosis of coronary arteries in sudden, unexpected death. *Circulation* 1975;**52**:27–33.

Roberts W, Bethesda M. Major anomalies of coronary arterial origin seen in adulthood. *Am Heart J* 1986;**111**:941–62.

Scholl J, Benacerra F, Ducimetiere P. Compensation of risk factors in vasospastic angina without significant fixed coronary narrowing to significant fixed coronary narrowing and no vasospastic angina. *Am J Cardiol* 1986;**57**:199.

Shapiro L, Sugden P. Left ventricular hypertrophy. In: Julian D, Camm A, Fox K, Hall R, Poole-Wilson P (eds). *Diseases of the heart*, 2nd edn. London: WB Saunders, 1996; 438–55.

Taylor A, Rogan K, Virmani R. Sudden cardiac death associated with isolated congenital coronary artery anomalies. *J Am Coll Cardiol* 1992;**20**:640–7.

Teare D. Asymmetrical hypertrophy of the heart in young patients. *Br Heart J* 1958;**20**:1–8.

Thiene G, Nava A, Corrado D, Rossi L, Pennelli N. Right ventricular cardiomyopathy and sudden death in young people. *N Engl J Med* 1988;**318**:129–33.

Tio Ra, Van Gelder IC, Boonstra PW, Crijns HJ. Myocardial bridging in a survivor or sudden cardiac near-death: role of intracoronary Doppler flow measurements and angiography during dobutamine stress in the clinical evaluation. *Heart* 1997;**77**: 280–2.

Thomas AC, Knapman PA, Krikler DM, Davies MJ. Community study of the causes of 'natural' sudden death. *Br Med J* 1988;**297**:1453–6.

Topaz O, Edwards JE. Pathologic features of sudden death in children, adolescents, and young adults. *Chest* 1985;**87**:476–80.

Virmani R, Chun P, Goldstein R, Robinowitz M, McAllister H. Acute take offs of the coronary arteries along the aortic wall and congenital coronary ostial valve-like ridges: Association with sudden death. *J Am Coll Cardiol* 1984;**3**:766–71.

Virmani R, Burke AP, Farb A, Smialek J. Problems in forensic cardiovascular pathology. In: Schoen FJ, Gimbrone MA (eds). *Cardiovascular pathology – clinicopathological correlations and pathogenetic mechanisms*. Baltimore: Williams and Wilkins, 1995; 173–93.

Warnes C, Roberts W. Sudden coronary death: comparison of patients with those without coronary thrombus at necropsy. *Am J Cardiol* 1984;**54**: 1206–11.

NINE

DEATHS FOLLOWING CARDIAC SURGERY AND INVASIVE INTERVENTIONS

INTRODUCTION

Post mortem examination is essential in any patient who dies unexpectedly after a cardiac surgical procedure and should be requested by the clinician or referred to the coroner or the county examiner. In general experience, 10–15% of deaths after cardiac surgery are due to unexplained poor right or left ventricular function after bypass. On the other hand, 15% of cardiac autopsies reveal important and unsuspected findings which alter the cause of death as determined clinically. Therefore, it is essential to seek autopsies in all cardiac surgical cases dying within 30 days of surgery, and even later, in order to assess the long-term effects following cardiac procedures.

POST-OPERATIVE DEATHS: APPROACH TO THE AUTOPSY

Post mortem techniques

Clinical records

It is essential that all the clinical records are available to the pathologist before the autopsy is done so that details of all operations, procedures and complications are carefully noted. The operative reports should be read carefully and details of intravenous fluid administration, urine output and changes in urea and creatinine noted. The most recent clotting test results such as prothrombin time should also be studied.

The body

Almost all operations on the heart using cardiopulmonary bypass ('open' operations) are done through a midline skin incision and a median sternotomy is always a long sternal scar. Drains scars are usually in the epigastrium. Coronary artery bypass procedures often involve the use of either one or both long saphenous veins, so that there will be long scars on the medial aspect of the legs. Some centres use tissue glue to stick the incision together and no sutures are present in these cases. Occasionally veins from the arms are used when saphenous veins are unavailable (previous operation) or are unsuitable (varices), and the internal thoracic arteries are increasingly being used as grafts.

Operations in which cardiopulmonary bypass is not used (the so-called 'closed' procedures) are generally performed through a lateral thoracotomy. As with median sternotomy, drains are inserted after lateral thoracotomy. The latter is approached through the bed of the third to the fifth rib and the rib is excised to allow closure of the wound. Operations performed through a left thoracotomy include closed mitral valvotomy (now obsolete in the West as a first operation for mitral stenosis – except as an emergency procedure during pregnancy – but still commonly performed in the Middle East and India), resection of coarctation of the aorta (irrespective of the technique employed), closure of patent ductus arteriosus, pericardiectomy, and many of the 'shunt' operations to increase circulation to the lungs in congenital cardiac malformations causing cyanosis. The thoracotomy is always drained, leaving additional small scars marking the respective positions of the drains. Patients who have had an operation to replace the mitral valve may have had closed mitral valvotomy in the past, so that their bodies carry the scar of a left thoracotomy as well as the median sternotomy. Previous median sternotomy is less obvious, as the midline is incised anew and a patient can have repeated midline sternotomy for bypass grafting or valve operations. Right thoracotomy is almost entirely confined to palliative operations for cyanotic congenital heart disease.

In addition to the surgical wounds there are usually some skin punctures (the sites of venous and arterial lines) and, in early post-operative deaths, there may also be small wounds in the chest wall where pacemaker wires have been removed, either on the ward or in the operating room. All of these lines and wires, including the chest drains, should either be left *in situ* or cut short, but such attachments are often cut or removed before the body reaches the autopsy room. If the sternum has been left open, check for drains in the pleural and pericardial cavities and check the opetative and post-operative notes for blood loss from these drains.

Check all surgical anastomoses and cotton pledgets and pericardial or synthetic Dacron inserts before any organs are removed from the body. Remember that clumsy manipulation of a surgical suture line at autopsy can cause artefactual breakdown. Check surgical site, drains and groins for significant haemorrhage. A certain amount of haemorrhage may occur after uncomplicated operations but a large collection of blood should be measured or weighed. Gelfoam at the operative site may be mistaken for blood clot or cotton swabs but will disintegrate in your hand and has a jelly-like consistency. Swabs usually have a radio-opaque marker on them so that the body should be X-rayed if there is such a possibility.

Take blood cultures from the heart or a spleen swab, after searing the surface to eliminate contaminants. Look carefully for signs of sepsis in the sternum, around the operative site, for subphrenic and pelvic abscesses and, in thoracic procedures, for empyema.

Examine the lungs and pulmonary vessels in detail for respiratory tract infection, consolidation and pulmonary embolism or infarcts. Post-operative pneumonia occurs in about 20% of all patients who have had thoracic or abdominal operations and is increased in patients with chronic respiratory disease. Other risk factors are obesity, age over 70 years and operations lasting longer than 2 hours. Histology is useful in diagnosing adult respiratory distress syndrome, pneumonia, and pulmonary hypertension.

The heart

If the heart is dissected by one of the commonly used techniques, following the flow of blood for example, it will probably be unrecognisable to the surgeon. It is advisable to have the surgeon present when you dissect the heart and the method of dissection will depend on the cardiac operation performed. His detailed knowledge concerning the operation and the problems that arose during the operation are invaluable when deciding on the immediate cause of death following surgery. He will also tell you about the problems that developed intra- or post-operatively in patients dying within one month of surgery. Often the notes may not appraise you of all the complications and discussing the whole case with the surgical/intensive care team is invaluable in setting the scene for the autopsy. It is advisable to retain the heart for fixation in all patients who die within a month of cardiac surgery. It is much better to cut the heart after fixation, because it is easier to obtain the correct blocks in a well-fixed specimen dissected at leisure. Pathologists working away from regional cardiothoracic centres may wish to refer hearts from patients dying soon after surgery to specialist pathologists in their region; this is especially important in cases when death occurred after heart or lung transplantation.

POST-CARDIAC PROCEDURE COMPLICATIONS

Today cardiologists carry out many invasive procedures in the investigation, assessment and treatment of patients with cardiac disease. These include catheterisa-

tion of the coronary arteries, percutaneous transluminal coronary angioplasty (PTCA), insertion of stents into the coronary arteries and intraaortic balloon pump insertion.

Cardiac catheters, angioplasty and atherectomy

Catheterisation is used to assess the coronary arteries in patients with symptoms of ischaemic heart disease such as unstable angina or cardiac failure. This procedure may simply destabilise the patient, particularly those in whom there is severe three-vessel disease. Often one finds that the infarcted area is in the subendocardial region or else crosses all three regions, so it is a general problem with hypoperfusion (Fig. 9.1). When death occurs it is essential to review the angiography tapes with the cardiologists. Bleeding from the vascular access site in the groin is a common problem (Fig. 9.2). Some patients develop ventricular tachycardia or fibrillation and there is a small risk of coronary artery dissection and cardiac perforation with haemopericardium. The major coronary artery branches are usually visible on angiograms and these help to localise the precise site at which the catheter lodged or other procedures were undertaken. There is often no actual mechanical problem with the catheterisation, i.e. blockage of an ostium or a thrombus breaking off to embolise into distal vessels. Look for platelet emboli in distal vessels in such circumstances. Antibodies to the platelet IIB/IIIA receptor is very useful in delineating these platelet emboli. It is important to remember that platelet emboli can occur spontaneously and do not need interventions to the coronary circulation to occur. However, cholesterol emboli occur acutely in the setting of catheterisation, intra-aortic balloon pump, angioplasty or coronary artery bypass grafting. There is usually general diffuse disease with ectatic vessels in

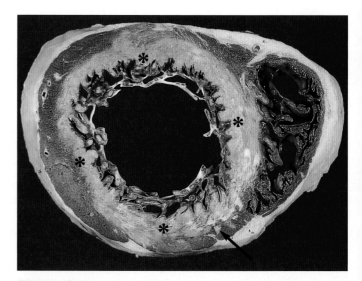

Figure 9.1
Case of ischaemic heart disease with fibrosis of the interventricular septum and anterior wall due to previous infarction (arrow). There is a large subendocardial infarct (*) due to poor ventricular output with peripheral collapse following coronary artery bypass grafting.

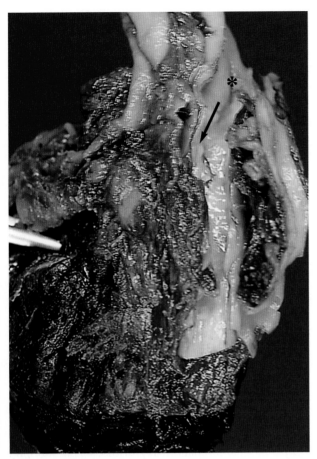

Figure 9.2
Dissection of thigh muscles and femoral artery to show extensive haemorrhage into the thigh muscles. Note the division of the artery into superficial and deep vessels (*) with an incision wound in the superficial vessel (arrow) due to insertion of a catheter for angioplasty.

these circumstances. They can also be found in the context of redo operations because the old venous grafts are filled with cholesterol and are manipulated during surgery. Contraction band necrosis is common

in the myocardium with this, indicating irreversible myocyte death (Fig. 9.3). Look carefully at intramyocardial vessels for the cholesterol clefts and the associated platelet emboli (Fig. 9.4). One should study the case and the angiography/angioplasty procedure with the cardiologist in detail for evidence of dissection of the coronary artery or plaque rupture with thrombosis. However, it is often impossible to tell if the catheter caused the dissection or the thrombosis unless evidence can be deduced from the angiogram itself. The patient is very likely to already have plaque rupture with overlying thrombosis in unstable angina and symptoms of a transmural or subendocardial infarct while undergoing catheterisation. These are well-recognised complications associated with cardiac catheterisation, but the mortality is less than 0.2%.

Although bypass grafting is currently the most common surgical treatment for coronary artery disease, it is increasingly being replaced by angioplasty techniques. These may be performed either percutaneously or under direct vision at surgical operation. Percutaneous transluminal coronary angioplasty (PTCA) is becoming very common and can take as long as a bypass operation (2–3 hours). It involves the balloon dilatation of stenotic segments of major coronary arteries or occasionally coronary artery bypass grafts which have become chronically occluded. When the technique was first developed, it was thought that patency was restored by simple compression of the atheromatous lesion. It is now clear from both clinical and experimental studies that tears and splits are produced around the edges of atheromatous plaques which then allow stretching of the underlying muscular media. Sometimes these tears extend to produce a dissection. Acute complications of angioplasty include rupture, thrombus formation, pericarditis, acute adventitial inflammation and distal embolization of atheromatous debris. Restenosis occurs in up to 30% of cases, largely as a result of fibrous intimal proliferation. In most centres the

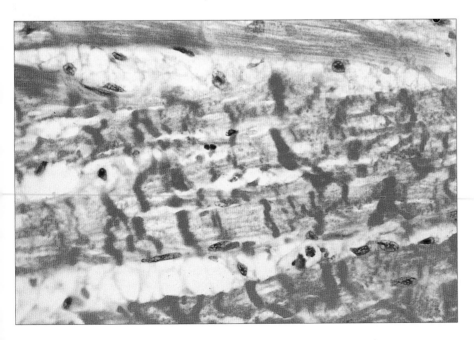

Figure 9.3
Haematoxylin and eosin stained section of myocardium showing contraction bands within the myocytes. Note that they are irregular, of variable thickness and dense compared to the normal endplates with which they can be confused.

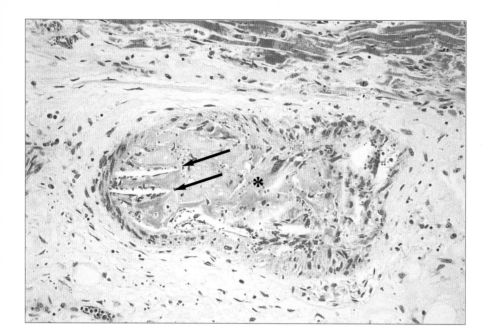

Figure 9.4
Haematoxylin and eosin stained section of myocardium showing an intramural artery containing cholesterol clefts (arrows) with surrounding platelets and fibrin (*) with an inflammatory reaction in the wall of the vessel. Patient had redo coronary bypass grafting with post-operative infarction.

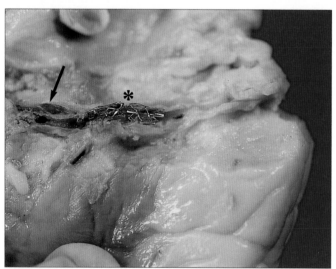

Figure 9.5
Metallic stent which has been inserted into the right coronary artery after angioplasty (*). Note the plaque which shows fragmentation distal to the stent at the site of angioplasty (arrow).

tip studded with diamond particles (Rotablator) is designed to grind atheroma into particles small enough to enter the circulation and to be phagocytosed in the reticuloendothelial system. Catheters with a laser beam at the tip have been used for the treatment of both peripheral and coronary artery disease but is still only used in specialist centres. The theoretical advantage of laser angioplasty is that the atheromatous debris is 'vaporised'. There are some difficulties in controlling the direction of the laser beam, and arterial perforation may be a more common complication than with other techniques. In early death following laser angioplasty the surrounding area is oedematous and may be haemorrhagic. The artery itself may be punctured which was a complication in the early work, when the beam hit the nearest bend in an artery, but it is uncommon now as modifications to the tip of the fibreoptic disperse the beam. The more usual finding is a variable degree of thermal injury, ranging from microscopically detectable to frank charring, readily recognised with the naked eye. The surrounding tissue granulates after a few days.

Intra-aortic balloon pumps are inserted into the aorta to help with the peripheral circulation in cases of left ventricular failure but there may be thrombosis associated with its insertion (Fig. 9.6)

Thrombolytic therapy

The central event of fibrinolysis is the generation of plasmin which cleaves fibrin and fibrinogen with the release of fibrin and fibrinogen degradation products. Free plasmin is rapidly inhibited by its inhibitor, alpha-2–antiplasmin. Fibrinolytic activity is initiated by the plasminogen activators, tissue plasminogen activator (tPA) and urokinase (u-PA) which convert plasminogen to the active serine protease plasmin. To limit necrosis of myocardium from acute infarction, thrombolytic drugs such as recombinant tissue plasminogen activator (rt-PA)

immediate mortality associated with the procedure is now less than 1%, but up to 4% of patients develop an acute myocardial infarction and 4–6% may require emergency coronary artery bypass grafting. Metallic stents to maintain patency are now being commonly applied to vessels following angioplasty and the results are superior to angioplasty alone (Fig. 9.5).

Directional coronary atherectomy is used to excise atheromatous debris from arteries, rather than simply compressing and rupturing plaques. The procedure causes more physical damage and the wall can rupture. The material extracted may be submitted for histological examination. As yet there is no evidence that atherectomy produces better long-term results than balloon angioplasty alone. A catheter with a rotating

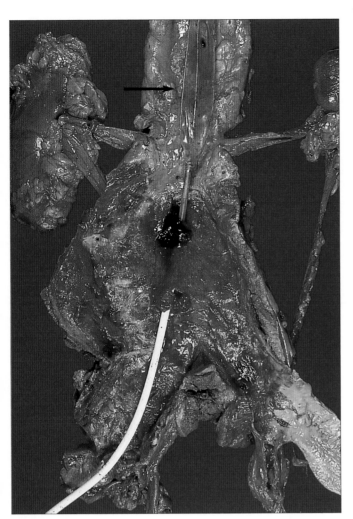

Figure 9.6
Abdominal aorta which contains an intra-aortic balloon pump (arrow). Note the thrombosis around the line in the infrarenal position which led to occlusion of the aorta.

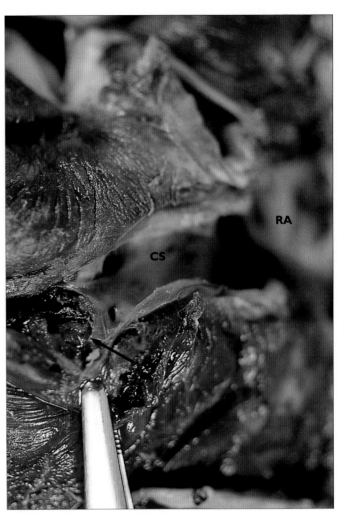

Figure 9.7
This shows the opened coronary sinus (CS) leading into the right atrium (RA). There is rupture of the vein distally (arrow) with haemorrhage associated with retrograde cardioplegia.

and streptokinase are administered early within 4–6 hours of the onset of symptoms and have been shown to improve patient outcome by re-establishing coronary artery patency. The risk of haemorrhagic complications, the most serious of which is intracranial haemorrhage, is the major adverse effect of these drugs. The risk of bleeding was 5.7% in a recent study, of which 1% were intracranial bleeds (Lauer *et al*. 1995). The most common location of significant bleeding is the gastrointestinal tract, followed by the arterial puncture site used during catheterisation, usually the groin. The risk is greater with women, elderly patients and those with hypertension. Obviously the use of catheterisation and angioplasty will increase the risk of systemic haemorrhage in patients with myocardial infarction. Thus, a pathologist must check carefully for internal haemorrhage in these patients and inspect wound sites as well as the groin carefully, to look for a large haematoma (Fig. 9.2).

Bypass procedures

The heart has to be arrested and perfused during bypass and valve operations and this can be a vulnerable situation, especially where there is coronary artery disease

and poor left ventricular function. A combined approach using antegrade and retrograde cardioplegia in conjunction with systemic hypothermia is commonly used. Initial electromechanical quiescence can be rapidly established using antegrade administration of 300–400 ml of cold blood cardioplegia delivered into the aortic root. Maintenance cold blood cardioplegia can then be delivered retrograde by a nearly continuous coronary sinus infusion. Review of the literature supports combined antegrade and retrograde cardioplegia delivery. In complex valve operations the overall mortality rate can be as high as 12.5%; if concomitant coronary artery bypass grafting is performed, the mortality rate rises to 15.2% when only antegrade cardioplegia is used. The high mortality rate demonstrates inferior myocardial protection achieved with only antegrade cardioplegia in this subset of complex patients. Recent clinical reports employing a combined antegrade and retrograde approach demonstrate greatly reduced mortality rates of 2.8% to 6.2% (Chitwood *et al*. 1995). The advantages and disadvantages show that antegrade cardioplegia delivered by way of the aortic root or coronary ostia is a relatively easy technique that permits rapid administration of cardioplegia solutions and produces rapid

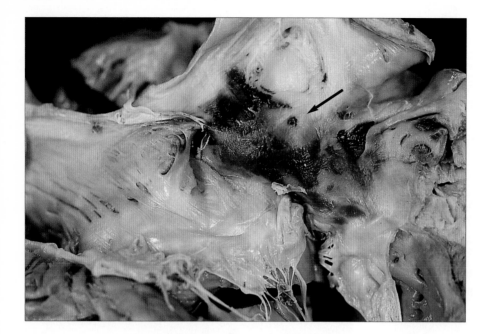

Figure 9.8
Right atrium showing extensive bleeding into the triangle of Koch (arrow) which led to complete heart block in this case of mitral valve replacement.

arrest. However, this technique is frequently associated with variable distribution, particularly in the presence of severe coronary artery occlusive disease. Furthermore, incomplete distribution can occur as a result of aortic insufficiency, as 42% of patients undergoing coronary artery bypass grafts have pre-existing or transient aortic insufficiency. Finally, antegrade cardioplegia is frequently associated with coronary embolism of atherosclerotic debris in reoperative coronary procedures. The advantages of retrograde cardioplegia include less operative interruptions, reduced risk of aortic root air, flushing of air and debris from the coronary arteries, and more even distribution of cooling, particularly in the presence of coronary artery disease. However, large volumes of cardioplegia solutions are required, as only 30% of coronary veins are nutritive, and arrest frequently occurs slowly. Further, because the coronary sinus drains the left ventricle preferentially, there is a question regarding the adequacy of distribution to the right ventricle, the posterior left ventricular free wall, and the septum. Because each approach is associated with specific merits and shortcomings, a physiologically tailored approach that applies the benefit of each technique to the individual patient is best. Typically, antegrade cardioplegia alone is sufficient in the patient with good left ventricular function undergoing uncomplicated coronary revascularisation. For patients having complex operations (valve repair, coronary artery bypass grafting and a valve operation, multiple-valve procedures, aortic reconstruction) or those with severely impaired ventricular function, a combined approach is best. Antegrade cold blood cardioplegic arrest with intermittent to nearly continuous coronary sinus maintenance provides superb myocardial protection during generally long arrest times while facilitating the operative aspects by minimising protective manipulation. This combined technique is not difficult technically and is associated with a low incidence of complications (Chitwood *et al.* 1995). Finally, retrograde cardioplegia alone can be used in reoperative coronary procedures to minimise the potential of microembolism or macroembolism. With each form of cardioplegia, the risk of myocardial infarction and arrhythmias leading to cardiac arrest are obvious. The longer the procedure, the effects of prolonged bleeding and the presence of severe coronary artery disease all predispose to myocardial ischaemia with cardioplegia. Small foci of necrosis are always demonstrable after cardiopulmonary bypass irrespective of discrete infarction, particularly with prolonged complicated operations. Large areas of myocardium are susceptible if cardiac output is low for prolonged periods. In addition, with retrograde cardioplegia there is a large risk of rupturing the coronary venous sinus during the procedure itself (Fig. 9.7).

GENERAL POST-OPERATIVE COMPLICATIONS

General complications occur in 0.8% of cases. They result from embolism and/or anoxia, hypoperfusion, exacerbation of pre-existing disease, iatrogenic factors and stress. They include haemorrhage from cannulation sites and multi-organ failure with cerebral anoxia, acute renal tubular necrosis, acute pancreatitis and adrenal cortical infarction. Subcutaneous fat necrosis in children has been described. Systemic and coronary emboli may occur. Embolised material includes thrombi, fat, bone marrow, air, calcium, atheroma, talc, silicone, platelets and other debris from the perfusion apparatus. Hypoperfusion can lead to cerebral infarction or ischaemic damage to the bowel, without there being thrombosis or emboli present in these organs.

Post-operative arrhythmias

These are common but their cause is often uncertain. Up to 25% of all patients with a previously normal rhythm develop transient atrial fibrillation after thoracic surgery.

Increasing age and obesity are important predisposing factors. Sudden unexplained deaths after cardiac surgery are usually attributed to ventricular arrhythmias, but evidence for this is as scant as in sudden deaths in the community. Reperfusion damage may play a part. In our experience, 10–15% of deaths occurring within 30 days of surgery are due to unexplained left or right ventricular failure with possible arrhythmias. Heart block is common with valve replacement operations, where the triangle of Koch or membranous septum may have extensive bleeding (Fig. 9.8). Surgical treatment of arrhythmias associated with myocardial infarction may utilise cryoablation, cautery, resection or encircling ventriculotomy. The site of cryoablation is difficult to identify unless it is marked at the operation by a suture. It appears as a lesion of 1 cm diameter or less, and looks like an area of infarction. Deep thermal injury is confined to this size, and although it results in necrosis, this does not spread as it does in coagulation necrosis due to ischaemia. The lesion heals to a small scar. Ablation of an arrhythmic focus using cautery also causes damage and heals in the same way as the cold burns, but leaves a slightly larger scar. Encircling ventriculotomy is made using either cautery or a knife. In the latter case the resulting wound is sutured with a thin raised scar and sutures may still be visible.

Infection

This is the most important non-cardiac complication of open heart surgery and may double the time patients stay in hospital. Sternal and mediastinal infections are particularly difficult to manage but only occasionally contribute to death (Bray *et al.* 1996).

CNS damage

There is a low but significant incidence of neurological and neuropsychiatric abnormalities after bypass procedures. Most are transient and there is evidence that transient brain swelling occurs in the first hours after uncomplicated bypass surgery. The risk of permanent damage is less than 1%. Intracerebral haemorrhage may be precipitated by poor anticoagulant control (Lauer *et al.* 1995).

Lung damage

The risk of adult respiratory distress syndrome is increased after prolonged cardiopulmonary bypass, perhaps due to lodgement of microaggregates of platelets and leucocytes in the pulmonary circulation. The patients are often elderly smokers and chronic obstructive airway disease can predispose to bronchopneumonia and pulmonary thromboemboli. Look also for evidence of pulmonary emphysema and hypertensive changes in the pulmonary arterial branches.

Haemorrhage

Coagulopathies are common after cardiac surgery. It is of utmost importance for the pathologist to check the haematological findings in cases of excess bleeding associated with cardiac surgery. During cardiac surgery patients are put on cardiopulmonary bypass and given heparin continuously to prevent clotting during the procedure. Hyperfibrinolysis occurs when fibrinolytic activity is potentially greater than fibrin formation such that clot integrity is threatened. Cardiopulmonary bypass is one of the major surgical procedures to induce a hyperfibrinolytic state, characterised by increased tissue plasminogen-activator (t-PA) concentrations during bypass and is responsible, in part, for the perioperative bleeding diathesis seen in cardiac surgery patients. Hyperfibrinolysis may be iatrogenic, due to the use of fibrinolytic agents in removing thrombus after arterial or venous thromboembolism. t-PA is released by endothelial cells, has a short half life of three to five minutes and is regulated by specific inhibitors, plasminogen activator inhibitors (PAI) types I and 2. PAI-1 is the main systemic inhibitor and is produced by several cell types including endothelial cells, smooth muscle cells, fibroblasts, and hepatocytes. Platelets are the source of 90% of the circulating PAI-I antigen, which is released at the site of a forming thrombus. Hyperfibrinolysis occurs when the balance of fibrinolytic activators to their inhibitors is disturbed.

The consequences of hyperfibrinolysis affect other aspects of haemostasis. Increased plasmin may reduce platelet adhesion and aggregation by degradation of receptor glycoprotein Ib and platelet fibrinogen receptor glycoprotein IIb/IIIa. The consumption of clotting factors due to the direct effect of plasmin and the formation of fibrinogen degradation, which inhibit fibrin polymerisation, result in poor fibrin generation. Chronic liver disease is a common cause of hyperfibrinolysis and these patients are poor risks for cardiac surgery. There is reduced clearance of t-PA, and reduced concentrations of alpha-2–antiplasmin, due to diminished protein synthesis. Measurement of fibrinolytic activity are used routinely as a quick marker of increased fibrin activity. However, they are crude and in situations such as post-operative bleeding are not useful, because concentrations are increased post-operatively in all patients. The thromboelastograph is the most useful instrument used in the surgical setting to determine the fibrinolytic status of a patient during surgical bleeding. If clinical bleeding is attributed to hyperfibrinolysis then an antifibrinolytic agent such as aprotinin is given continuously perioperatively, which is very effective in reducing bleeding during cardiac surgery. Heparin can also cause a thrombocytopenia due to the production of antibodies with a heparin-platelet receptor complex, which can lead to extensive bleeding and/or clotting due to platelet aggregation. All details of such drug administration must be made known to the pathologist if bleeding is the cause of death.

During surgery, it is usually at the surgical site that bleeding occurs, with generalised oozing from all anastomosis sites which may be sucked out during the procedure. The pathologist is unaware of the extent of

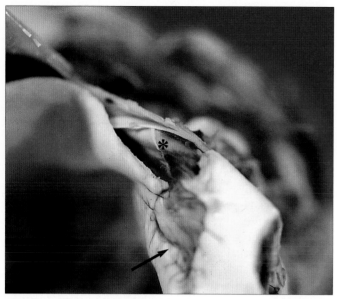

Figure 9.9
Edge of ascending aorta with the sutured opening of a proximal vein graft (arrow). Note that there is a line of dissection (*) leading away from this opening in a case of post-operative bleeding.

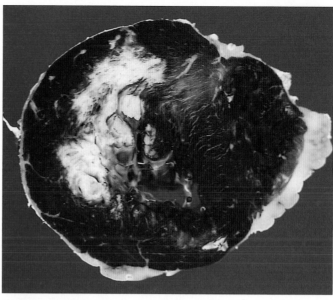

Figure 9.10
Nitro-blue-tetrazolium stain in fresh transverse slice of heart which shows an infarct in the anterior and lateral free wall of the left ventricle. Note the marked left ventricular hypertrophy in a case of ischaemic heart disease and hypertension. Patient had undergone bypass grafts to the anterior descending and posterior descending coronary arteries.

this bleeding, and needs this information from the surgeon or anaesthetist. If there is a drain *in situ* check the amount of blood present. The surgical team will provide details of the amount of drainage both during the operation and post-operatively. Post-operatively if there is a sudden loss of blood from a drain, the surgeon will re-explore the operative site, locate the source of bleeding and oversew the area so that it may be impossible to localise a specific site for bleeding if the patient dies during the procedure. The surgeon is the best person to state the exact site and should demonstrate this at the autopsy (i.e. dissection at aortic anastomosis site after coronary artery bypass operation (Fig. 9.9)). If a drain has been removed and the patient continues to bleed with low haemoglobin, again it is often due to generalised oozing at the operative site and a specific site of bleeding is rarely identified.

Infarcts after surgery

The leading cause of death after cardiac surgery is myocardial infarction. Operative myocardial infarction is extremely rare in patients with no previous evidence of ischaemia, but occurs in up to 5% of patients with ischaemic heart disease. Perioperative infarction and those occurring early in the post-operative period, can be difficult to confirm by the usual means. While in 'medical' patients confirmation of the diagnosis of infarction generally presents no difficulties, virtually none of the diagnostic criteria, e.g enzymes, ECG changes, are reliable in patients who have just undergone operations under cardiopulmonary bypass. Non-fatal myocardial infarction accounts for considerable

morbidity; it may be silent in up to 25% of cases, and it is associated with poor outcome. In a recent study, 4.1% of patients with a history of coronary heart disease suffered perioperative infarcts. Patients over 75 years of age and those with pre-operative evidence of cardiac failure are at particular risk. Perioperative infarcts are especially common after operations for peripheral vascular disease and pre-operative electrocardiographic monitoring is a useful method for assessing cardiac risk (Lee 1997). The clinical diagnosis of post-operative infarction is notoriously difficult. The pain is often masked by analgesic drugs or is confused by the discomfort of the surgical procedure itself. The majority of post-operative infarcts occur 1–3 days after the surgical procedure and the reason for this timing may be uncertain. Prolonged bypass/bleeding are obvious factors which can lead to infarction. Many cases have no single cause and it is considered that the combination of severe coronary disease with ventricular hypertrophy, ischaemic fibrosis etc, may precipitate an irreversible episode of ischaemia. Hypoxia during anaesthesia and intraoperative blood loss have been implicated in the past, but oximetry shows little variation in oxygen tension during most surgical procedures. Myocardial perfusion cannot be measured directly, but is influenced by both diastolic blood pressure and heart rate. A fall in either of these during the induction of anaesthesia may induce myocardial ischaemia, especially in patients with pre-existing coronary heart disease or in cardiac failure. Continuous electrocardiographic monitoring of patients undergoing surgery for peripheral vascular disease has demonstrated a high incidence of arrhythmias in the post-operative period and these correlated with perioperative ischaemia. Up to 50% of episodes of 'long-duration' ST segment depression occur after, rather than before or during, operations (Mamode *et al.* 1996).

Careful macroscopic and histological examination of the myocardium is essential and it is easy to overlook or misinterpret the early macroscopic features of myocardial infarction. Blocks should be taken from all areas of the myocardium, the anterior, lateral and posterior left ventricle, the interventricular septum and the right ventricle. Histology is important in establishing the cause of death and is of particular value in the diagnosis and dating of myocardial infarction. Several cases interpreted macroscopically as acute infarction because of vague colour differences or softening may have no histological evidence of infarction.

Macroscopic changes, beginning with the appearance of haemorrhagic areas, are evident after about 12 hours. Discrimination between regional and diffuse necrosis in the early post-operative period is possible. Diffuse often subendocardial necrosis is a common finding in patients with previous low cardiac output (Fig. 9.1), but regional necrosis will be confined to the area supplied by the coronary artery branch involved in the procedure (Fig. 9.10). Myocardial necrosis can be demonstrated by a number of techniques, including staining of slices of fresh tissue with nitro-blue-tetrazolium (Fig. 9.10). Unaffected tissue takes up the stain, and is uniformly blue, while dead myocardium is unstained due to loss of mitochondrial dehydrogenase in the dead fibres. Fibrous tissue appears white.

It is impossible to identify myocardial necrosis of less than 6 hours duration, but dead myocytes (stained with haematoxylin and eosin) fluoresce when examined in ultraviolet light and will fluoresce even in unstained material. This phenomenon occurs immediately, as the edges of a myocardial biopsy will show, and is independent of autolysis and long-term storage. Contraction band necrosis confined to one area of the myocardium is the earliest histological evidence of irreversible myocyte death and points to ischaemia in that area (Fig. 9.3). Dead myocardial fibres are fuchsinophilic for about 12 hours after death, and a number of special stains based on both acid and basic fuchsin are available. They all have the disadvantage of technical complexity and are indiscriminate, in that myocytes dead from any cause, e.g. anoxia, are stained, especially in the subendocardium.

Pre-operative infarction in the immediate pre-operative period is an increasing indication for emergency operation, and death is relatively common despite urgent revascularisation of the heart. Mortality is increased when grafting is performed as an emergency procedure, usually in patients with unstable angina, recent infarction or after an unsuccessful angioplasty. In these cases the myocardium should be sampled with particular care and attention to the age and areas of infarction. When acute infarcts occur after coronary artery bypass grafting, almost all are in the territory supplied by the vessel into which the graft has been inserted (Fig. 9.10).

Cardiac failure

Pre-operative pump failure as a cause of death can be defined to include patients who were receiving inotropes, or had an intra-aortic balloon pump, or no spontaneous cardiac output when they went to theatre, and in whom poor ventricular function persisted after coming off cardiopulmonary bypass until death. Pre-operative cardiac failure is the most common cause of death after emergency procedures in both ischaemic and valvar heart disease.

All too frequently when acute infarction, sepsis, haemorrhage and pulmonary embolism have been excluded, all that remains to explain the death of the patient is pulmonary oedema. Non-cardiac conditions such as raised intracranial pressure, renal failure and intravenous fluid overload ('houseman's lung') should be considered, but cardiac failure is the commonest cause. There is good correlation between the development of post-operative pulmonary oedema and pre-operative evidence of heart failure. Nevertheless, more than 50% of patients over 65 years of age who develop post-operative heart failure, as opposed to myocardial infarction, have no previous clinical evidence of myocardial disease. Perioperative atrial fibrillation may contribute to cardiac failure and is more common in elderly and obese patients. Histological changes of pulmonary hypertension, intra-alveolar haemosiderin accumulation and hepatic venous congestion may be evidence of long-standing heart failure.

There is difficulty in defining cardiac failure, especially in the post-operative period. It is common to use a clinicopathological definition, and pulmonary oedema is the major pathological feature, although this may be a terminal event. In the majority of patients there is substantial ischaemic or valvar heart disease with extensive hypertrophy, fibrosis or thinning of the myocardium (Fig. 9.11). The patients often have a stormy operative course with prolonged bypass. However, there are often no new histological lesions to explain the post-operative poor ventricular function.

Cardiogenic shock is a clinicopathological diagnosis, defined as failure of the left ventricle with lack of perfusion of distal organs. Patients have hypotension and oliguria, and are usually inotrope-dependant or have had an intra-aortic balloon pump inserted prior to death. There is often a history of cardiac failure or acute infarction prior to surgery and the ventricle is usually thin-walled and dilated. Other patients have a history of hypertension or aortic stenosis with marked left ventricular hypertrophy (Figs. 9.10 and 9.11). Patients go on to develop multi-organ failure with adult respiratory distress syndrome, or may simply die with pulmonary oedema.

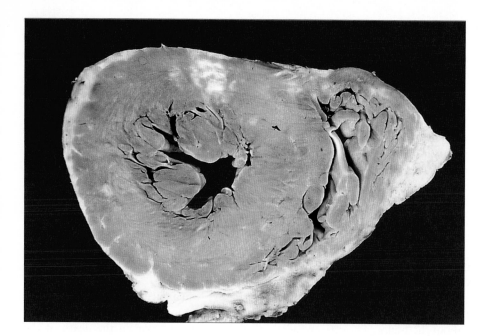

Figure 9.11
Transverse section of both ventricles showing marked hypertrophy of the left ventricle with fibrosis in the anterior wall. Case of pump failure after aortic valve replacement.

CORONARY ARTERY BYPASS GRAFTING (CABG)

Coronary artery bypass grafting is now the commonest cardiac surgical procedure in both North America and Europe. The techniques used are continually changing. The long-term patency rates for saphenous vein grafts between the aorta and coronary arteries are about 60%. More recently, arterial grafting is combined with vein grafting to give better long-term results since arteries do not occlude as fast as vein grafts. A systemic artery is dissected as a pedicle and anastomosed either end-to-side or side-to-side to a distal coronary artery. The left internal mammary artery is now the graft of choice for arteries on the anterior surface of the heart, but right internal mammary grafts are also increasingly used. In some centres the gastroepiploic artery is brought up through the diaphragm to arteries on the inferior surface of the heart and the epigastric artery is dissected from the anterior abdominal wall and used as a free graft in the same way as a saphenous vein (Fig. 9.12). When the internal mammary artery is anastomosed to the left anterior descending branch, it is often a small vessel embedded in fatty tissue and can easily be ripped out during removal of the sternum. Always check what exactly was anastomosed and where, from the notes or surgeon. Obviously in coroners' cases this detail may not be available and one has to procede carefully with removal of the sternum to check for this vessel. The presence of leg wounds obviously identifies patients who had vein grafts, so these should be carefully documented. If the long saphenous veins are unavailable (previous operation) or unsuitable (severe varices), arm veins or man-made grafts or, less commonly, bioprostheses in the form of umbilical veins are utilised instead. Although the left internal mammary artery is used for up to three-quarters of grafts to the left anterior descending branch, internal mammary artery grafts account for only about one-quarter of all the bypass grafts done in the UK, so that vein grafts still constitute most of the surgical cases. Vein grafts are anastomosed proximally into the ascending aorta singly, sometimes quite close to each other with a separate stoma for each (Fig. 9.9). The anastomoses are made with continuous suture and generally cause no problems with bleeding. The distal anastomoses vary a little. They may be applied singly to a coronary branch, in which case the vein is tailored so that the anastomosis is slightly enlarged end-to-side. Alternatively, a longer length of vein may be used for sequential anastomoses, known as 'snake', 'sequential' or 'horseshoe' grafts, or trouser leg grafts to two branches (Fig. 9.13). In these, the anastomoses are made side-to-side. Grafts to the obtuse marginal branches are often passed through the transverse sinus of the pericardium to reach their destination. This manoeuvre has a threefold advantage: it reduces the risk of compression when the chest is closed, the shorter length of vein has better flow and it saves vein. The distal anastomoses, like the proximal ones, are made with a fine monofilament suture (6/0 or less) which can leak, but this is rare

Study of the most recent post-operative coronary arteriograms is the ideal aid to the examination of the heart, as they identify the location of the grafts. In specialised centres, the full extent of the saphenous vein grafts are best visualised radiographically. It is usual to inject all of the vein grafts simultaneously and radiograph them before injection of the coronary arteries. This enables more detailed study of the native coronary arteries distal to the grafts as well as at the coronary graft anastomosis. Measurements of lumen diameters may be made from the radiographs. In those cases in which the internal mammary artery is anastomosed to the left coronary system, the internal mammary artery is injected from where it has been severed during removal of the heart. The native coronary arteries are injected, fixed, and radiographed to evaluate the extent of disease.

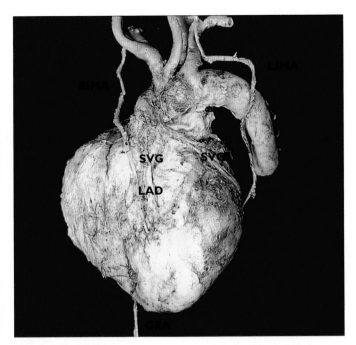

Figure 9.12
Anterior view of the heart which shows right internal mammary arterial graft (RIMA) extending from right subclavian down to anastomose on the left anterior descending coronary artery (LAD). The left internal mammary artery (LIMA) anastomoses to an oblique marginal branch of the circumflex. Gastroepiploic artery (GEA) comes up posteriorly behind the heart to anastomose to the posterior descending artery. Two saphenous vein grafts (SVG) extend down from the aorta to anastomose with diagonal branch of LAD and an oblique marginal branch of the circumflex. Note the adhesions on the epicardial surface of the heart.

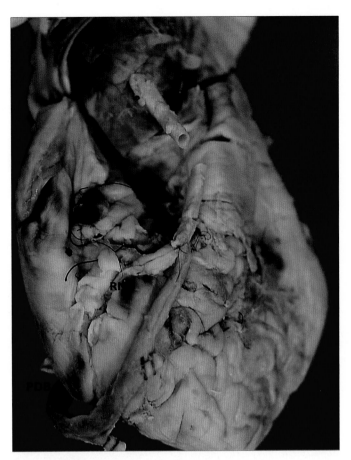

Figure 9.13
Saphenous vein graft to the right coronary artery with clips to tie off the side branches. There is a trouser-leg division which supplies the right marginal branch (RMB) and the posterior descending branch (PDB).

After recent CABG operation, care is needed to examine the operative site and avoid damaging the proximal and distal anastomoses. The pericardium is left open and blood accumulates with pericardial adhesions which makes it difficult to identify structures and a graft can easily be avulsed (Fig. 9.14). Although time consuming, it is better to use blunt dissection with the fingers. It is helpful to have available some means of magnification for the distal anastomoses. Even an ordinary magnifying glass will suffice, but the task is made much easier if an illuminated magnifying glass is available. Although the grafts are often very difficult to see, particularly on the right, they may be palpable. It is helpful to try to locate them by palpation before removing the pericardium, as considerable damage to them can result from the sharp dissection which is often necessary for this manoeuvre.

In CABG cases where the original operation took place several years before, because of early arterialisation and the almost inevitable intimal hyperplasia, the grafts feel firm to the touch, even when widely patent. A graft to the right coronary artery is often invisible as it quickly becomes buried in fat in the right atrioventricular sulcus so that it resembles a native artery. Those to the anterior branches of the left system are usually visible and resemble large, firm native arteries. Grafts passing through the transverse sinus, like those to the right, are invisible for much of their length. In the case of vein grafts, early occlusion causes the vein to atrophy, so that it may be impossible to locate on the heart. Sometimes the surgeon places a radio-opaque marker at the aortic end to facilitate post-operative arteriography, and this may be a clue to the site of the graft. The tributaries of the vein are ligated with thread or clips and their remnants sometimes identify the site. Internal thoracic artery grafts also fail and atrophy, in which case they are impossible to find unless there are still either a few suture ends visible from the anastomosis or the metal clips used to ligate the branches of the artery can be found. In late deaths, occlusion, if present or suspected, is usually throughout the length of the vessel. The site of occlusion can be found more easily if the angiogram or the report is available. Grafts can be sectioned either longitudinally or transversely (the latter enables better assessment of the patency but longitudinal section keeps the specimen together, particularly if the grafts are not firmly adherent to the epicardial surface).

Often there are adhesions with haemorrhage over the visceral pericardium because of the recent procedure or dense fibrosis if the grafting was done in the distant past. A longer segment of the ascending aorta is left in continuity with the heart to enable examination of vein grafts from the aortic orifice to distal anastomosis. We

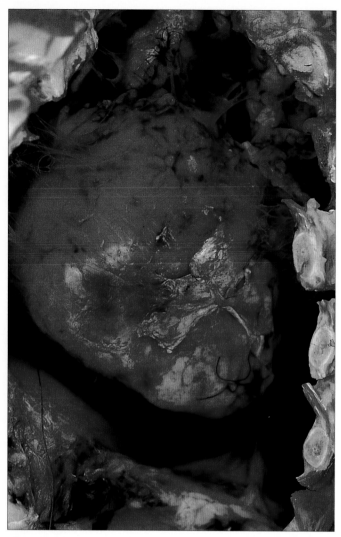

Figure 9.14
Operative site with opened pericardium in a case of bypass grafting with death shortly after the operation. There is haemorrhage with pericardial adhesions making it difficult to trace the bypass grafts on the surface of the heart.

find it useful to trace the origin of the saphenous vein grafts within the ascending aorta and probing is useful when the grafts are embedded in dense fibrous tissue. The proximal ends of the grafts are, fortunately, usually easy to see, so that the graft can easily be traced from its origin. In this way one can easily detect occlusion with recent or old thrombosis and atherosclerosis within the vein grafts. Recent thrombosis renders the graft solid, which can be palpated before probing (Fig. 9.15) in the fresh state. The grafts and native arteries may then be removed from the heart, radiographed, and cut at 5 mm intervals to determine the extent of luminal narrowing, the presence or absence of thrombi, and/or extent of atherosclerosis in vein grafts and coronary arteries. In most routine cases, the heart is fixed in 10% buffered formaldehyde overnight before dissection of the grafts and native vessels.

It can be useful to follow the anatomy of the coronary arteries in vein grafts in order to check for the most likely distal anastomosis sites, particularly when one does not have any operative details. The right coronary artery originates in the right coronary sinus and passes in the right atrioventricular sulcus to the acute margin of the heart, giving a variable number of right ventricular branches (which cannot be grafted). At the acute margin there is a fairly constant branch, the acute marginal branch, which is sometimes grafted (Fig. 9.13). The right artery usually continues in the atrioventricular sulcus until the crux of the heart where it loops into the myocardium and the main artery divides into a posterior descending branch, which is a very important vessel for grafting, and may continue as the posterolateral branch, which also can be grafted. Less commonly, the posterior descending branch originates at the right acute margin to pass obliquely across and gain the posterior interventricular sulcus. The pathologist must be aware of these variations in the anatomy of the right coronary artery when looking for grafts. The left coronary artery originates in the left (anterolateral)

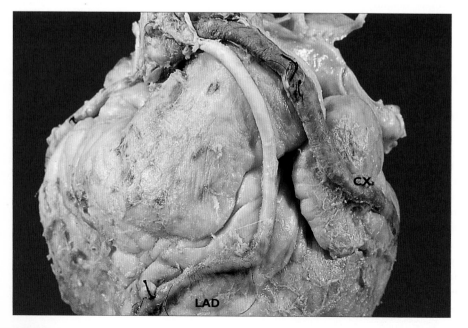

Figure 9.15
Two saphenous vein grafts supplying an oblique marginal branch of the circumflex (CX) and the anterior descending branch of the left coronary artery (LAD). There is thrombosis of the entire length of the graft to the obtuse marginal branch and thrombosis at the distal anastomosis site of the LAD graft.

aortic sinus and passes undivided for up to 2.5 cm as the left main coronary artery and this is usually not grafted. Lesions of the left main stem preferentially undergo balloon angioplasty. The anterior descending branch passes in the anterior interventricular sulcus towards the apex and during its course it gives a variable number of branches (diagonal branches) to the left ventricle. These, together with their parent branch, are important for grafting (Fig. 9.12 and 9.15). The circumflex branch of the left coronary artery occupies the left atrioventricular sulcus and is not graftable because of its inaccessibility in the left atrioventricular groove, but gives a variable number of branches called obtuse marginal branches, which are grafted.

COMPLICATIONS FOLLOWING VEIN/ARTERIAL GRAFTING

Early post-operative death

The most common causes of death early in the post-operative period are:

1. Cardiogenic shock leading to peripheral circulatory failure.
2. Acute myocardial infarction.
3. Left/right ventricular failure.
4. Technical problems associated with the operation.

Technical problems include overlong grafts which can kink, cutting off the flow. The grafts may be compressed by the sternum or, rarely, by a chest drain. This is not easy to identify in the post mortem room as the chest drain has invariably been taken out before the body arrives, but it may have left an impression on the surrounding tissues. The veins themselves may accidentally have been narrowed during ligation of the tributaries, causing poor 'run-off' to the downstream myocardium. The technical problems outlined above are very rare. Patency of the grafts can be confirmed quite simply because when fully patent they are flat. A useful method of checking patency is to inject water into the grafts from the aorta and watch them fill which will also help to trace the grafts distally.

Haemorrhage

This is a major technical problem and side suture lines in the aorta, and graft anastomoses and ligatures around side branches must be inspected carefully (Fig. 9.9). Blocks must be taken for histological examination of the anastomosis, the proximal and distal coronary artery and left ventricular muscle supplied by each graft. When there are no lesions identifiable, grossly random sections of the entire length of the grafts should be taken. Anastomotic sites are sectioned in different ways depending on whether the connection is end to end or end to side.

Acute thrombotic event

In the early post-operative phase thrombosis causes total and irreversible graft occlusion (Fig. 9.15). The presence of ante-mortem thrombus leads to poor run-off and usually to new infarction. If this area is examined by sectioning it transversely, beginning at the anastomosis, it will usually reveal that the distal artery is either very small or that there is diffuse distal atherosclerotic disease which is common in diabetic patients. This, and prolonged periods of low-output failure permitting stasis, are the causes of thrombosis within grafts in the early post-operative period. Grafting combined with atherectomy of the distal coronary vessel has a high risk of thrombosis. Synthetic grafts are not used for coronary artery bypass surgery because of the very high risk of thrombosis. Redo coronary artery grafts have a much higher mortality than first operations.

Dissection of the aorta

At the site of proximal anastomosis acute dissection is a rare complication (Fig. 9.9). The aorta may have the changes of cystic medial necrosis in the wall which can predispose to dissection, particularly if the patient is hypertensive or has Marfan's syndrome.

Arterial grafts

There are several complications which may be associated with internal mammary artery grafts. The dissection at operation to collect the artery may cause bleeding, especially in obese people, and many surgeons consider obesity to be a contraindication to the procedure for this reason. Some surgeons measure the flow through the artery before implanting it and discard it if the flow is poor. Thus, the patient has all the disadvantages of having the artery prepared for grafting, without benefits of an arterial graft. (Poor flow is often associated with arterial spasm during dissection; this is largely overcome by manoeuvres such as wrapping the graft in a swab moistened with papaverine to lessen the spasm.) Arterial grafts do badly in the early post-operative period because they are of small lumen and take time to expand – up to one month – and they are liable to spasm. As a result it is usually only the left internal mammary artery which is anastomosed to the left anterior descending artery, while venous grafts are used on the other vessels which open early and establish rapid blood flow

Infections

Other complications include local and systemic infection including infective endocarditis. Patients who have had revascularisation operations without other procedures are not especially susceptible to endocarditis. If there are prosthetic valves put in at the same time, the risks of endocarditis are the same as those of valve replacement alone.

Reperfusion injury

An important early cardiac complication, which may follow bypass surgery or interventional procedures such as angioplasty, is global myocardial dysfunction. The underlying mechanism may be free radical damage and alterations in intracellular calcium as a result of reperfusion/exacerbated enzyme leakage with calcium and sodium overload. These changes may worsen irreversible

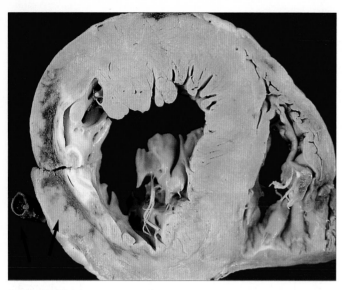

Figure 9.16
Transverse section of the ventricles in a case of ischaemic heart disease with evidence of an old healed infarct in the left lateral free wall with hypertrophy of remaining left ventricle wall. There is reperfusion haemorrhage in an area of infarction in the lateral wall associated with a thrombosed vein graft (arrows) to an oblique marginal branch of the circumflex. Patient had acute infarction associated with thrombosis of the circumflex and emergency CABG.

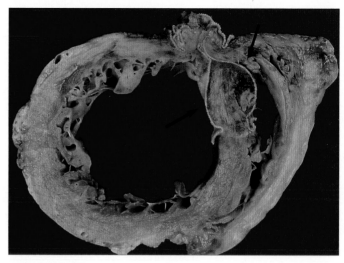

Figure 9.17
Transverse section of both ventricles showing an anterior infarct associated with an anterior VSD which has been repaired on both ventricular aspects with cotton pledgets, which have also been applied to the anterior wall of the heart (arrows). Patient was in cardiogenic shock and did not survive the operation.

myocardial damage already present, or precipitate arrhythmias and myocardial stunning. There is often reperfusion haemorrhage in infarcted areas of the myocardium following revascularisation procedures (Fig. 9.16). No specific morphological changes are known to occur with reperfusion arrhythmias or myocardial stunning. The latter is diagnosed on echocardiography as an area of myocardial hypokinesia during a period of reduced blood flow which returns to normal gradually over hours to days or weeks following the restoration of blood flow. The diagnosis is confirmed and recovery aided by a response to inotropes. Mechanical support (intra-aortic balloon pump, left ventricular assist device) may be required during the recovery phase.

Tamponade

When drains are removed post-operatively, there may be torrential bleeding into the opened pericardium due to ventricular rupture subsequent to pre-operative or perioperative infarction. A common cause of tamponade is leakage from the aortotomy site or due to a suture cutting out of a distal anastomosis. Graft disruption due to overwhelming infection is a very rare event.

Concomitant procedures

Endarterectomy

Removal of atheromatous debris with the intima may prepare a vessel for grafting, particularly the right coronary artery, but the left system is less amenable to this. However, there is a high risk with removal of plaque which may damage the arterial wall, particularly if there is calcification, and dissection or early post-operative thrombotic occlusion may result.

Ventricular aneurysmectomy

Removal of dilated fibrosed ventricular wall may be performed at the time of grafting and often the patients are in cardiac failure, so mortality is high.

Closure of VSD

Closure of of ischaemic ventricular septal defect (VSD) is increasingly being done in the acute phase. The defects are usually located posteroapically, among the trabeculae. There is usually no distinct morphology, the defects consisting only of perforations due to necrosis. Closure is effected by direct suture, usually over pledgets of felt or similar material (Fig. 9.17). In these patients, with poor myocardial function, the haemodynamic derangement caused by the sudden left-to-right shunt in the presence of low cardiac output may be the prime contributor to death. A frequent finding is occlusion of the proximal part of the posterior descending coronary artery in individuals with poor or absent collateral circulation. Thus, people with dominant left coronary artery are especially at risk, as are those with previous anterolateral or apical infarction. There may be little to see from the right ventricle, as the rupture is usually a breakdown of the trabeculae carneae posteriorly. If the operation included closure of VSD, a degree of breakdown of the closure can result from spreading necrosis despite the most meticulous attention to excision of necrotic myocardium at operation.

Late death

Myocardial revascularisation does not arrest the underlying disease. Thus, patients who die late after operation (which can be repeated a number of times to relieve symptoms) may or may not have patent grafts, but they will have progression of the underlying disease in the coronary vessels. As there are so many people with bypass grafts, the causes of late death among them are legion, but ischaemic heart disease with evidence of cardiac failure is probably the most common.

Late graft failure is associated with occlusion, which is often due to exaggerated healing with fibrosis of the intima and atherosclerosis. When the vein is removed from the leg it loses much of its adventitia and it is exposed to arterial blood pressure. As a consequence, the intimal endothelium, deprived of its blood supply from the vasa vasorum, is lost as well. The changes which take place to repair this damage initiate the process of healing. The loss of the endothelium produces oedema and a transient, acute inflammatory cell reaction in the intima and subjacent media. Microthrombi and fibrin are deposited on the intima, and these, together with proliferating smooth muscle cells, fibroblasts and endothelial cells, form a new, pseudointima by the end of 4–6 weeks. This new surface reaches its maximal thickness after 4–6 months. During the ensuing 6 months the new surface condenses and fibroses. The media also loses its blood supply at transplantation from the leg, so that many smooth muscle cells die and are replaced by fibrous tissue. The surviving myocytes hypertrophy, causing the media to become relatively thick and firm. The adventitia is replaced by scar tissue which eventually revascularises; by the end of a year the graft is arterialised, i.e. it has a firm, thickened wall and a patent lumen. The 'healed' graft may have a lumen lined with mature fibrous tissue covered by endothelium which is called a neointima, but the lumen may be lined with other material, for example fibrin and/or collagen. When this happens, the lining is a pseudointima. Smooth muscle cells acquire some of the characteristics of endothelial cells when they are exposed to the bloodstream, so that positive identification of a neointima depends on identifying some product of endothelial cells, e.g. factor VIII.

Slight graft–artery mismatch can cause jet lesions close to the anastomosis, but much more commonly there is exaggerated fibrosis of the new intimal layer, which is often concentric throughout the length of the graft. This condition is called fibrointimal hyperplasia and may continue to develop until the lumen of the graft is occluded. This explains the superior patency rate of internal thoracic artery grafts, but these too may develop the changes described, although usually to a much lesser degree. Other materials used for aortocoronary grafts usually develop a pseudointima, but man, in contrast to some other species, has little ability to heal long lengths or large areas of prosthetic material. It has been stated that up to a third of patients have stenoses in their vein grafts by the end of the first year. Thrombosis is a rare cause of late graft failure and becomes more so the longer the patient survives. Most thrombotic occlusions of the graft occur within the first post-operative year. Graft occlusion is due either to progressive intimal hyperplasia or to atheromatous disease progressing in the grafts. Rarely, a slightly too-long graft, and therefore usually kinked, is 'suddenly' occluded by intimal hyperplasia. Patients who had endarterectomy at operation are especially affected, as the damaged arterial wall is stimulated by platelet activity to intimal hyperplasia. In a recent study 19% of the examined vein grafts showed occlusion as the result of an organised fibrotic thrombus. In 81% the stenosis was the result of a myo-intimal thickening and an associated luminal accumulation of foam cells and mural thrombi (Underwood and Coumbe 1994). Transverse sections should be made through each of the anastomoses and examined carefully for thrombus formation.

CARDIAC VALVE SURGERY

Valvuloplasty

In some patients who are not fit for formal replacement of stenotic rheumatic or calcified aortic or mitral valves, balloon valvuloplasty will allow an increase in haemo-

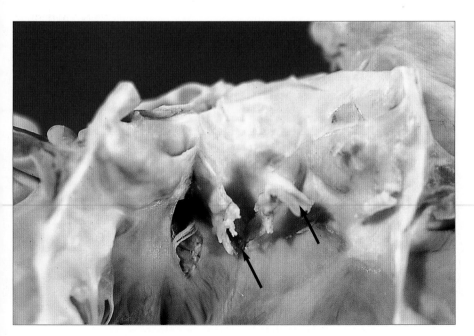

Figure 9.18
Balloon valvuloplasty in a case of aortic calcific stenosis showing the ruptured cusp which is the right coronary cusp with fragments of calcium at the edge (arrows). Patient had severe respiratory insufficiency making an open operation unsuitable.

dynamic output (Fig. 9.18). This is commonly done in the Middle East and India for rheumatic valve stenosis. Some degree of damage to the calcified cusps is inevitable and debris may embolise into the systemic circulation.

Annuloplasty

In this operation (approached from above) the valve ring is reduced either by placing a purse-string around part of it (Wooler's operation), by placing a double purse-string around the annulus and adjusting the tension to the desired diameter (De Vega's annuloplasty) or by fitting a soft plastic ring and tailoring the valve to that (Carpentier's annuloplasty). The leaflets are also amenable to refashioning. This is most commonly done for tricuspid regurgitation or less commonly mitral regurgitation

Leaflet resection

In addition to the above, there is another procedure especially suitable for mitral valve regurgitation due to floppy change, which is the commonest cause of regurgitation seen in surgical series in the West. A section of the valve is excised as a rectangle of tissue comprising the affected chordae, the adjacent leaflet and a small segment of annulus (Fig. 9.19). The edges of the remaining annulus and leaflet are apposed and sutured so that competence of the valve is restored.

All materials used inside the heart are 'permanent' in that they are non-absorbant. Contemporary suture materials are of man-made fibres and may be of even thickness (monofilament), stranded or braided. Several types of fabric exist which may be non-woven (felt), woven or knitted from synthetic yarns. Some woven cloths are manufactured as a cylinder and these are often crimped in a concertina fashion to allow greater freedom of movement for arterial grafts. Most of these have an X-ray detectable strip woven into them and many of the materials unravel when they are cut, necessitating care when examining at necropsy. Most of the commonly encountered materials are perhaps better known by their registered trade names rather than their composition: for example, Teflon felt and two-way-stretch Dacron for patching, and crimped Dacron Gore-Tex for grafts. Plastics are used to make parts of artificial valves and prosthetic devices for annuloplasty. In addition to the man-made products, there are several natural materials used in cardiac surgery. These may be taken from the patient at the operation (autologous tissue), from another human being (homologous) or from another species (heterologous or xenograft). Autologous tissues include saphenous vein, pericardium, pulmonary valve, and (now obsolete) fascia lata. Homologous tissues include aortic valves, pulmonary valves and umbilical veins. Heterologous tissues include pericardium, aortic valves and dura mater from bovine species in particular. The sternotomy is almost universally closed with stainless-steel wire.

PROSTHETIC HEART VALVES

Most prosthetic heart valves are used to replace aortic and mitral valves. Details of the type of heart valve inserted should be available to the pathologist. Examination of valve implants include determination of:

1. the type of implant as well as its size and position regarding annulus and chamber;
2. adequacy of movement of the valve apparatus;
3. presence of thrombi, vegetations, and paravalvar abscesses or leaks;
4. evidence of valve degeneration.

In particular, paravalvar abscesses may not be visible without careful inspection of the native annulus follow-

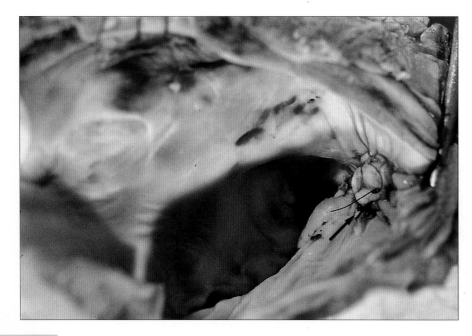

Figure 9.19
Repaired posterior leaflet of mitral valve (arrow) with sutures at the site of excision of a wedge of valve. Case of floppy mitral valve with regurgitation.

ing removal of the implant. Demonstration of any pathology may be enhanced using short-axis cuts through the atrioventricular junction. Post mortem clot commonly forms around prosthetic valves and must be carefully removed to expose true thrombus or dehiscence around the valve annulus.

Many prosthetic heart valves contain a cloth ring, metal and – more recently – purolytic carbon. Another non-metallic substance widely used in heart valves is silicone rubber for the ball or poppet. 'Plastic' rings are also used for both mitral and tricuspid annuloplasty.

CAGED BALL PROSTHESES

In 1960, Starr and his engineer colleague Edwards, both American, introduced the valve which bears their name. The original model had a silicone rubber poppet in a metal cage, with three struts for aortic prostheses and four struts for mitral ones. The sewing ring was (and still is) of silicone foam-rubber covered in knitted cloth. The original model was soon withdrawn because the composition of the ball (poppet) permitted the absorption of lipids into it, causing 'ball variance'. The adjustment of the silicone rubber during manufacture abolished ball variance permanently and the modified valve (model 1260) is in worldwide use today. The most common complication is thromboembolism, so efforts to reduce the incidence of thromboembolism in patients with Starr–Edwards valves produced numerous modifications to the basic design (Fig. 9.24). Among these have been: a hollow metal poppet in the original cage; covering the outside of the cage with cloth; covering the seat of the poppet as well as the cage and covering the seat only. Because the metal poppet has to be placed in the cage before the cage is completed, it is not fully closed at its apex, but the gap is very small. Other caged ball valves include the Braunwald–Cutter, the Macgovern (which was 'sutureless', being applied with a special instrument which released metal teeth from the valve into the aortic annulus) and the Smeloff–Cutter. They are all slightly different in appearance; for example, in the Braunwald–Cutter the apex of the cage is open with rounded struts.

TILTING DISC PROSTHESES

The first tilting disc valve was developed by the Swedish surgeon, Björk, and the American engineer, Shiley, in 1969. The slightly biconvex disc was plastic while the struts within which the disc tilted were of metal, as was the annulus. The sewing ring, as in all replacement heart valves, was covered in cloth. Like the Starr–Edwards, the Björk–Shiley valve has undergone modifications, both to improve its haemodynamic characteristics and to reduce the incidence of thromboembolism. The current model is made entirely of pyrolytic carbon (Fig. 9.21). There have been several other tilting disc valves but none has been as universally used as the Björk–Shiley. A few, such as the

Hall–Kast (Norwegian–American) introduced in 1979 are in use, but most such as the Hammersmith valve (1964) have long since become obsolete.

SPLIT DISC VALVES

These are also tilting discs but the disc is split into two equal halves so that when the valve is open the two flaps are at right-angles to the ring, giving a very large orifice. The discs are made of pyrolytic carbon. These are relatively new valves so they do not as yet have the multiplicity of model numbers reflecting modifications to the design which all the older ones have. Names include Duromedic, St Jude and Omniscience.

BIOPROSTHESES/TISSUE VALVES

The simplest of the bioprostheses is the 'free' or 'unstented' aortic valve homograft, the use of which was introduced by the New Zealand surgeon Barratt–Boyes. In addition to the natural valves, there are several prostheses fashioned from heterologous tissues. They are cut and shaped to resemble the leaflets of aortic valves and are then mounted into a stent. The Wessex Medical valve, for example, is constructed from bovine pericardium. The theory behind these is that they have the advantage of natural valves (lower thrombogenicity) without the restraints imposed by the size of natural ones. However, they are not made in sizes much above 40 mm overall diameter, as the semi-lunar design, when man made, does not suit larger sizes. Heterograft valves have as their usual source the pig, as the size range accords with that of man. These valves are marketed by various manufacturers; some carry the name of a surgeon (for example Carpentier–Edwards), whose ideas were incorporated into the product. The morphology of the stent varies a little according to whether the valve is to be used in the aortic or mitral position, those for the former having a more steeply angled sewing ring.

Human (homograft) valves are collected during necropsy and in the early days were sterilised in P-propriolactone or ethylene oxide gas before storage, either in a tissue culture medium or after freeze-drying. Today they are treated by immersion in an antibiotic solution for some days before either freezing or wet storage. Nowadays most aortic valve allografts come from transplantation programmes, and are often used fresh, without any *in vitro* treatment. Stented homograft valves are sewn into a frame (stent) before further processing.

MULTIPLE VALVE OPERATIONS

As the incidence of new rheumatic heart disease continues to decline, the necessity for multiple valve replacements declines with it. Although triple valve replacement is now a fairly rare procedure, aortic and mitral replacements still occur. The combination of aortic and tricuspid replacement is uncommon.

TRICUSPID VALVE OPERATIONS

Organic tricuspid valve disease is uncommon even as part of the spectrum of rheumatic heart disease, and is rare on its own. Replacement of the valve may be necessary in the treatment of end-stage rheumatic disease but, as already indicated, the need is decreasing steadily. Annuloplasty is performed whenever possible. When replacement is unavoidable, bioprostheses tend to be preferred to mechanical valves for the tricuspid position. This is partly due to the shape of the tricuspid annulus and right ventricle, and partly because the thrombogenicity of mechanical valves is increased in the tricuspid position. Tricuspid valve replacement may still be performed for infective endocarditis or for a congenital malformation. In the case of endocarditis, the tricuspid valve is commonly affected in abusers of drugs, especially those taking them intravenously. It is also at risk in patients with long-term intravenous lines and those with transvenous endocardial pacemakers.

COMPLICATIONS OF VALVES

Mechanical prostheses

Mechanical non-tissue valves have the advantage of greater durability but patients require lifelong anticoagulant therapy, with its attendant morbidity. Many late deaths are due to complications of anticoagulation, notably cerebral haemorrhage. Haemolysis is another disadvantage of mechanical valves. This is largely due to turbulence resulting from transvalvar pressure gradients, and is more severe in caged ball valves than in tilting disc models (Fig. 9.20). Mechanical prostheses are durable but more prone to thromboembolic complications than tissue valves (Fig. 9.21). Post mortem clot commonly forms around prosthetic valves and must be carefully removed to expose true thrombus or dehiscence around the valve annulus. They are less likely to degenerate over time than tissue valves. Structural failure of some types of Björk–Shiley valves has received much adverse publicity but human or porcine bioprosthetic valves are at least ten times more liable to fail. In contrast, perivalvar leaks and haemorrhagic complications of anticoagulation, especially blood-stained pericardial effusions, are more common with mechanical devices. Progress in the design and structure of mechanical prostheses over the years has led to a considerable improvement in their haemodynamic features and durability, such that they are now preferable to bioprostheses in many cases. However, their use is still burdened with the risk of complications, among which thrombosis is the most dreaded.

Although obstruction is most often thought to result from valve thrombosis, the role of chronic pannus (fibrosis) formation in causing obstruction is less well-established (Fig. 9.22) but occurs around the mechanical valve ring.

Ventricular rupture is associated with mitral valve replacement. The risk of rupture is increased when ischaemic or infarcted papillary muscle are involved. It is usually difficult to distinguish grossly between left ventricular rupture due to papillary muscle necrosis and that consequent upon pre-operative or perioperative infarction.

Bioprostheses

The latter have a limited span *in situ* (about 10–15 years) and deteriorate slowly, unlike mechanical valves, which, when they do fail, tend to do so suddenly, with results which may be fatal. The patient is spared the disadvantages of long-term anticoagulant therapy but irrespective of their source, tissue valves have a finite life-span, so that all but the oldest patients will eventually need another operation, with all the complications associated with reoperation. The site of implantation is not relevant to persistence *per se*. Bioprostheses are contraindicated in children and adolescents because the valves calcify early, sometimes within a year. This is usually attributed to a combination of enhanced calcium metabolism and rapid heart rate in young patients.

In the case of bioprosthetic valves in the aortic position, most living patients have a diastolic murmur by the end of the first year following operation, so that a degree of regurgitation is nearly always present. This regurgitation causes turbulence, which in turn causes a degree of haemolysis. Obviously, severe haemolytic anaemia necessitates a change of valve, and the hepatic, splenic and renal manifestations of subclinical haemolysis are often to be seen at necropsy. In unstented grafts there is no possibility for paravalvar leaks, as there is no paravalvar space, so that in the absence of infection, deterioration of the graft must be suspected as a cause of regurgitation. Valve failure is a slow and (usually) gradual process which is a late complication of tissue valve replacement and is due to degeneration of the prosthesis. This nearly always occurs as a result of thinning of the valve leaflet due to degeneration of collagen close to the 'hinge'. In stented valves, the thinning is more noticeable near the commissures, where there is the greatest anatomical distortion of the leaflets, due to hydrodynamic forces acting upon the valve as a whole. Thinning is often accompanied by calcification (Fig. 9.23). Rarely the leaflet (of an aortic valve replacement) may be holed by spicules of calcium from the adjacent mitral valve. However, sudden spontaneous leaflet rupture is a rare cause of late death in patients with tissue valves.

Endocarditis, both early and late, occurs in mechanical and bioprostheses, irrespective of their method of preparation and storage. This can lead to regurgitation due to perforation and paravalvar leaks (Fig. 9.24). Care must be taken to look for leaks and probe the

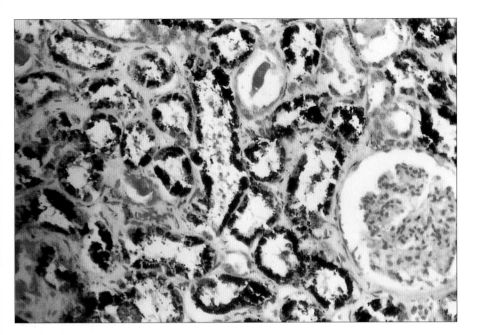

Figure 9.20
Perls stain showing deposits of iron as blue/black granules in the tubules of the kidney from a patient with a mechanical valve (Starr–Edwards) in the aortic position causing haemolysis with deposition of iron in several organs.

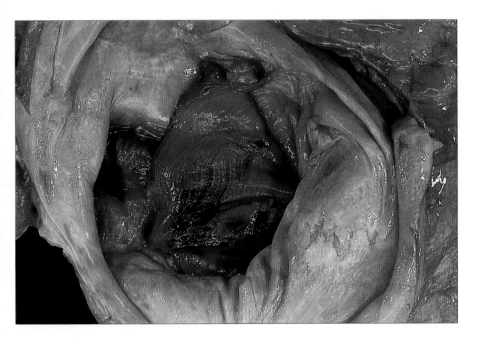

Figure 9.21
Left atrium viewed from above showing recent thrombus with lines of Zahn overlying a mechanical valve which is obscured by the extensive thrombosis.

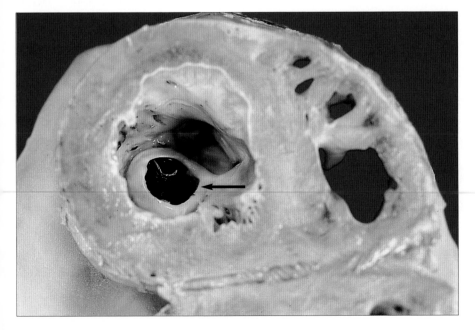

Figure 9.22
Case of mitral valve replacement with a Björk–Shiley tilting disc mechanical valve 10 years before for congenital mitral stenosis in a 12-year-old boy. Presented with mitral obstruction due to pannus formation (arrow) over the ventricular aspect of the valve with fibroelastosis of the left ventricular wall.
Death was due to left ventricular failure with extensive fibrosis of the wall.

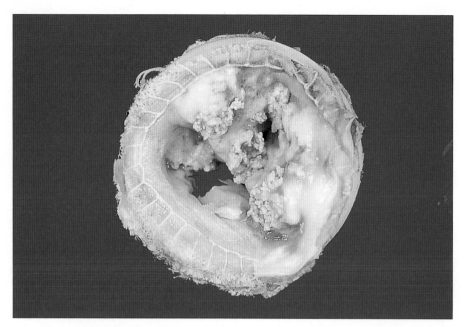

Figure 9.23
Bioprosthesis showing the synthetic cloth ring and the tissue cusps distorted and replaced by dense deposits of calcium causing stenosis of the valve with fibrosis and thickening. Carpentier–Edwards bioprostheses.

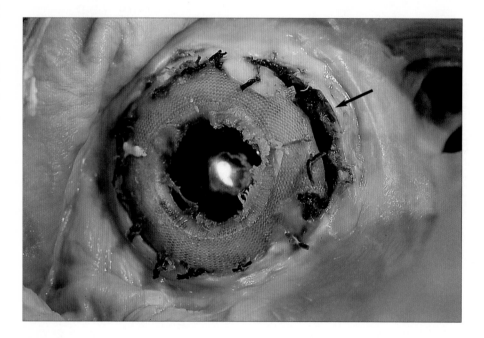

Figure 9.24
Acute dihescence (arrow) of a Starr–Edwards steel ball and cage mechanical valve due to endocarditis with small vegetations at the edge of the dehiscence.

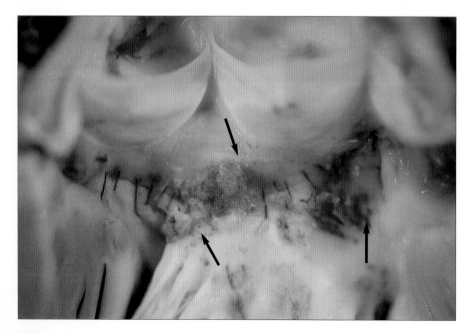

Figure 9.25
Aortic homograft showing vegetations (arrows) due to endocarditis on the lower suture line of the homograft.

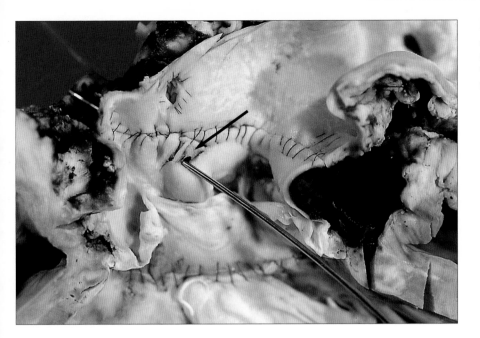

Figure 9.26
Aortic homograft showing rupture of sutures at the upper suture line (arrow) with dissection of the aortic wall causing fatal haemorrhage.

suture line and annulus carefully to check for this. Tissue valves in the atrioventricular position are obligatorily stented, adding to the prosthetic material in the heart and theoretically increasing the risk of endocarditis. Most valves for this purpose are heterograft (usually porcine) aortic valves, inverted and stented. Hence, they are of limited size, so that in all but the smallest patients there is likely to be a degree of stenosis.

Aortic homografts are liable to complications similar to the above including endocarditis (Fig. 9.25) and acute rupture due to suture breakdown (Fig. 9.26).

The dataset on more than 45 000 patients in The United Kingdom Heart Valve Registry (UKHVR) (Taylor 1997) show the trends in heart valve implantation. In the early years of the registry (1986–89) around 5000 artificial valves were implanted each year in just over 4500 patients. Since 1989 there has been a steady increase in numbers and, in 1994, 6000 valves were implanted in 5500 patients as first time operations. Closer inspection of the data shows that this 20% increase in activity has occurred principally in the elderly population (over 70 years of age at the time of their first valve replacement operation). The overall percentages of single valve versus double valve replacements has remained at 90% and 10%, respectively, each year since 1986. Aortic valve replacements have increased since 1986 from 54 to 64% compared with a fall in mitral replacements from 45 to 35%, probably reflecting two distinct phenomena. The increase in mitral valve repair procedures and the reduction in chronic rheumatic valve disease in the UK population.

The issue of patient age is a major influence on both heart valve replacement operations and on the short- and long-term results of surgery. In 1986, the mean age of patients having their first time valve replacement was 58.5 years (median 60). By 1994 this had risen to 63.4 years (median 65). In 1986, only 12% of patients were

older than 70 years at the time of their first valve replacement; in 1994 this figure had risen to 29%. Also there is an increased preference for mechanical versus bioprosthetic valves, shift from single leaflet to bileaflet mechanical valves, reduced use of pericardial bioprosthetic valves and increased use of stentless bioprostheses since 1992. Improved haemodynamics with the bileaflet design are a widely perceived benefit, and perhaps the much publicised strut fracture complication of the Björk–Shiley convexo-concave valve have been a powerful stimulus to change. Early (30 day) mortality for all first-time valve replacement operations has fallen steadily from 7.37% in 1986 to 4.33% in 1994. This fall in early mortality is despite the increase in elderly patients operated on during that time. Early mortality is consistently higher for mitral (7%) versus aortic sites (5%), for double valve replacements (9%) versus single (5%), for females (6.5%) versus males (5%), and for patients aged over 70 years (8%) versus younger patients (5%). Early mortality after reoperation is substantially higher than for first time procedures. From 1986–90 it remained at around 20–25%; however, during 1992–94 it fell to around 12%. Actuarial survival for all patients is around 60% at 10 years post-implantation. There are no differences between males and females, but site of valve implantation is significant: aortic (65%), mitral (57%), and tricuspid (31%). The major factor influencing survival after valve replacement surgery is patient age: 65% at 10 years for patients younger than 70 years at the time of valve implant compared with 42% for older patients.

LATE COMPLICATIONS OF CARDIAC SURGERY – POST PERICARDIOTOMY SYNDROME

This syndrome may occur several weeks to months after pericardial injury. It was first described following mitral valve commissurotomy and has since been reported after a wide variety of cardiac surgical procedures with an incidence estimated between 10 and 50%. Its features are identical to Dressler's syndrome following myocardial infarction. A small pericardial effusion may be detected by echocardiography. A pleural effusion occurs in 77% of cases, cardiac tamponade or constriction develops in 0.1–6% of patients. Coronary artery and bypass graft occlusion, unstable angina and persistent pericardial pain have been described. The majority of patients respond to anti-inflammatory agents, only a small proportion requiring pericardial drainage or pericardiectomy. Post-pericardiotomy syndrome is thought to result from immune complex disease. High blood titres of anti-heart antibodies and raised actin and myosin antibodies have been found in patients with the syndrome.

SUMMARY

A recent study of the necropsy findings in 108 of 123 (88%) patients who died in the early post-operative period after cardiac surgery for coronary and valvar heart disease found that the main causes of death were cardiac failure (52%), haemorrhage (14%), pulmonary emboli (5%), and cerebrovascular disease (6%) (Lee *et al.* 1997). The overall mortality figure was 4.4% which is very similar to the national figures for 1991 and 1993. The procedure with the highest mortality rate is repair of postinfarction ventricular septal defect. Fourteen of 37 patients (38%) died, but all procedures were performed as emergencies in the immediate postinfarction period. In the 1980s Schoen suggested that perioperative infarction occurred in 50% of patients dying after coronary artery bypass grafts, but is much less in more recent studies. It has been suggested that focal myocardial necrosis may reflect more widespread myocardial dysfunction. Fatal pulmonary emboli are less common after valve replacement operations than after coronary artery bypass grafting. There is conflicting evidence about whether deep venous thrombosis is more common in the leg from which saphenous vein grafts have been taken. Comparisons of pre mortem and post mortem diagnoses have been made since the beginning of the century. Despite modern laboratory and radiological investigations, important discrepancies continue to be found in 10–30% of cases, even in patients dying after surgery or on intensive care units. One necropsy study of children with congenital heart disease, some of whom had undergone surgery, showed

undiagnosed anomalies or surgical flaws in 17% (Sotaniemi 1995). Paediatric autopsy remains useful in delineating these complex cases (Gatzoulis *et al.* 1996). This recent study found major discrepancies between the clinical and pathological cause of death in 15% of patients, and in 6% these may have affected survival or treatment. Necropsy series of unselected patients have found pulmonary emboli, myocardial infarction, and infections, especially pneumonia, are the conditions most often missed in life. An incomplete or uncertain cause of death was found in 15 of 108 patients (Russell and Berry 1989). This compares with rates of between 3% and 9% in necropsies on unselected patients, patients dying in intensive care units and 'natural' sudden deaths. Thus, the role of autopsy in establishing death in cardiac procedures is extremely important, but we also need to clarify the uncertain cases in the future.

References

Bray PW, Mahoney JL, Anastakis D, Yao JK. Sternotomy infections: sternal salvage and the importance of sternal stability. *Canadian Journal of Surgery* 1996;39:297–301.

Chitwood WR, Wixon CL, Norton TO, Lust RM. Complex valve operations: antegrade versus retrograde cardioplegia. *Ann Thorac Surg* 1995;60:815–8.

Gatzoulis MA, Sheppard MN, Ho SY. Value and impact of necropsy in paediatric cardiology. *Heart* 1996;75:626–31.

Lauer JE, Heger JJ, Mirro MJ. Hemorrhagic complications of thrombolytic therapy. *Chest* 1995;108:1520–3.

Lee AHS, Borek BT, Gallagher PJ *et al.* Prospective study of the value of necropsy examination in early death after cardiac surgery. *Heart* 1997;78:34–8.

Mamode N, Scott RN, McLaughlin SC *et al.* Perioperative myocardial infarction in peripheral vascular surgery. *British Medical Journal* 1996;312:1396–7.

Russell GA, Berry PJ. Post mortem audit in a paediatric cardiology unit. *J Clin Pathol* 1989;42:912–8.

Sotaniemi KA. Long-term neurologic outcome after cardiac operation. *Annals of Thoracic Surgery* 1995;59:1336–9.

Taylor K. The United Kingdom Heart Valve Registry: The first 10 years. *Heart* 1997;77:295–6.

Underwood MJ and Coumbe M. Histological changes in venous grafts. *J Clin Pathol* 1994; 47:94–7.

INDEX

Note: page references in *italics* refer to figures; those in **bold** refer to tables